Family Caregiving for Older Disabled People: Relational and Institutional Issues

FAMILY CAREGIVING FOR OLDER DISABLED PEOPLE: RELATIONAL AND INSTITUTIONAL ISSUES

ISABELLA PAOLETTI
EDITOR

Nova Science Publishers, Inc.
New York

For permission to use material from this book please contact us:
Telephone 631-231-7269; Fax 631-231-8175
Web Site: http://www.novapublishers.com

Library of Congress Cataloging-in-Publication Data

Family caregiving for older disabled people : relational and institutional issues / Isabella Paoletti (editor).

p. ; cm.

Includes bibliographical references and index.

ISBN 1-59454-808-0

1. Caregivers. 2. Caregivers--Family relationships. 3. Older people--Care. 4. People with disabilities--Services for. 5. People with disabilities--Care. 6. Older people--Home care. [DNLM: 1. Home Nursing. 2. Aged. 3. Caregivers. 4. Cross-Cultural Comparison. 5. Disabled Persons. 6. Family Relations. WY 200 F1976 2006] I. Paoletti, Isabella.

RA645.3.F36 2006

362'.0425--dc22 2006000489

Published by Nova Science Publishers, Inc. ✦New York

CONTENTS

INTRODUCTION

This collection of essays is about dependent older people and their families, that is, older people who need help in their daily life: from the frail elderly who need mainly minor assistance in performing housework or for transportation, to severely disabled older people, bedridden or senile. The studies reported in this book offer a wide and informed overview of issues connected with caring for frail and disabled older people, whether carried out by family caregivers, paid helpers or formal caregivers. That the number of older people worldwide is increasing can certainly be considered a human achievement, but at the same time it generates a series of problems that must be faced.

THE AGING POPULATION

It is not news that the older population is increasing at a fast pace (ECE-UNFPA, 1992; Gavrilov and Heuveline, 2003; Stolnitz, 1994; UNDP, 1998; UNFPA, 1998; United Nations, 2001). This is the first time in history that societies have had to deal with a substantial change in the structure of their populations in relation to a growing number of older people. This is true in western countries, but developing countries also show this trend, although to a lesser extent. The United Nations (2002) graph of the changing structure of the population can be considered an icon of our times.

The alarming news is that governments are doing very little to face the challenges created by these structural changes in the population, in particular the growing number of dependent, frail and disabled elderly. It must be said that the great majority of elderly people (over 65 years old) are healthy and strong and lead independent lives; even in the eldest cohort 80 and over there are many people who are able to cope independently or with minimal help (Dooghe and Appleton, 1995; ISTAT, 1997; Savage, 1996; Walker, 1983). But frail and dependent older people are a reality, increasing exponentially (Wolfe, 1993; Gavrilov and Heuveline, 2003).

Not only are support services for disabled older people and their families scarce even in some of the most developed countries (Gori, 2002; Katz-Olson, 2003), but also in countries that have an established tradition of state support services for the elderly, drastic cuts in welfare spending are undermining both those services and long established rights (see Gustafson and Pyysiäinen in this volume).

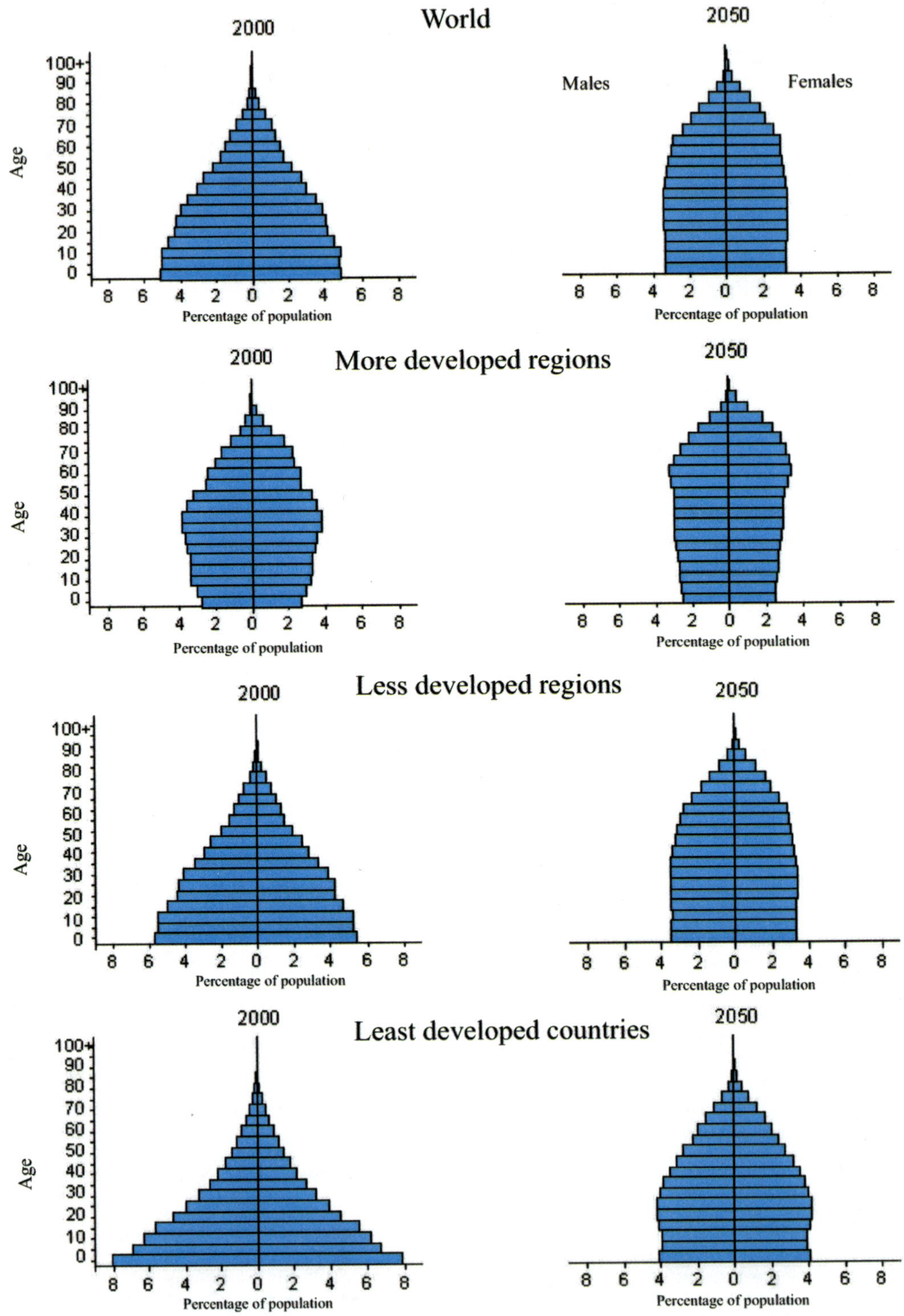

Figure 1. Population pyramids: age and sex distribution, 2000 and 2050.
Source: The Sex and Age Distribution of the World Populations: 1998 Revision, Volume II: Sex and Age (United Nations publication, Sales No. E.99.XIII.8), medium variant projections.

In fact, worldwide, most caregiving is carried out by close relatives (Aronson, 1990; Baldassarre, 1995; Caro and Leventhal-Stern, 1995; Jenkins, 1997; Stoltz, Udén and Willman, 2004) and these relatives are usually women.

THE GENDER ISSUE

The percentage of women aged 65 and over in all European countries, Russia, USA, Canada and Japan, is impressively higher than that of men and the difference increases with age (Council of Europe, 1997; Dooghe and Appleton, 1995; EUROSTAT, 1995; 1996; Gavrilov and Heuveline, 2003; Houdart-Blazy, 1997). Indeed, of the frail elderly, the majority are women; The following graphs (Gavrilov and Heuveline, 2003) illustrate very vividly this issue.

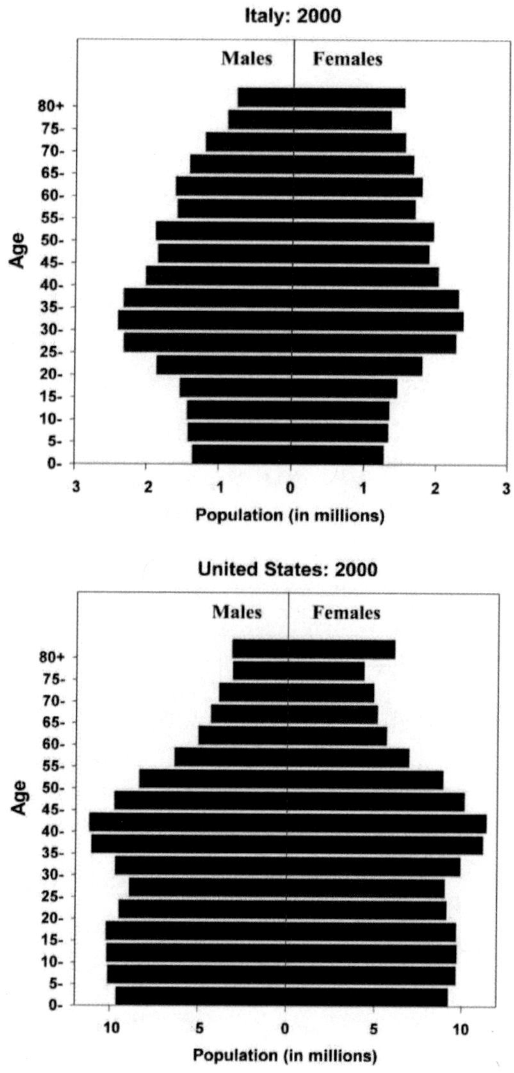

Figure 2. Aged population.

If we look at the other side of the caring relationship, again we find women in greater number, providing the bulk of care in terms of number of tasks performed and amount of time devoted to caring. Family caregivers are mainly women (Clarke, 1995; Facchini and Scortegagna, 1994; Jenkins, 1997; Katz-Olson, 2003; Martin-Matthews and Campbell, 1995; Mengani and Lamura, 1995; Najafizadeh, 2003; Neal, Ingersoll-Dayton and Starrels, 1997; Rose and Bruce, 1995; Walker, 1983; Zhan and Montgomery, 2003) and, more often than is generally thought, they are elderly women (Arber and Ginn, 1991). On the other hand, male caregivers are also a reality and their number is increasing. Husband are as likely to care for their disabled spouse as wives are (see Walters this volume). In fact, there is a lack of studies on the specific challenges encountered by male caregivers (Arber and Gilbert, 1989).

The Hidden Costs of Family Caregiving

Caregiving is hard work physically and psychologically (Aronson, 1990; Haley and Perkins, 2004; Taccani, 1994), lasting, at times, for decades. It can entail the carrying out of heavy tasks such as lifting and handling bed-ridden elderly and coping with mentally impaired elderly or with angry and resentful disabled people. It also involves a complex array of sentiments and emotions connected with the kin relationship (Dalley, 1993; Pohl, Boyd and Given, 1997; Paoletti, 1999; Raschick and Ingersoll-Dayton, 2004; Taccani, 1994), and feelings of moral obligation and identification issues (Finch and Groves, 1983; Joshi, 1995; Paoletti, 2001; 2002). Caring often involves contradictory feelings (Pohl, Boyd and Given, 1997); as Aronson (1990) points out: "qualitative studies are revealing the complexity of caregivers' experience which may simultaneously include strongly held wishes to support a relative, stress and resentment" (page 63).

Many carers become severely stressed and ill because of their caring commitments (Baldassarre, 1995; Jenkins, 1997; May, 1994; Paoletti, 1999), and it is the lives of women that are mostly affected by caring for disabled older relatives. They experience proportionally greater stress (Neal, Ingersoll-Dayton and Starrels, 1997) and greater negative consequences on their employment (Joshi, 1995) compared to men. The actual strain produced by the heavy load of daily tasks that caregiving implies is often increased by a construction of the caring relationship that excludes any alternative solution. The caregiving experience can have devastating effects on the overall wellbeing of the family involved, undermining positive family relationships, the financial stability of the household and endangering the physical and psychological health of their members (see Paoletti and Oddone and Aguirre in this volume).

Community Care

Personally, I believe that frail and disabled older people are better cared for in their community, in the surroundings in which they have spent their lives and where they have ties and interests. Moreover, home care services are highly cost-effective compared to institutionalized care (Caro and Leventhal-Stern, 1995). Saying this does not mean endorsing conservative discourses aimed at suppressing any form of help for older disabled people and their caregivers, nor upholding the idea that family caring should weigh only on women's shoulders. Since the early 1990s, "Family care", "community care" and de-institutionalization discourses are strongly supported by the new right in various countries as a means of justifying drastic cuts to social services budgets (Walker, 1995). We risk seeing elderly people abandoned in the community, instead of cared for in it. But "community care" can and should mean the provision of a number of services such as nursing homes for temporary admissions, day centers, home help, home medical assistance, meals-on-wheels, laundry services, the provision of aids such as wheelchairs, hoists, special beds and mattresses, etc. An integrated and multi agency approach to the support of older people is necessary (Foote and Stanners, 2002). The fear that providing services could imply the withdrawal of family support for their older members is baseless (Caro, Leventhal-Stern, 1995). Various studies "provide evidence that informal care may be supplemented, but it is rarely replaced, by formal care" (Williams, Lyons and Rowland, 1997, 112). Community services could flexibly combine with the existing informal support networks (Caro and Leventhal-Stern, 1995; Cristini and Cesa-Bianchi, 2003; Foote and Stanners 2002; Saccomani, 2001; Stalker, 2002; Taccani et al 2002; Trabucchi et al., 2002; Walker, 1995); a more shared model of caring should be implemented (Equal Opportunities Commission,1982), together with adequate legislation to foster the conciliation of working and family life. Not only would these changes provide a better life for older disabled people and make life bearable for caregivers, but also prevent the hidden costs that unsupported family caregiving often entails.

FACING THE CHALLENGES

This book puts the challenges posed by an increasing number of frail and disabled older people in the spot light. It aims to alert scholars, politicians, policy makers, health and social services managers and practitioners in the health and social service sectors to specific problems related to family caregiving.

The book will illustrate, with a wealth of ethnographic details, the many indirect social costs of delegating the care of older people to their families: the health, financial and relational implications of caregiving for the caregivers and their families. Providing efficient, reliable and affordable support services to family caregivers should be a priority for governments and would prevent very significant social costs. Organizing support services, however, does not assure that they will be used. Family caregivers often do not seek help, nor accept it when it is offered (Paoletti 1999; Taccani 1994). It is important to understand the complex relational and identity issues connected with caregiving. Above all, it should be pointed out that caregiving is not just a job, that is, a series of discrete tasks, but rather is centered around a core of emotional labour, respect, support, work towards reacquiring independence. Whether at home or in institutions, the quality of caregiving is measurable in terms of these rather intangible characteristics of caregivers' work. A specific effort should be put towards bridging the gap between the culture, order of priorities and structural necessities of institutions and the culture, order of priorities and specific needs of users. Then there is the simple fact that services are not used if the public does not know they exist. Services need to be publicized intensively; informing the public of their existence should be an integral part of their functioning.

In discussing central issues of family caregiving at relational and institutional level, this essay collection presents specific and innovative methodological approaches. Attention is drawn to the cultural dimension of caregiving in several essays, and the presence of case studies, from various countries worldwide, emphasizes its relevance to caregiving: the cultural dimension from an anthropological perspective, that is, the specific attitudes, habits, customs, in relation to caregiving in a specific ethnic group; the cultural dimension from a sociological perspective, that is, the different institutional cultures, order of priorities and needs of different agencies. Other essays point out the relevance of adopting a network perspective in studying family caregiving, avoiding a dyadic perspective. Furthermore, the usefulness of focusing on the changes over time in the care relationship is also stressed. Caregiving is not a linear, unchanging activity, it is a process of adjustment to an evolving situation. Adopting this perspective can bring many benefits in terms of understanding the specific needs of family caregivers. Let us look at the content of the following chapters in more detail.

The book is divided into two volumes: the first volume focuses on the complexity of the caring relationship, with its inextricably interwoven relational, moral, identity and cultural issues; in the second volume, institutional issues related to support services for family caregiving and home care are discussed.

THE FORTHCOMING CHAPTERS

Volume I: Relational Issues

In chapter 1, I introduce the subject of relational issues of family caregiving, focusing on its complexity. The intricacy of moral, relational, gender, financial and housing issues are highlighted, exploring the discursive construction of caring. A case study of a family caregiver in Italy is reported, showing how caregiving poses great strain and pressure on the carer and her family. Caring duties are constructed conversationally as bound to kin and gender membership as a moral imperative, but also financial and housing issues are implicated. Serious family conflicts are generated in relation to caring commitments.

The moral imperative of providing care to close kin is further discussed by Saija Katila, in Chapter 2, in relation to a very different cultural and social context: Finland. In fact, the Finnish welfare society provides universal care for the sick and the elderly regardless of their material wealth. Thus, the majority of the population use the services provided by society. It is, however, still common that farming families in Finland do not make full use of the services provided. Based on an ethnographic study, this chapter demonstrates that the value of taking care of the preceding generation is part of the system of values and norms that constitute the moral order of Finnish farming families. The study indicates that taking care of the elderly at home is a taken-for-granted fact in the families under study. In this context, which prioritises family welfare over narrow self-interest, relying on institutional care is not considered an appropriate expression of individuality. The study further highlights the gendered nature of caregiving on the farms, and the potential masculisation of care because of farmers' difficulty in finding wives. The study also suggests that the emotions of guilt, shame and love play important roles in family caregiving relationships. The study emphasizes that the "rationality" of caregiving by farm business families cannot be understood in purely utilitarian terms.

The interwoven relational, financial and housing implications of family caregiving are also the focus of María Julieta Oddone and Mónica Beatriz Aguirre, in chapter 3. They seek to identify specific difficulties experienced by families who take care of their elderly family members with health problems in Argentina. Their study describes the strategies that families develop to meet the needs of the dependent elderly and the costs--economic, emotional, and health-related--that these strategies imply for the caretakers. They explore in detail the support networks involved in the caring, the position of the main caretaker (spouse, son/daughter, grandchild, etc.), the tensions within the family, financial aspects (the weight on the family budget) and the role of community resources. The responsibilities of the family and the state are also discussed.

In chapter 4, Richard Cheung Lam shows the contrasts between the traditional Chinese value of social piety and structural constraints. He focuses on the Hong Kong sandwich generation, showing how it perceives and performs its informal caregiving roles towards its elderly, and on the structural constraints such as living arrangements and family income that affect its caregiving performance. In this survey study, most respondents, who internalize the traditional Chinese value of filial piety, are willing to take care of their elderly and perform the caregiving role. However, respondents do not perform all the domains of the caregiving role that accord with their perception of filial piety. Cross-tabulation with selected variables indicates that the structural constraints such as living arrangements, family income, as well as the ability of care-receivers to take care of themselves have limited the sandwich generation in performing different domains of the caregiving role. It seems that the effect of the structural constraints plays a more important role than internalized filial piety in affecting caregiving performance.

Joanie Sims-Gould and Anne Martin-Matthews, in chapter 5, strongly suggest the usefulness of looking at caregiving from a network perspective. They point out that family caregiving research has largely been focused on studies of the “primary” caregiver, and typically emphasizes the motivation and costs associated with caring for an older family member. This focus has generated a surplus of research on individual caregiver stress and burden but has done little to advance knowledge and understanding of the roles, responsibilities and relationship dynamics when multiple family members contribute to the care of elderly kin. Current research in caregiving suggests that systemic analyses of the ways in which groups of people with social or kin ties to older adults organize themselves to provide care have rarely been conducted. This chapter furthers the current understanding of family caregiving through an examination of longitudinal data from a survey study in Canada, with a focus on understanding the nature of caring relationships and the relative contributions of women, men, family and friends. Their analysis compares and contrasts the responsibilities of primary caregivers and helper caregivers (“helpers”). Empirical findings are linked to the Canadian context and implications for gerontological research, practice, policy and education are emphasized in their conclusions.

The Finnish context is the focus of chapter 6, that discusses the process of becoming a carer. Jaana Pyysiäinen and her colleagues examine how much room for manoeuvre a daughter who cares for an elderly parent has within the care arrangement. This is done by looking carefully at the negotiation process of the care arrangement. The analysis shows that the daughters become carers through a natural, gradual process without making a conscious decision. The reputations and moral identities of the family members are found to guide this process. After the commitment is formed, the room for manoeuvre can be modified through negotiations of the care arrangements. It is, though, rarely possible to negotiate completely openly about the different aspects of care. Indirect negotiations have the important function of maintaining the needed independence of the parent and the proper distance between the carer and elderly parent.

These studies show that caring for close kin is a major concern of family members world wide, and that it has many hidden social costs in terms of financial and relational stability of the family involved and in terms of negative effects on the health and employment of the caregivers. Family caregiving cannot be considered just a job; on the contrary, it involves complex relational, moral, gender and cultural issues.

In the second part of Volume 1 some special problems related to family caregiving are discussed. Lesley Baillie (chapter 7) explores caregiving for older relatives where there is a poor relationship, a little addressed dimension of caring. The chapter starts by analysing policy documents and their assumptions about caregiving relationships in Great Britain. A literature review reveals instances of caregiving where relationships are poor, but these are generally afforded little prominence. To examine this sensitive issue, case studies were examined. These case studies confirm that some caregivers do have a poor relationship with those they care for, and the discussion examines motives for caregiving, in particular, obligation and reciprocity. The chapter concludes that while this is a difficult topic to raise and pursue, health and social care professionals should be alert to caregivers who may care for, but not about, the person they are caring for. Clearly this is an area where more research is needed, but there may be reluctance to discuss the subject openly, rendering accessibility to study participants problematic. It is necessary to find more indirect forms of access to the study of this problem.

For some family caregivers, caregiving is a life long commitment. In this book we do not confront the dramatic issues of parents looking after their disabled children, as this is not the focus of the book. Among disabled older people, however, there are some whose health problems started at quite an early age; among those, there are people suffering from multiple sclerosis. Elizabeth A. Watson (chapter 8) considers the situation of a group of older married men caring for a partner with multiple sclerosis in Australia. The chapter focuses on the ways in which MS has shaped and continues to shape both the life of the carer and of his wife, the impact on their immediate family and friends and especially upon the marriage. The chapter considers how these men explain their caring and why they are doing it. It explores some of the choices these couples confronted following diagnosis – about paid work, where to live and whether to move house or modify their present home - and the costs associated with these choices, both the financial costs and the less tangible costs involved in being distant from family and old friends and from services and support. The impact of these choices is most acutely felt as the couple grow older and the chronic illness takes its toll.

Another group of caregivers that demands special attention is those who care for senile older people, and in particular those looking after relatives suffering from Alzeimer's disease. Catherine Ward-Griffin and Nancy Bol, in chapter 9, stress the fact that, in order to understand the complexities of the care process in dementia, research needs to focus on caregiving as a dyadic process. Grounded in the feminist interpretive and life course perspectives, their qualitative study explores the subjective perceptions and experiences of 25 adult daughters and their mothers with Alzheimer's Disease. The data analysis reveals five inextricably linked phases of the mother-daughter relationship: recognition, negotiation, regulation, compensation and isolation. With respect to the daughters' perspective, five interconnected themes emerged: becoming aware/stepping in, finding a balance, leading the way, carrying the load, holding on/ letting go. As well, findings illuminated how mother-daughter relationships within AD care changed over time, and how this care process influenced the health and well-being of adult daughters and their mothers. With the increasing emphasis on home care in Canada, study findings offer insights for health promotion, program planning and public policy development related to caregiving within AD and other related dementias.

Finally, issues of long-distance caregiving are discussed in chapter 10. Loretta Baldassar and her colleagues point out how nowadays it is increasingly common to find family members caring at a distance. Their study focuses on adult children in Australia who care for their relatives back home in Europe. Geographic distance separates a large number of aging parents in Europe from their potential sources of support: their adult children who migrated to Australia in previous decades when the parents were healthy and independent. This study shows how migrants in Australia care for their parents back home when they become more dependent and frail and how they respond to their increased need for support. They argue that, in spite of the difficulties that are created by distance, migrant children overseas do provide care from a distance to their disabled parents, by developing strategies for communicating with and otherwise supporting their aging relatives. However, none of this support is automatic, and it is always informed by the cultural expectations of caregiving, specific family contexts, and the history of migration and its effect on family relationships. In a series of detailed case studies, they examine the ways in which migrants mobilise and supplement the aged care services locally available to their parents, and the concerns and strategies of aged care that are specific to family members living at a distance.

Volume II: Institutional Issues

In the second volume, institutional issues related to support services to family caregiving are discussed in detail. Institutions have orders of priorities and demands related to the structural features of the organization. Limited funding and resources, work shifts and timetables, socio-political accountability and visibility are some examples. In support services to family caregiving, this institutional order of relevance can conflict at times with the needs and priorities of caregivers and their cared for. In this second volume, such issues are confronted in a series of detailed empirical studies in different countries in the world. The tendency towards a reduction of support services to family caregiving is shown in some countries, but support service non-use also appears as a central and puzzling aspect of institutional problems in relation to support to family caregiving.

Diana L. Gustafson (chapter 11) explores the reconstitution of individual need for home care services following a time of sweeping health care restructuring in Ontario, Canada in the mid-1990s. Using a method of social inquiry called institutional ethnography, this retrospective investigation compares the documentary practices used at two distinct historical moments for assessing an elderly, disabled person's home care needs. The analysis reveals how the discourses of family caregiving and cost containment converge in ways that reconstitute need and disqualify or limit eligibility for home care services. The study supports calls for federal Home and Community Care legislation that would enshrine the principles of universality, accessibility, comprehensiveness, portability, and public administration. Such legislation would ensure that no elderly, disabled person or their family would be denied adequate support because of inability to pay or to participate in care. This study helps to illuminate the alarming tendency of making cuts in services provision for older disabled people, and how this is done in terms of specific institutional practices.

In the United States today, the vast majority of caregiving for the frail elderly is undertaken by family members. Accordingly, the wellbeing and needs of the family caregiver are crucial determinants of quality in eldercare. Julie Walters and Connie L. McNeely, in chapter 12, characterize this highly complex situation in terms of the emotional and psychological needs, the physical needs and the financial needs of the caregiver, exploring their general implications and the degree to which they are met or unmet relative to caregiver wellbeing and effective eldercare, and delineating sources from which support might be drawn. Moreover, recognizing and defining family provided eldercare as a public concern, they consider relevant policy initiatives and approaches at different levels of analysis to assess the nature and availability of external support and involvement. By examining the needs of family caregivers relative to both within-family and broader social dynamics, they contribute to a deeper understanding of the relationship between their wellbeing and successful eldercare in general.

Chapter 13 is focused on care homes. Care homes are in a way in the background of family caregiving. Temporary admittance to a care home or the decision to enter one are possibilities that are often discussed by cared for and caregivers. To be able to rely on high quality and affordable institutional care, if needed, that is, having a feasible alternative, is very important psychologically for both the cared for and the caregiver. Ingrid Eyers describes how formal caregivers are crucial to the quality of life experienced by older people who for health and social care reasons are living in a care home. In a comparative study of 50 formal caregivers in England and Germany, Eyers identifies time as an important factor in the interface/interaction between formal caregivers and an old person. In addition to the obvious physical bodywork involved, vital invisible, intangible and non-measurable skills were being used. Such skills are taken for granted, as they are perceived to come naturally to every woman in this female dominated field of employment. Skilled formal caregiving is a combination of time-budgeting abilities coupled with an understanding of the medical and social needs of older people living in a care home. The findings presented in this paper indicate that it is important to establish governmental policies that take into greater consideration the time factor in the provision of care. Furthermore, it is important that caregivers are trained to specifically meet the requirements of older people and that such work is respected and rewarded.

In Sweden, family caregiving is to a certain extent institutionalised. The municipalities have the ultimate responsibility for the elderly, ill and disabled. Even so, most caring takes place within the family. Ann-Britt M Sand, in chapter 14, examines in detail an institutional practice that consists in the municipality employing as caregiver a relative of the person in need of care. This study discusses some of the advantages, and problems, of this type of employment. One conclusion that can be drawn from this investigation is that employment and a salary are appreciated forms of support. A salary is compensation for work effort, and also provides the opportunity of giving up other work, or reducing the time spent on it, in order to handle the caregiving. Apart from the bread-winning aspect, a salary has another important significance – it is regarded as recognition of the work. The majority of the kin care providers are contented, although many of them want better employment terms and higher wages. More specifically, they want conditions that correspond to other care work, and a salary which corresponds to the effort.

In chapter 15, Pirjo Nikander focuses on the allocation of financial support to relatives taking care of elderly family members still living at home in Finland, specifically, on the decision making process. The chapter approaches caregiving through the eyes of social and health care professionals and focuses on interprofessional meeting interaction during which members of different professional groups make practical decisions concerning support to carers. The data were video taped and allow direct access to decision making episodes and face-to-face interactions of professionals in elderly care. The meetings under examination were attended by representatives of home help teams, doctors, nurses and a secretary. The chapter starts out with the notion that the on-going discourse in meetings can be analyzed as the practical and empirical site where various controversies, dilemmas and the morality of elderly care and help allocation come into being in analysable ways. One of the key claims is that discursive analyses of interaction excerpts from institutional settings enable the study of professional logic in the making. The analyses describe professional practices of client categorisation and description, and outline details of professional advocacy talk and argumentation. Particular attention is given to the ways in which life course ideals and imagery are used when describing elderly clients and their carers.

In the second part of this volume some specific issues in relation to conflicts between support services and caring family are discussed. Saarenheimo and her colleagues (chapter 16) provide insight into the cultural process and dynamics of family care in Finland by focusing on the different "microcultures" involved in the process. The data consist of qualitative interviews that were carried out during home ethnographies in the respondents' homes. The focus of the research was family care as a practical, day-to-day activity and the caregivers' own conceptualizations of care and related issues. The data reveal three domains within which the "microcultures" of family care were examined in detail. The domains were changes within the domestic culture, the social networks of the caregiving families and encounters between families and service providers. The main findings show that the interpretations given of home and intimate relationships, as well as the conceptualizations of support, play an important part in the carer's adjustment to the needs of the disabled spouse. Focusing on the meanings given by the caregivers themselves, the authors outline some of the considerable underlying conflicts between the families and the service system. Finally, the findings and their implications are discussed in the larger cultural context.

Community services designed to support carers can significantly improve their health and welfare. Formal services complement rather than substitute for informal care; however, Patricia Hill and her colleagues in chapter 17 point out that few Australian carergivers make use of the formal services on offer. There appears to be a significant number of carers who would benefit from the support of formal services but do not take them up. This chapter uses the 1998 Australian Survey of Disability Ageing and Carers to explore the characteristics of carers who may be isolated from appropriate formal support networks, specifically highlighting the care situations of carers who do not access formal services and the reasons why people report not using services. The research also focuses on the non-use of services by carers who may have more need of support, such as carergivers who are burdened or in poor health themselves and young carers. For primary carergivers, take up of formal services increases as the number of hours of support provided per week increases. Men and women providing care make use of different combinations of services. Australians from culturally and linguistically diverse backgrounds are less likely to use services. The findings of this research may assist in more appropriate targeting of resources to support these isolated carers.

Conflicts between service providers and family caregivers and the cared for are highlighted by Katharine Jeary and Olive Stevenson, in chapter 18. This case study, concerning an elderly, severely disabled African woman living in an English city, is drawn from a wider qualitative research project in which case conferences, convened to consider allegations of abuse against vulnerable adults, were examined. The case raises complex and challenging issues in relation to ethnicity and caregiving. These center upon the relationships between the woman herself, family members and the paid 'carers' from the statutory services. Case analysis suggests that the social services offered were adversely affected by uncertainty and confusion about the dynamics of the family and culturally significant factors. In consequence, it is arguable that the woman was neglected, which is one of the forms of abuse which is recognized in official definitions.

Concluding Comments

This book deals with one of the most serious problems posed by the growing older world population: the disabled elderly' s need of care and the social impact this has. Old age is often associated with decrement, poor health and loss of mental and physical capabilities, and the healthy and active elderly are considered the exceptions; now these images are no longer socially sustainable. We need cultural changes that acknowledge the hope and the reality of healthy and socially productive later years for the majority of the population. We must invent a new life for ourselves after 60 years of age and make a space in society for a portion of the population, the elderly, that was not there before. There is the need to rethink all the structures of society with this new section of population in mind. If, on the one hand, everything possible should be done in order to include older people in society as active and important members, on the other hand we have to recognize older people's frailty and their need of care when this occurs. It is necessary that we provide adequate social services to face this challenge.

Bibliography

Arber, S. Ginn, J. (Eds.) (1991) *Gender and later life*. London: Sage.

Arber, S. and Gilbert, G.N. (1989) Men: The forgotten carers. *Sociology*, 23, (1), 111-118.

Aronson, J. (1990) Women's perspective on informal care of the elderly: Public ideology and personal experience of giving and receiving care. *Ageing and Society,* 10, 61-84.

Baldassarre, G. (1995) Il ruolo della famiglia nell'assistenza all'anziano non auto sufficiente: problemi, risorse, proposte *Il Giornale di Gerontologia,* 43, 303-311.

Caro, F.G. and Leventhal-Stern, A. (1995) Balancing formal and informal care: Meeting needs in a resource-constrained program. *Home Health Care Services Quaterly*, 15, (4), 67-81.

Clarke, L. (1995) Family care and changing family structure: Bad news for the elderly? In I. Allen and E. Perkins (Eds.) (1995) *The future of family care for older people*. London: HMSO, 19-49.

Council of Europe (1997) *Recent demographic development in Europe*. Strasbourg: Council of Europe Publishing.

Crisitini, C. and Cesa-Bianchi, G. (Eds.) (2003) *Il centro diurno integrato per anziani :una risorsa per la qualità della vita.* Milano: Angeli.

Dalley, G. (1993) Caring: a legitimate interest of older women. In M. Bernard and K. Meade (Eds) *Women come to age: perspectives on the lives of older women.* London: Arnold, 106-190.

Dooghe, G. and Appleton, N. (Eds). (1995) *Elderly Women in Europe*. Bruxelles: Centrum vor Bevolkings.

ECE and UNFPA (1992) *Changing population age structures 1990-2015. Demographic and economic consequences.* Geneva: United Nations.

Equal Opportunities Commission (1982) *Who care for the carers*. Manchester: EOC.

EUROSTAT (1996) Statistiche generali dell'Unione Europea 33° Ed. Lusemburgo: Ufficio delle Pubblicazioni Ufficiali della Comunità Europea.

EUROSTAT (1995) Les femmes et les hommes dans l'Union Européenne. Portrait statistique. Luxembourg: Offices des Publications Officeles des Communites Européennes.

Facchini, C. and Scortegagna, R. (1994) Italia: Alternative all'istituzionalizzazione e ruolo centrale delle donne. In F. Lesemann and C. Martin, (Eds.) *Assistenza a domicilio, famiglia, anziani*. Milano: Angeli, 33-109.

Finch, J. and Groves, D. (Eds.) (1983) *A labour of love: Women, work and caring*. London: Routledge and Kegan Paul.

Foote, C. and Stanners C., (2002) *Integrating care for older people.* London: Jessica Kingsley Publishers.

Gavrilov L.A., Heuveline P. (2003) Aging of Population. In: Paul Demeny and Geoffrey McNicoll (Eds.) *The Encyclopedia of Population*. New York, Macmillan Reference USA, from http://www.galegroup.com

Gori, C. (Ed.) (2002) *Il welfare nascosto: il mercato privato dell'assistenza in Italia e in Europa.* Roma: Carocci.

Haley, W E. and Perkins, E A. (2004) Current Status and Future Directions in Family Caregiving and Aging People with Intellectual Disabilities. *Journal of Policy and Practice in Intellectual Disabilities* 1 (1), 24-30.

Houdart-Blazy, V. (1997)Age become her, older women in the European Unions. *The Women of Europe Dossier* n. 45, Buxelles.

ISTAT, (1997) *Anziani in Italia*. Bologna: Il Mulino.

Jenkins, C.L. (1997) Women, work, and caregiving: How do these roles affect women's well-being? *Journal of Women and Aging*, 9 , (3), 27-45.

Joshi, H. (1995) The labour market and unpaid caring: Conflict and compromise. In I. Allen and E. Perkins (Eds.) *The future of family care for older people*. London: HMSO, 93-118.

Katz Olson, L. (2003) *The not-so-golden years: Caregiving the frail elderly, and the long-term establishment.* Lanham, MD: Rowman and Littlefield.

Martin-Matthews, A. and Campbell, L.D. (1995) Gender roles, employment and informal care. In S. Arber and J. Ginn (Eds.). *Connecting gender and ageing. A sociological approach.* Buckingham: Open University Press,129-143.

May, M.P. (1994) Il lavoro di cura. In P. Taccani, (Ed.) (1994) *Dentro la cura.* Milano: Angeli, 25-86.

Mengani, M. and Lamura, G. (1995). Elderly women, family structure and care patterns in Italy. In G. Dooghe and N. Appleton (Eds.) *Elderly Women in Europe.* Bruxelles: Centrum vor Bevolkings.

Najafizadeh, M. (2003) Women's empowering care work in post-soviet Azerbaijan. *Gender and Society*, 17, (2) 293-304.

Neal, M.B., Ingersoll-Dayton, B. and Starrels, M.E. (1997) Gender and relationships differences in caring patterns consequences among employed caregivers. *The Gerontologist*, 37, (6), 804-816.

Paole tti, I. (1999) A half life: women caregivers of older disable relatives. *Journal of Women and Aging*, 11, (1), 53-67.

Paoletti, I. (2001) Membership categorization and time appraisal in interviews with carers of disabled elderly, *Human Studies,* 24, 293-325.

Paoletti, I. (2002) Caring for older people: a gendered practice. *Discourse and Society*, Special Issue on Language and Gender 13, (6), 805-817.

Pohl, J.M., Boyd, C. and Given, B.A. (1997) Mother-daughter relationships during the first year of caregiving: A quality study. *Journal of Women and Aging*, 9, (1/2), 133-149.

Raschick, M. and Ingersoll-Dayton, B. (2004) The costs and rewards of caregiving among aging spouses and adult children, *Family Relations,* 53, 3.

Rose, H. and Bruce, E. (1995) Mutual care but differential esteem: caring between older couples. In S. Arber and J. Ginn, (Eds.) *Connecting gender and ageing.* Buckingham: Open University Press,129-143.

Saccomani, R. (2001). *Le reti della solidarietà: l'assistenza domiciliare nella terza età.* Milano: Hoepli.

Savage, A. (1996) *Qui prendra soin d'eux. Perspectives d'avenir de les familiae aux personnes agées dans lUnion européenne.* Dublin: Foudation Europeénne pour l'amélioration des conditions de vie et de travail.

Stoltz, P. Udén, G. and Willman A. (2004) Support for family carers who care for an elderly person at home - a systematic literature review. Scandinavian Journal of Caring Sciences, 18, (2).

Stalker, K. (Ed.) (2002) *Reconceptualizing work with « carers ». New directions for policy and practice.* London: Jessica Kingsley Publishers.

Stolnitz, G.J. (1994) *Social aspects and country reviews of population aging. Europe and North America.* Economic Studies n. 6, New York: United Nations.

Taccani, P. (1994) Le relazioni familiari. In P. Taccani (Ed.) *Dentro la cura.* Milano: Angeli, 109-170

Taccani, P. Tognetti, A., De Bernardinis, S., Florea, A., Credendino, E. (2002) *Curare e prendersi cura.* Roma : Carrocci.

Trabucchi, M., Brizioli E. and Pesaresi, F. (Eds.) (2002) *Residenze sanitarie per anziani* Bologna: Il Mulino.

UNDP (1998) *Human Development Report 1998*. New York: Oxford University Press.

UNFPA(1998). The state of the world population 1998. Press summary, from *http://www.unfpa.org/SWP/swp98/pressumary2.htm*

United Nations (2001). *World population prospects: the 2000 revision.* New York: United Nations.

Uneted Nations Department of Economic and Social Affairs, (2002) World Population Ageing: 1950-2050, from *http://www.un.org/esa/desa.htm*

Walker, A. (1983) Care for elderly people: A conflict between women and the state. In J. Finch and D. Croves (Eds.) *A labour of love: Women, work and caring*. London: Routledge and Kegan Paul, 106-128.

Walker, A. (1995) The family and the mixed economy of care – can they be integrated? In I. Allen and E. Perkins (Eds.) (1995) *The future of family care for older people*. London: HMSO, 201-220.

Williams, J., Lyons, B. and Rowland, D. (1997) Unmet long-term needs of elderly people in the community: a review of literature. *Home Health Care Services Quarterly*, 16, (1/2), 93-119.

Wolfe, J.R. (1993) *The coming health crisis : who will pay for care the aged in the twenty-first century?* Chicago: University of Chicago press.

Zhan, H.J. and Montgomery, R.J.V. (2003) Gender and elder care in China. The influence of filial piety and structural constrains. *Gender and Society*, 17, (2), 209-229.

In: Family Caregiving for Older Disabled People
Editor: Isabella Paoletti, pp. 1-18
ISBN 1-59454-808-0

Chapter 1

THE INTRICACY OF GENDER, MORAL, RELATIONAL, FINANCIAL AND HOUSING ISSUES

Isabella Paoletti
University of Bologna, Italy

INTRODUCTION

This chapter aims to describe the intricacy of moral, relational, gender, financial and housing issues that are connected with caring for older disabled relatives, exploring the discursive construction of caring, in order to understand the complexity of the caring relationship and plan effective support services to family caregivers. The data analysed in this study consist of interviews with family caregivers, conducted as part of a larger research project, by a gerontological research centre in Italy.

Qualitative studies have explored the complexity of the caring relationship and its pregnancy in relation to moral, emotional and identity issues (Abel, 1990; Aronson, 1990; Dalley, 1993; Finch and Groves, 1983; Pohl, Boyd and Given, 1997; Taccani, 1994). Caregiving is a demanding job physically and psychologically (Aronson, 1990; Jenkins, 1997; Matthews and Campbell, 1995; Silverman and Huelsman, 1990; Taccani, 1994; Walker, 1995), lasting for decades in some cases. Not only can it imply the fulfillment of tiring tasks such as lifting, handling bed-ridden elderly, coping with mentally impaired elderly or with angry and resentful disabled people, but it involves a complex array of sentiment and emotions connected to kin relationship (Dalley, 1993; Pohl, Boyd and Given, 1997; Taccani, 1994), feelings of moral obligation and identification issues (Finch and Groves, 1983; Joshi, 1995; Rose and Bruce 1995). Caring often involves contradictory feelings, (Pohl, Boyd and Given, 1997); as Aronson (1990) points out: "qualitative studies are revealing the complexity of caregivers' experience which may simultaneously include strongly held wishes to support a relative, stress and resentment" (page 63). Moreover, the caring is often not the responsibility of just one person, but different tasks are distributed among family members. A very complex structure of caring arrangements is organized around a disabled older person and often this means re-negotiating all the family relationships (Taccani, 1994, 109). In particular, feminist studies have highlighted the relevance of caregiving to gender identification, providing care to close kin is described as a distinctive feature of femininity (Graham 1983). The task of caring within the family is not only very hard work, but a very symbolically, morally, emotionally loaded task.

Since the beginning of the project in the pilot phase, I started noticing puzzling aspects of the caregiving relationship. I was impressed by the effects I was observing of caring on caregivers' health (Paoletti, 1999b). In particular, daughters assisting their long-term disabled mothers showed signs of severe health problems, in one case, the life of the carer seemed at risk. Caregiving can be a very demanding and exhausting job, physically and psychologically, no doubt about this, but I could notice a supplementary amount of tension, stress and suffering whose source did not appear justified by the caring task load in caregivers' tales. In particular, a puzzling perception of time was noticeable: some carers were describing caring as occupying all their time even if they received substantial help (Paoletti, 1999b; 2001). The sense of pervasiveness and ineluctability of caring seemed to be an actual source of stress for caregivers. In particular, the way in which caregivers constructed their situation appeared as relevant as their material condition in relation to their ability to cope, that is, there are instances in the data in which similar material situations (disability of the cared-for, amount of help received etc..) were constructed in polarized ways and resulted in very different types of lives for caregivers (Paoletti, 1999b; 2001).

What makes caring such an overwhelming burden in some cases, so that carers' health and even their lives can be threatened? Why are different solutions not sought? What tangle of emotions, moral obligations, strong identification processes is effecting carers? I have been sincerely puzzled talking with some caregivers on the verge of a nervous breakdown who firmly refused to seek or accept help (Paoletti 1999b). The difficulty of some caregivers in seeking help has already been highlighted (Taccani, 1994). How could carers be helped? In other instances caregivers were receiving help, but they did not feel relieved by it, in fact they saw their time and all their thoughts occupied, pervaded by caregiving, with no life left for themselves (Paoletti, 2001; Paoletti , 1999b). How can some caregivers manage to cope? Is the relevance of caring in relation to feminine identity connected to the greater stress women derive from caregiving?

The Discursive Construction of Caring

In this study I explore the discursive construction of caring. I argue that "the women's will to care" is not just the product of socialization in childhood, but of something more cogent, pressing and pervasive. Caring is almost always attributed to women in ordinary conversation. Conversationally, men are not made accountable for caring commitment, if they perform any caring task they are appreciated for it, women providing care to elderly relatives just do what it is expected of them. In fact they can be exempted from it only for serious motives. In this study I look at how caring is constructed conversationally and how it is related to gender categorizations and moral identification work. I draw on the work undertaken on membership categorizations (Baker, 1997; 1984; Day, 1998; Hester and Eglin,1997; Jayyusi, 1984; Sacks, 1992, Watson, 1997) and on identification work (Antaki and Widdicombe, 1998; Garfinkel, 1967; Paoletti, 1997; 1998a; 1998b) within the ethnomethdological approach.

To study categorization work allows analysts to observe how commonsense knowledge of the social world is employed, made visible and made relevant in relation to specific settings and course of affairs in ordinary interactions (Sacks, 1992: 40). Naming a category evokes a whole domain of interrelations with other categories, with category-bound activities, category-bound knowledge, sets of duties, obligations and rights, identity attributions (Antaki and Widdicombe, 1998; Sacks, 1972; 1992; Jayyusi, 1984; 1991; Hester and Eglin, 1997). They are observably reciprocally implicative; that is, naming a category evokes sets of category-bound activities; but the reverse is also true: naming an activity that is clearly bound to a category mobilizes the corresponding categorization process. Let us make an example, using the category "doctor" would activate a field of related categories, such as patient, nurse etc, and category-bound activities: visiting patients, writing prescriptions etc. Category-bound knowledge, (anatomy; neurology, etc.) would also be mobilized, as well as sets of duties and obligations, for example, to provide help in emergencies.

Exploring the moral dimension of categorization work is practically rewarding in relation to the understanding of specific caregivers' problems, and theoretically in relation to the understanding of aspects of social order. The social order has a moral character, it rests on moral imperatives. We are morally accountable for making sense, for replying to questions, answer greetings and in generally cooperate in the orderly conduction of ordinary activities. We are able to interact meaningfully with interlocutors because we behave in cooperative and finely synchronized ways, that is we feel morally obliged to do so and we are morally accountable not to do so. Garfinkel's (1967) breaching experiments showed very effectively the moral accountability bound to social practices. Departure from the ordinary acceptable course of behavior were met with a request of explanation, sanctions, that is, they were treated as illegitimate and morally reproachable. Garfinkel (1967, 35) says: "A society's members encounter and know the moral order as perceivable normal courses of action-familiar scenes of everyday affairs, the world of daily life known in common with others and with others taken for granted. They refer to this world as the 'natural facts of life' which, for members, are through and through moral facts of life. For members, not only are matters so about familiar scenes, but they are so because it is morally right or wrong that they are so". Social interaction relies on the basic fact that members will act cooperatively "as matter of moral necessity" (Heritage, 1984, 82). Moral accountability is also a resource that is used by members to explain, justify reasons, choices and behaviors. Above all categorial work, that is the way in which members are described for various practical tasks in the course of ordinary activities, has pervasively a moral character. As highlighted by Jayyusi (1984, 6): descriptions "are embedded in the contexts of rights, obligations, practical interests and moral conventions that we can and do presuppose, or take for granted".

Caring appears to be a membership-bound activity to kin and gender membership categories, with strong moral connotations. "Being a daughter", "being a son", etc., are good enough reasons for becoming a carer, that is, the use of the category mobilizes strong moral imperative in relation to providing care for close kin, see the next chapter for the relevance of the moral accountability of caring in a completely different social and cultural context. In the interview interaction, interlocutors display an orientation towards the production of a moral order in which duty and responsibilities are allocated on the basis of gender distinction. Males are generally not made responsible for caring tasks, except for situations in which females are absent or sick, that is, for "serious motives". Caregivers' perception of the time devoted to caring is pervasive, most carers describe caring as occupying all their time (Paoletti, 2001), but gender differences are noticeable. Caring tasks are recognizable as gender specific practices, therefore, failing to carry out these tasks is morally sanctionable when referred to women, but not so much, when referred to men. We could talk of a gendered moral order. But there is nothing monolithic about social constructions, in this same data I found instances of distancing from caregiving as a female practice (Paoletti, 2004), as it will be discussed later on, moreover Katila, in chapter 2, and Watson, in chapter 8, discuss issues related to male caregivers, that are often overlooked in the literature (Arber and Gilbert, 1989).

In this chapter I highlight how moral accountability is made relevant in caregivers' talk. Caring duties are bound to kin and gender membership, but also financial and housing issues are frequently implicated. The caring task is constructed in the course of the interview as a woman's duty, inscribed in a gendered moral order. Caring tasks often pose great strain and pressure on caregivers and their families, serious family conflicts are often generated in relation to caring commitments. In this chapter I analyze transcripts taken from the interview with Anna who assists her mother-in-law. Caregiving is having a negative effect on Anna's life and her family. Moral accountability in relation to providing care, bound to kin and gender membership, is shown to be the base on which this family drama rests. To explore the moral dimension of the caring relationship is crucial to the understanding of the complexity of such a relationship. I argue that in order to help caregivers it is important to provide community services that can relieve their heavy load of caring tasks, but also to understand these complex relational and identity issues that, in some cases, make material help useless.

The Study

This study is part of a wider research project, "The role of women in the family care of disabled elderly", conducted by the Department of Social and Economic Studies of INRCA (National Institute for the Cure and Care of Older People), Ancona, Italy, supported by a grant of CNR (Italian Research Council) (Paoletti, 1998c; 1999a; 1999b; 2001; 2002). This study project comprised a survey study and an action research project. After the pilot phase (22 interviews conducted by professional researchers), the action project was articulated in three phases. 1) Women from the Pensioner Trade Unions in Ferrara were initially involved in interviewing caregivers of older disabled relatives in order to understand their problems and needs (33 interviews). 2) Support initiatives for caregivers were planned and implemented on the basis of these interviews. 3) At the end of the project I conducted feedback interviews with some of the caregivers who received help (9 interviews). The interviews lasted between twenty minutes and three hours, all the interviewers were provided with a list of topics to cover in the interviews. The data analyzed in this chapter are taken from the first phase of the action research project.

Researchers in various sociological traditions use interview data to provide relevant information in relation to the object of study or to gather the subjective perspective of the interviewee on a specific topic. This study refers to the ethnomethodological use of interview data to document identity work (Antaki and Widdicombe, 1998; Baker, 1984; Garfinkel, 1967; Paoletti, 1997; 1998a; 1998b; Watson and Weinberg, 1982). The interview data are treated as "moral tales" (Baruch, 1981; Silvermann, 1987, 1993), that is, ways for members to display their moral responsibility and a morally adequate image of being a caregiver.

Interviews were transcribed and then analyzed. Transcribing is anything but a neutral and mechanic work; it is part of the analysis and of the interpretative work (Ochs, 1979), spoken expression are often unclear, repetitious, incomplete. The translation of the transcripts from Italian to English implies further choices and adjustments (see Moerman, 1996 and Day, 1998, for the complex issue of working with translated transcripts). Therefore, I conducted the analysis on the original transcript in Italian.

Through a detailed conversation and categorization analysis (Atkinson and Heritage, 1984; Sacks 1992), I looked at how caregiving is constructed conversationally as a moral duty connected to kin and gender membership. I analyzed an interview with a caregiver, Anna (the name of the woman interviewed has been changed to preserve confidentiality), who very lucidly describes the effects that caring for her mother-in-law has on her life and on her family. In the analysis I will show how relational issues are interrelated with financial and housing issues, but primarily with moral issues connected to kin and gender membership. I will start the analysis, describing how Anna became a carer.

THE ANALYSIS

Becoming a Carer

Anna is a good-looking woman in her late forties. When Anna's father-in-law died, her husband decided that they would go to live with his mother. After some time, her mother-in-law had a stroke and became bedridden and senile. Anna assisted her mother-in-law for several months while she was in hospital. Talking about that period, she says that it was really very hard. In fact, she kept her job, had the housework and the caring and got very little help from her husband, who works long hours, or from her husband's siblings. Then her husband's brothers insisted on putting their mother in a nursing home. Now she is in a home for severely disabled people, paying a thousand and three hundred Euros a month. Until the time of the interview, it had been possible to pay the nursing home with the mother's savings, but these were rapidly disappearing. In the following transcript Anna explains how she became a carer. Kin membership categories are mobilized in her account.

Anna	at his death (0.7) she collapsed (1.6) my husband didn't want to leave her alone (in this thing)	alla morte (0.7) lei ha avuto un crollo (1.6) e::: mio marito non ha voluto lasciarla sola (in questa cosa)
I	you mean she collapsed psy[chologically	cioè un crollo a livello psi[cologico
Anna	[physically psychologically also physically probably (0.5) she probably needed [somebody	[fisico psicologico anche fisico probabilmente era andata molto giù non mangiava più (0.5) aveva bisogno di qualcuno [probabilmente
I	[of course	[certo
Anna	and my husband felt let's say being the last child she was counting on him (0.3) on my husband (0.4) because he was always here also before heh (0.7) and she asked us (0.6) she asked us if we wanted to go to live with her (0.4) since there was room and we were paying rent	e mio marito si è senti:to diciamo essendo l'ultimo dei figli lei era molto appoggiata (0.3) a mio marito (0.4) perché lui era sempre qui anche pri:ma: eh (0.7) e:: c'ha chiesto (0.6) c'ha chiesto se volevamo andare ad abitare con lei (0.4) visto che il posto c'era noi eravamo in affitto il posto c'è venite lì

	there is room come here	
I	I see	certo

From the beginning and all through the interview, Anna attributes the decision to take on caring responsibilities to her husband who felt responsible to help his mother after his father's death, *my husband didn't want to leave her alone (in this thing).* The relational pair child/parent (Sacks, 1967) is mobilized by the use of the category "child", together with all the obligation of mutual care implied in the categorization, that, in this case, are strengthened by her husband's particular position within his family, *being the last child.* Anna highlights her husband's closeness to his mother describing his supportive relationship with her, *she was counting on him (0.3) on my husband (0.4),* and probably alluding to cohabitation before getting married as the only child left, *he was always here also before.* In this tale, Anna's husband's moral accountability to provide care to his mother is used as a resource to justify and explain their decision to move into the house.

The decision to move into her mother-in-law's house is constructed as a consequence of a precise request of hers, *she asked us (0.6) she asked us if we wanted to go lo live with her.* But housing and financial issues are also reported as having determined this decision, in fact it is constructed as a convenient solution for both parties, *since there was room and we were paying rent.* This is quite a common occurrence, housing issues are often related to caring arrangements (Taccani, 1994) see also Watson in chapter 2, for a detailed description of the house restructuring connected to caring for a disabled person. The accommodation is exchanged with provision of care, as in this case, or different housing arrangements become necessary because new needs of the cared for (Paoletti 2002). In this case, moral duty and financial convenience seem interrelated.

Shortly after the interview Anna explains further motives of her mother-in-law's wish to share her house with them and these are precisely connected to caring expectations.

Anna	it was she who asked us to come here after all [I think also to secure to herself a comfortable old age	è stata lei che ci ha voluto qui insomma [anche io credo per assicurarsi la sua vecchiaia
I	[( )	[( )
Anna	she manage to wring a promise out of my husband I hhhh! (0.8) I'll do anything you like as long as you don't put me in a nursing home (0.9) she said when she had her wits	e si è fatta strappare anche una promessa da mio marito io::: hhhhh! (0.8) faccio tutto quello che vuoi purché tu non mi porti al ricovero (0.9) lei diceva quando era in ragione
I	of course	certo
Anna	heh we did it while it was possi[ble this	eh::::: l'abbiamo fatto finché è stato possi[bile questo qui
I	[well of course (1.3) and so and didn't your husband take the fact of having to put her in a nursing home very well?	[bè certo (1.3) e quindi e:: suo marito l'ha vissuto male questo fatto di:: ricoverarla?
Anna	heh not much (1.7) it was a period a little he had a period that ((whispering)) it was a period for all [a bad period for all	eh: insomma (1.7) è stato un periodo un pochettino ha avuto un periodo che:: ((bisbigliando))è stato un periodo per tutti [un brutto periodo per tutti
I	[hah well ( ) very hard things=	[a bè ( ) cose molto pesanti=
Anna	=hard yes	=pesanti sì

Anna reiterates her remark, underlying that her mother's-in-law made the first move, proposing them to cohabit, *it was she who asked us to come here.* Then she highlights a possible secondary aim of her mother-in-law's proposal concerning caring needs, *after all [I think also to secure for herself a comfortable old age.* Anna reports a promise made by her husband to his mother that is constructed as having forcedly obtained from him, *she managed to wring a promise out of my husband.* Such a promise related to caring arrangements: avoiding being in a nursing home. Being in a nursing home is constructed as a very undesirable caring solution, such as the mother is prepared to do anything in order to avoid it, *1 hhhh! (0.8) 1'll do anything you like as long as you don't put me in a nursing home.* This construction is supported by the interviewer, *of course (line 10).* In particular the expression: "*we did it while it was possi[ble this*" highlights Anna's will to meet her obligations, projecting a positive moral image for her and moral accountability over the present situation, that is her mother-in-law's admittance in a nursing home needs to be explained and justified. It is not an ordinary caring solution. The interviewer reinforces the ordinariness of this moral tale, *well of course.* The interviewer also points out a possible psychological consequence of the present nursing home admittance of her mother-in-law on her husband, *didn't your husband take the fact of having to put her in a nursing home very well?* Anna answers in the affirmative, saying: *it was a period for all [a bad period for all.* This is above all a moral tale (Silvermann, 1987;1993; Baruch, 1981), in which duties and responsibilities are distributed according to kin membership, moral accountability is interactionally produced in the course of the narration: being her husband the last child, the promise, having used the house are the "good reasons" to take up the caring. Becoming a carer is seldom a matter of conscious choice, but it is often a gradual process, that does not imply open negotiation as Pyysiäinen describes in details, in chapter 6.

A history of family relationship, financial and housing issues and her husband's promise are the strings of the net from which the caring responsibilities are shown to have originated and to have fallen on Anna. Here gender membership becomes relevant. The ordinariness of the gender character of the moral order (Paoletti, 2001; 2002) appears evident in this account in which neither Anna nor the interviewer make in any way visible and relevant the fact that it is Anna's responsibility and not her husband's to take up the role of caring. This occurrence is constructed as a matter of course, no news, just as things ought to be. The strength of the gendered moral order rests precisely on this invisibility. In the analysis of the transcript that follows, the complexity of the caring relationship is further highlighted looking at the conflicts among siblings and the consequences they have for caring arrangements.

Siblings Conflicts

In the next transcript Anna explains how they came to the decision to put her mother-in-law in a nursing home, in spite of her husband's unwillingness; a mixture of financial and relational as well as moral issues are reported.

Anna	there are the brothers that they seem that I don't know (0.7) let's say as if (1.6) we have I don't know how to explain it (0.9) you have to be inside the situation to understand it (1.2)	Anna ci sono i fratelli che sembrano che: non so (0.7) diciamo come::: (1.6) abbiamo non so come spiegarla: (0.9) bisognerebbe esserci dentro per capire (1.2)
I	heh no try [to explain it to me	eh no mi provi [a spiegare
Anna	[they think that we are we exploited the situation let's say so (0.5) the situation till (0.3) we exploited it and now we have to ta- (0.8)	[ritengono che noi siamo: f::- abbiamo sfruttato diciamo così (0.5) la situazione finché::: (0.3) l'abbiamo sfruttata e adesso ci dobbiamo::::: a:: accon- (0.8)
I	to take [the consequences too ( )	accollare [anche le conseguenze ( )
Anna	[to take also the thing let's say the negative part of this thing here (0.7) we have to manage it by ourselves (1.2) we have to (0.8) heh (1.4) my husband would have followed Rossi's suggestions to keep her in the hospital of (0.9) of (0.8) not to accept discharge from the hospital (0.7) while there was the possibi- well while this person was in need of care (0.4) but but (1.2) the brothers no they pushed to the extreme to get us to put her in a place (0.6) where she'd be cared for (0.5) because I believe this is my thing probably also a bad one because they do not want (0.8) they don't want to know about they don't want to be involved and so there she is settle (0.6) they don't need to go to see her when I have some problems or I can't go (0.8) mm [( )	[accollare anche le cose:: diciamo negative di questa cosa qui quindi (0.7) ce la dobbiamo gestire noi (1.2) ce la dobbiamo (0.8) eh::: (1.4) mio marito avrebbe (0.7) avrebbe seguito diciamo così i consigli di Rossi quello di lasciarla in ospedale di (0.9) di:::: (0.8) di non accettare le dimissioni (0.7) fino a che c'era:::: la possibi- 'nsomma fino a che questa persona ha bisogno di questa assistenza (0.4) però (1.2) i fratelli no::: hanno premuto fino all'esasperazione perché la mettessimo in un posto (0.6) dove fosse assistita (0.5) perché io credo questa è una cosa mia anche cattiva forse perché loro non vogliono (0.8) n:::on ne vogliono sapere cioè non vogliono essere coinvolti e quindi là è a posto (0.6) non hanno più bisogno di andarla:::::: a vedere quando io ho dei problemi o non posso andare (0.8) um:: [( )
I	[hah you mean because in the hospital there was (1.5) [this fact that at least his sister	[ah cioè perché in ospedale c'era (1.5) [questo fatto che almeno sua sorella::
Anna	there was th[is fact	c'era que[sto eh questo fatto
I	your husband's sist[er ( )	la sorella di suo mari[to ( )
Anna	[yes ( ) also the one in Bologna the other sister who lives in Bologna every now and then she came down (0.7) then she staid here two or three days and then she of course she went home because she also had a family (1.1) heh (1.5) then I think that they (0.4) pushed in this direction because (0.3) to not to free themselves from this commitment (0.5) I mean heh to not have the duty (1.3) that I think it was a duty for them as children (1.0) to care for her	[sì ( ) anche quella di Bologna l'altra sorella che abita a Bologna ogni tanto veniva giù (0.7) poi stava qui due o tre giorni e poi andava a casa naturalmente perché anche lei aveva la sua famiglia (1.1) eh::: (1.5) allora penso che abbiano (0.4) premuto in questo senso perché (0.3)per non per liberarsi di questo impegno (0.5) cioè eh::::: di non avere più l'obbligo (1.3) che::: credo che sia stato un obbligo per loro in quanto figli (1.0) di dover assisterla

Anna shows a certain difficulty and embarrassment in talking about the issues relating to the conflicts within the family. Notice the edging, before starting the tale, and the several small pauses, *I don't know (0.7) let's say as if (1.6) we have I don't know how to explain it*

(0.9) you have to be inside the situation to understand it (1.2) conveying uncertainty: She is constructing the topic as a delicate and embarrassing matter.

On the interviewer's request to attempt an explanation, Anna states the point of view of her husband's siblings on the matter; she refers to her family using her mother-in-law's house for free, as the motive for the siblings' lack of involvement in the caring, *they think we are we exploited the situation let's say so (0.5) the situation till (0.3) we exploited it and now we have to ta- (0.8).* Again the several pauses and the edging, *let's say so,* (line 8), indicate the delicacy of the issue at hand. Then she stops in the middle of a word briefly. The collaborative completion (Sacks, 1992, 651) produced by the interviewer, *to take [the consequences too ( ),* is different from the one projectable from Anna's turn, in fact, "accollare" that is "to take up", has a different meaning from "accontentare", that is "to be satisfied" that is clearly inferable from Anna's last part of the turn (*accont-*). Anyway, the completion is endorsed by Anna in her next turn, *to take also the thing let's say the negative part of this thing here.*

The caring arrangement initially prospected by her husband was keeping his mother in the hospital since it was possible, *my husband would have followed Rossi's suggestions to keep her in the hospital.* Rossi is a doctor, evident institutional conflicts within the health system are highlighted in this passage, in fact this doctor's advise is to oppose an institutional decision, *not to accept of (0.9) of (0.8) not to accept discharge from the hospital (0.7).* The initial formulation, *while there was the possibi-,* is changed in, *well while this person was in need of care (0.4),* indicating different framing of the caring needs: institutional priorities versus patient's order of relevance.

The siblings are saddled with the responsibility of the decision to admit their mother to a nursing home, *the brothers no they pushed to the extreme to get us to put her in a place (0. 6) where she would be cared for (0.5).* Anna attributes the motivation for this decision to their lack of interest in their own mother. Notice the framing of her account, the prefacing: *because I believe this is my thing probably also a bad one,* is a negative evaluation of her thoughts on the sibling intentions; this is a self-accusation that contributes to construct the gravity of what is coming, *because they do not want (0.8) they don't want to know about they don't want to be involved and so there she is settled.* Not caring for one's own mother is a serious charge. This is a moral tale (Baruch, 1981; Silverman, 1993) in which blame and praise are attributed in relation to caring commitment for a close relative. She specifies the limited contribution the siblings are giving to caring for their own mother, *they do not need to go to see her when I have some problems or I can't go (0.8).*

The interviewer solicits then an account of the sibling's contribution to the caring while their mother was in the hospital and she mentions a sister, *because in the hospital there was (1.5) [this fact that at least his sister.* Anna mentions the help received by a husband's sister leaving in a different town, *every now and then she'd come down (0.7) then she'd stay here two or three days.* The limited help is justified by other caring commitments, *and then she of course she went home because she also had a family.* The relevance of gender in this account is striking: the interviewer mentions a female member among the siblings. Anna speaking of her husband's sister constructs an "ordinary female" which primary duties are caregiving duties (Finch and Groves, 1983). Caregiving is attributed to women in conversation as a matter of course (Paoletti, 2001; 2002).

In the last part of the transcript, the duties bound to kin relationship are spelled out. The category "children" is evoked as entailing the caring, *I mean heh to not have the duty (1.3) that I think it was a duty for them as children (1.0) to care for her*. Caregiving is constructed as a moral duty bound to the membership category "children". Her husband's siblings are made accountable for not providing care for their mother. In the next transcript Anna discusses the consequences that caregiving had on her health and family life.

The Effect of Caring

Anna tells how, particularly in the first period in which she was caring for her mother-in-law, she became very stressed and started to lose weight, she says: *I couldn't sleep at night because often she was causing confusion she had always (0.3) and I lost ten kilos (all of a sudden)*. Moreover, her caring commitment had an effect on her employment too, in fact she points out: *without my awareness probably (0.9) my job suffered from it too because there was a shortage of work (0.6) and I was the first one to be sent home.* Then she gradually started to cope better, but caring for her mother-in-law has been having an effect that seems to be reaching well beyond the time of assistance. Anna tells of the effects that the caring had and still has on her married life, although her mother-in-law is now in a nursing home.

Anna	and then I was always fighting with my husband terrible hah apart the burden [of this thing here	E poi si litigava sempre con mio marito 'na cosa:: ah:: oltre al peso [di questa cosa qui
I	[heh well of course	[e bè infatti
Anna	always because then after (0.3) arguments would arise and well (0.3) one with his nerves on edge(0.2) and we'd be always arguing always arguing (0.3) therefore (0.5) always in a bad mood	sempre perché dopo poi (0.3)nascevano delle discordie e lì (0.3) uno con i nervi tirati (0.2) e si litigava sempre sempre a litigare (0.3) quindi (0.5) sempre di malumore
I	[of course	[certo
Anna	[this thing here that was always pressing heh heh [(it is)	[questa cosa qui che ti premeva sempre eh:::: eh::[(è)
I	[which were the main motives for the arguments if there was any argument?	[qual erano i motivi de: di dissidio maggiori se:: c'erano dei motivi::?
Anna	with my husband?=	con mio marito?=
I	=yes=	=sì=
Anna	=(well thi-) mine was I mean I (0.2) mm (0.4) that I couldn't cope by myself (1.0) [( )	=(bè que) il m:io era cioè io (0.2) em:: (0.4)che non ce la facevo da sola (1.0) [( )
I	[you were complaining [let's say	[lei si lamentava [diciamo
Anna	[I was complaining that I couldn't cope by myself and he would say that there was no other way of doing it (0.5) because as I told you they had made such a drama of it also his brothers when we tried to involve them a bit (1.1) and therefore it must be so (0.4) it must be [(and then)	[io mi lamentavo che da sola non ce la facevo e lui diceva che non ci non c'era altra maniera di fare (0.5) perché::: come le ho detto ci sono state delle tragedie anche con i fratelli quando abbiam cercato di coinvolgerli un po' (1.1) e quindi::: doveva essere così (0.4) doveva essere [(e allora)
I	[therefore the motive of your let's say family arguing was precisely the caring	[quindi proprio l'assistenza era il motivo della:: della discordia diciamo familiare
Anna	yes I would say so	sì direi di sì
(2.5)		

Caring was a reason for constant quarrelling with her husband, *I was always fighting with my husband.* This fact is constructed as very negative together with the caring itself, *terrible hah apart from the burden [of this thing here.* The caring commitments were both the motive of the discussion and the reason of her tiredness and edginess, *arguments would arise and well (0.3) one with his nerves on edge (0.2).*The picture of the family tensions is efficaciously rendered by the repetitions, *and we'd be always arguing always arguing (0.3) therefore (0.5) always in a bad mood.* Notice that the words caring, caregiving are not used by the interviewee, caregiving is hinted by expressions such as: *this thing here that was always pressing* (lines 12-13), *apart the burden [of this thing here* (lines 2-3). Caregiving is constructed as an unbearable burden. It is precisely the fear of being left alone with this burden that was the main reason for Anna's arguing with her husband, *=(well thi-) mine was I mean I (0.2) mm (0.4) that I couldn't cope by myself (1.0) [( ),* the preface, the small pauses project the issue as delicate and controversial. The interviewer constructs such accounts as "complaints", *[you were complaining [let's say,* construction that is promptly endorsed by the interviewee, *[I was complaining that I couldn't cope by myself.*

We can sympathize with Anna's frustration at her husband's reply, *and he would say that there was no other way of doing it.* Nevertheless, her husband's siblings' uncooperative behavior did not allow a better prospect, *they had made such a drama of it also his brothers when we tried to involve them a bit.* The repetitions effectively project the ineluctability of her forced commitment to caring for her mother-in-law, *therefore it must be so (0.4) it must be.* Caregiving is spelled out as the cause of family conflicts by the interviewer, *[therefore the motive of your let's say family arguing was precisely the caring,* and acknowledged by Anna, *yes I would say so.* A significant pause follows, *(2.5)*, then Anna starts to talk again producing accounts and justifications for her complaints.

1 2 3 4 5 6 7	Anna	I mean the the the the my (0.3) my fear of not being able to cope of having to (0.6) look after all these things and not being able to cope (0.8) probably it was me who was complaining too much then you know how it goes (0.3) then you complain and other things come out	cioè il:: il::: il:: il mio (0.3) la mia paura di non farcela di dover (0.6) stare dietro a tutte queste cose e di non farcela (0.8) ero io probabilmente che mi lamentavo troppo poi sa com'è (0.3) dopo uno si lamenta:: e vengono fuori delle altre cose
8	I	yes yes of course [then	sì sì certo [poi
9	Anna	[mm	[um
10 11	I	as you just said one is stressed tired (0.5) irritable (0.9) [then	uno appunto come diceva lei è teso è stanco (0.5)nervoso (0.9) [poi
12	Anna	heh[it is easy heh	eh:: [fa presto eh
13	I	a motiv[e	il motivo:::[:::
14	Anna	[also [( )	[anche [( )
15	I	[for arguing	[per discutere::
16	Anna	triv[ial	bana[le
17	I	[you find it	[si trova
18	Anna	hh! you find it you find it	hh! si trova si trova
19	I	I mean when you are in a difficult situation=	cioè quando la la situazione::: è pesante=

The pause, *(2.5),* (line 36 previous transcript) is attributable to the interviewer, in fact, in an interview situation, when the interviewee's turn appears clearly finished, as in this case, the floor passed invariably to the interviewer (Frankel, 1990). The absence of a new question is interpreted by Anna as an invitation to continue, to account and justify her complaints. What is Anna doing in this passage? My understanding is that she interprets as a criticism the interviewer's framing of her tale as "complaints" and she produces an account in order to justify herself and produce a positive moral image of herself. The several repetition indicates the need of a time to thing and organize her reply, *I mean the the the the my (0.3) my fear of not being able to cope of having to (0.6) look after all these things and not being able to cope.* She reiterates her feeling overwhelmed by the task. Then a self accusation follows, *probably it was me who was complaining too much.* Anna feels the need to justify herself for her complaining about caregiving, because caregiving is a precise duty of her, but she is also justified in part on her complaints because she is left by herself in the caring and this is not right. Moreover the cared-for is not her mother, but her mother-in-law. The gradable properties of moral accountability of kin membership categories, in relation to the duty of providing care, are mobilized in this account: children are more morally bound to providing care to their own parents than children-in-law, daughters more than sons. This is the cultural knowledge background on which this account becomes significant and understandable.

In a minuet of overlapping turns at talk interviewer and interviewee construct an ordinary psychological account for the generation of arguments among partners. Anna starts acknowledging the ordinariness of the occurrence, *you know how it goes (0.3)* and then producces thc dcscription of how conflicts get generated, *then you complain and other things come out.* The interviewer produces some acknowledgment tokens, *yes yes yes of course*, then she mentions the psychological causes of getting into arguments previously (line 7 of the previous transcript) pointed out by Anna, *as you just said one is stressed tired (0.5) irritable.* At first sight the following sequence of overlapping sentences could appear as a delayed completion sequence (Lerner, 1989, 169), and a distancing move could be inferred. In fact, we could look at the interviewer's turn, *a motiv[e ... [for arguing ... [you find it*, as interrupted by Anna's attempted cooperative completion moves *[also [( ) ... triv[ial,*that were resisted though delayed completion, but at a closer look the cooperative qualities of the passage appear evident.

Overlapping is not always connoted as interruptive in conversation in the Italian culture, it can denote for example excited participation or support as in this case. Interviewer's turn, *a motiv[e*, is specified by Anna's turns, *[also [() ... tri[vial*, and completed by the interviewer, *[you find it.* Anna's prompt acknowledgment underlies the aligning character of the move, *you find it you find it.* As well as the content of interviewer's next turn, *I mean when you are in a difficult situation=,* appears clearly a supportive move, expressing understanding for Anna's difficult situation. In my view this passage denotes alignment.

The situation is changed, Anna's mother-in-law is now in a nursing home, the difficulties with her husband, though, still persist.

Family Conflicts with No Solution

In the next passage Anna describes how the present situation is still very difficult, although her mother-in-law is now in a nursing home. She keeps quarelling with her husband in particular over the frequency of the visits to his mother who is fading away and is no longer able to recognise them. Anna wishes to go back to normal life, but her husband insists in spending all weekends with his mother.

Anna	=even now (we) still argue (0.5) about this thing (0.7) ((whispering)) (because) now (0.3) my husband although his mother is (0.5) let's say cared for (0.6) and that she's not (0.5) for what she can (0.5) have ehm let's say she is confortable (0.5) even if we don't go there one Saturday or one Sunday (0.5) even if we miss a visit (1.1) it's not that what does she lose (0.7) she isn't even able to recognise us	=anche adesso (noi ci) litighiamo ancora (0.5)per questa cosa qui (0.7) ((bisbigliando)) (perché) adesso (0.3) mio marito nonostante sua madre si:a (0.5) diciamo assistita (0.6) e che non (0.5) per quello che può (0.5) a:vere diciamo eh::m:: non gli manca nulla (0.5) anche se noi non c'andiamo una:: un sabato o una domenica (0.5) anche se saltiamo (1.1) non è che: gli viene cosa cosa gli viene a mancare a lei (0.7) che non ci conosce neanche
I	of cour[se	cer[to
Anna	[but he must (0.3) go to see anyway he is very close to his mother (0.3) he was and he still is now (0.4) and now now more more than before I can say	[però lui deve (0.3) andare a vedere lo stesso lui è molto legato a sua madre (0.3) lo è stato e lo è tuttora (0.4) e adesso:::: adesso più più di prima posso dire
I	of course	certo
Anna	because he probably sees that she is getting worse (0.8) I would like to let her go a bit to loo-(0.3) to loosen a bit [wouldn't it	perché adesso forse vede che:::: sta peggiorando la cosa (0.8) io sarei per lasciarla un pochettino allen- (0.3)allentare un pochettino [no
I	[of course	[certo
Anna	now that we have for a few months we have managed let's say to have a little freedom (0.3) I'd like to go out mm	adesso che abbiamo::: siamo riusciti da qualche mese diciamo ad avere un attimo di libertà (0.3) mi piacerebbe andare fuori um::::
I	[of course	[certo
Anna	[but no (0.8) but no (1.3) we have to it seams that (1.2) this agony has to go on (1.1) mm? [let's say	[e invece no (0.8) e invece no (1.3) bisogna mi pare che (1.2) bisogna che continui questa agonia (1.1) um? [diciamo
I	[yes yes yes	[sì sìsì sì
Anna	ours and hers (0.9) beacouse til- (0.3) I believe that it will always be (1.4) it'll always be worse (1.0) because you can see it week by week that she is getting worse	nostra e sua (0.9) perché fin- (0.3) io credo che sarà sempre (1.4) sarà:: andrà sempre in peggio (1.0) perché si vede in settimana in settimana che peggiora

The mother-in-law goes on being a motive for arguments between husband and wife, even though she is in a nursing home, *=even now (we) still argue (0.5) about this thing (0.7).* All their free time is spent visiting her in the hospital, *even if we don't go there one Saturday or one Sunday (0.5) even if we miss a visit (1.1) it's not that what does she lose (0. 7) she doesn't even recognise us*. The concreteness of Anna's point of view is contrasted with her husband's, *[but he must (0.3) go to see anyway,* and his feeling of closeness to his mother, *he is very close to his mother (0.3) he was and he still is now (0.4,),* in particular at the time in which she is fading away, *and now now more more than before 1 can say ... because he probably sees that she is getting worse.*

Anna wishes to go back to normal life; she constructs the issue as delicate when she hesitates in pronouncing "loosen" and makes it follow from a tag question, *I would like to let her go a bit to loo-(0.3) to loosen a bit [wouldn't it.* The interviewer promptly produces an alignment token, overlapping with her turn, *[of course.* Anna continues, expressing her desire to go out, to go back to ordinary life, *now that we have for a few months we have managed let's say to have a little freedom (0.3) I'd like to go out mm*. Such a desire is acknowledged by the interviewer. Very effectively she pictures their situation, *this agony has to go on (1.1) mm? let's say ... ours and hers (0.9)*. The prefaces, several pauses and the edging contribute to produce the delicacy of the issue. It is an agony that is burying their marital relationship. Her husband's closeness and his moral accountability towards his mother appear to be the insuperable obstacles Anna is fighting against. A little further on in the interview, Anna very lucidly and dramatically refers to her mother-in-law's death as a liberation.

1	I	what might help you	che cosa l'aiuterebbe
2	Anna	me?=	per me?=
3	I	=yes	=sì
4	Anna	for me [personally (0.9)	per me [personalmente (0.9)
5	I	[yes	[sì
6 7 8 9 10	Anna	hah it's awful to (say it) (0.4) but (3.2) I don't know when I was home I used to say (0.4) I felt guilty because I said (0.6) while she lives I'll never feel good again (1.4) and (0.4) the solution for me was her death	ah:: è brutta a (dirselo) (0.4) però (3.2) non so io quando ero a casa dicevo (0.4) mi sentivo in colpa perché dicevo (0.6) finché vive io non starò mai bene (1.4) e:: (0.4) la soluzione per me era la sua morte
11	I	of cour[se ((whispering))	cer[to ((bisbigliando))
12 13 14 15		[then she went into hospital different problems but (0.3) she wasn't in the house at least (0.3) there was no longer (0.7) this (0.6) this presence always	[dopo è andata in ospedale altri problemi però (0.3) mancava qui in casa perlomeno (0.3) non c'era più (0.7) questo:: (0.6) questa presenza sempre

The feelings of guilt are clearly expressed not only by the explicit reference to it, *I felt guilty*, (line 8), but also by the preface, *hah it's awful to (say it) (0.4)*, (line 6). The noticeable pause that follows, *but (3.2)*, and the edging, *I don't know*. All these conversational objects are prefacing and announcing the fact that something terrible and reproachable is coming. *While she lives I'll never feel good again (1.4) and (0.4) the solution for me was her death.* The agreement token pronounced by the interviewer with a barely audible voice, *of cour[se (whispering)*, is a weak agreement and conveys disagreement (Pomerantz, 1984). It contributes to constructing the dramatic force of the expression. Anna is left alone with her guilt. The interviewer's supportive attitude all through the interview do not overcome this trial. Anna continues, constructing the caring as an obsession with no escape, *she wasn't in the house at least (0.3) there was no longer (0.7) this (0.6) this presence always*. Again the several pauses convey the delicacy of the matter.

The moral accountability of providing care to close relatives becomes evident in the interview interaction, not only through what is narrated, but also though the interaction itself in which caregiver's moral accountability is actively negotiated between the interviewer and the interviewee.

This analysis could appear to reinforce the common sense assumption of caregiving as pertaining to women. This is not my objective. I showed how the attributions of caregiving duties to female kin are very powerful commonsense assumptions, finely engrained in ordinary conversation, a matter of course, on which background understanding is achieved by interlocutors. In another study (Paoletti, 2004) I have shown how these assumptions are actively contrasted in caregivers' talk. There is nothing "natural", "absolute", "essential" about common sense assumptions. They can be changed, they are regularly changed, but we cannot forget that they are very powerful. Social reality holds together because of them.

Conclusion

Caring is not only a time-consuming and physically demanding job, it is also a task in which complex moral and emotional issues are involved. Duties related to kinship, strong relational bonds and gender identification processes are involved in the provision of care to order family members. Moreover complex financial, housing issues are at times related to the caring arrangements as it was illustrated in this study.

In this chapter I showed how strongly caregiving can affect a caregiver's life and health and family. In some cases not even the admittance in a nursing home can resolve the family conflicts generated from caring for a dependent relative. It is essential to understand the complex moral, emotional and identity issues related to caring as well as financial and housing issues in order to organize support services that are really effective in helping family caregivers. I support entirely Abel's (1991, 66) perspective when she says in relation to respite care and support services for caregivers: " The overriding issue is not how to relieve stress but how to organize society to make care for the dependent population more just and humane."

Recommendations

- For any government, particularly in Western Countries, a first priority should be the organization of support services to family caregivers, in relation to facing the issue raised by the increasing older population.
- Support services should be flexible and cover a vast array of possible needs: support personnel (home helpers, nurses, physiotherapists, doctors etc.) financial support, counseling, respite services (temporary admittance in hospitals or nursing homes, day care centers), provision of technical devices (while chairs, lifting devices, etc..), house structural modifications, help in changing house etc..
- Caregiver/s and cared for should be involved in the decision making pertaining the allocation of support services.
- Respite services (temporary admittance in hospitals or nursing homes, day centers) should planned to provide useful services to the person in need of care, such as for example: check up, rehabilitation, occupation therapy etc. They shouldn't be planned as parking sites for the elderly.
- Personnel, at any level working in support services, should be trained to be flexible, to strive to look at the whole picture of the caregiving situation from the point of view of the people involved, to be aware of gender issue related to caregiving.
- Policies should be developed that aim to limit the damages on female employment in relation to caregiving commitments.

Transcript Notations

. or,	Stop or pause in the rhythm of the conversation
?	Rising intonation
!	Excited tone
( )	Word(s) spoken, but not audible
(dog)	Word(s) whose hearing is doubtful
((laugh))	Transcriber description
[	Overlapping utterances at this point
=	No gaps in the flow of conversation
(0.4)	Pause timed in seconds
.....	elongation

Bibliography

Abel, E.K. (1990) Daughters caring for elderly parents. In J.F. Gubrium and A. Sankara (Eds.) *The home care experience: Ethnograph policy* (pp. 189-206) Newsbury Park. CA: Sage.

Abel, E.K. (1991) *Who cares for the elderly? Public policy and the experiences of adult daughters*. Philadelphia: Tample University Press.

Antaki, C. and Widdicombe, S. (Eds.) (1998) *Identities in talk*. London: Sage.

Arber, S. and Gilbert, G.N. (1989) Men: The forgotten carers. *Sociology*, 23, (1), 111-118.

Aronson, J. (1990) Women's perspective on informal care of the elderly: Public ideology and personal experience of giving and receiving care. *Ageing and Society,* 10, 61-84.

Atkinson, M.J. and Heritage, J. (Eds.), (1984). *Structures of social action. Studies in conversational analysis.* Cambridge: University Press.

Baker, C. (1984) The "search for adultness": membership work in adolescent-adult talk. *Human Studies*, 7, 301-323.

Baker, C. (1997) Membership categorization and interview accounts. In D. Silverman (ed.) *Qualitative research. Theory, method and practice* (pp. 130-143). London: Sage.

Baruch, G. (1981) Moral tales: parents' stories of encounters with the health profession. *Sociology of health and illness*, 3, (3), 275- 296.

Dalley, G. (1993) Caring: a legitimate interest of older women. In M. Bernard and K. Meade (Eds.) *Women come to age: perspectives on the lives of older women* (pp. 106-1990). London: Arnold.

Day, D. (1998) *Being ascribed and resisting membership of an ethnic group*. In C. Antaki and S. Widdicombe (Eds.) *Identities in talk* (pp. 151-170). London: Sage.

Finch, J. and Groves, D. (eds.) (1983) *A labour of love: Women, work and caring*. London: Routledge and Kegan Paul.

Frankel, R. (1990) Talking in interviews: A dispreference for patient-initiated questions in physician-patient encounters. In G. Psathas. (Ed.) *Interaction competence* (pp. 231-262). Washington: Interactional Institute for Ethnomethodology and Conversation Analysis and University Press of America.

Garfinkel, H. (1967) *Studies in ethnomethodology*. Englewood Cliffs, N.J.: Prentice-Hall.

Graham, H. (1983) Caring: A labour of love. In J. Finch and D. Groves (Eds.) *A labour of love: Women, work and caring*. (pp. 13-31). London: Routledge and Kegan Paul.

Heritage, J. (1984) *Garfinkel and ethnomethodology.* Cambridge: Polity Press.

Hester, S. and Eglin, P. (eds.) (1997) *Culture in action. Studies in Membership Categorization Analysis.* Washington: International Institute for Ethnomethodology and Conversation Analysis and University Press of America.

Jayyusi, L. (1984) *Categorization and the moral order.* Boston: Routledge and Kegan Paul.

Jayyusi, L (1991) Values and moral judgment: communicative praxis. In G. Button (Ed.) *Ethnomethodology and the human sciences* (pp. 227-251). Cambridge: Cambridge University Press.

Jenkins, C.L. (1997) Women, work, and caregiving: How do these roles affect women's well-being? *Journal of Women and Aging*. 9, (3), 27-45.

Joshi, H. (1995) The labour market and unpaid caring: Conflict and compromise. In I. Allen and E. Perkins (Eds.) *The future of family care for older people* (pp. 93- 118). London: HMSO.

Matthews, A.M. and Campbell, L.D (1995) Gender roles, employment and informal care. In S. Arber and J. Ginn, (Eds.) *Connecting gender and ageing* (pp. 129- 143). Buckingham: Open University Press,.

Moerman, M. (1996) The field of analyzing foreign language conversations. *Journal of Pragmatics,* 26, 147-158.

Ochs, E. (1979) Transcription as theory. In E. Ochs and B.B. Schieffelin (Eds.). *Developmental pragmatics*. (pp. 43-72) New York: Academic Press.

Paoletti, I. (1997) La produzione dell'identità nell'intervista con anziane, In A. Macarino, (Ed.) *Analisi della Conversazione e prospettive di ricerca in etnometodologia.*(pp. 235-247). Urbino: Edizioni Quattroventi.

Paoletti, I. (1998a) Handling "incoherence" according to the speaker's on-sight categorisation. In C. Antaki and S. Widdicombe (Eds.) *Identities in talk.* (pp. 171-190). London: Sage.

Paoletti, I. (1998b) *Being an older woman. An interpretative study in the social construction of identity.* Hillsdale, NJ: Lawrence Earlbaum.

Paoletti, I (1998c) Indicazioni per la modifica del questionario per le assistenti" Rapporto di Ricerca: Dipartimento di Ricerche Gerontologiche, INRCA, Ancona Italy.

Paoletti, I. (1999a) Caring women, cared women: The discourse of caregiving in Italy. In Judd, K., Ash de Pou, J., Tavares-Bucher, Sikoska, T. and Solomon, J. (Eds.) *Ageing in a gendered world: Women's issues and identitie* (pp. 133-152). Santo Domingo: INSTRAW.

Paoletti, I. (1999b) A half life: women caregivers of older disable relatives. *Journal of Women and Aging*, 11, (1), 53-67.

Paoletti, I. (2001) Membership categorization and time appraisal in interviews with carers of disabled elderly, *Human Studies,* 24, 293-325.

Paoletti, I. (2002) Caring for older people: a gendered practice. *Discourse and Society,* Special Issue on Language and Gender 13, (6), 805-817.

Paoletti, I (2004) La resistenza ad assunti di senso comune in interviste con assistenti familiari agli anziani disabili, *Rivista Italiana di Psicologia Applicata*, 2-3, 95-109.

Pohl, J.M., Boyd, C and Given, B.A. (1997) Mother-daughter relationships during the first year of caregiving: a quality study. *Journal of Women and Aging*, 9, (1\2), 133-149

Pomerantz, A. (1984) Agreeing and disagreeing with assessments: some features of preferred/dispreferred turn shapes. In M.J. Atkinson and J. Heritage. (Eds.) *Structures of social action. Studies in conversational analysis* (pp. 57-101). Cambridge: Cambridge University Press.

Rose, H. and Bruce, E. (1995) Mutual care but differential esteem: caring between older couples. In S. Arber and J. Ginn, (Eds.) *Connecting gender and ageing*. Buckingham: Open University Press.

Sacks, H. (1967) "The search for help: No one to turn to". In J. Schneidman (Ed.) *Essays in self-destruction*, (pp. 203-223) New York: Science House,.

Sacks, H (1972) On the analyzability of stories by children. In J Gumperz and D Hymes (Eds) *Directions in Sociolinguistics: The ethnography of communication.* (pp.329-345) New York: Holt, Rinehart and Winston.

Sacks, H. (1992) *Lectures on conversation vol. I and II,* Cambridge, MA: Blackwell.

Silverman, D. (1993) *Interpreting qualitative data*. London: Sage.

Silverman, D. (1987) *Communication and medical practices*. London: Sage.

Silverman, M. and Huelsman, E. (1990) The dynamics of long-term familial caregiving. In J.F. Gubrium and A. Sankara (Eds.) *The home care experience.* Thousand Oaks: Sage.

Taccani, P. (Ed.) (1994) *Dentro la cura*. Milano: Angeli

Walker, A. (1995) The family and the mixed economy of care In I. Allen and E. Perkins (Eds.) *The future of family care for older people*. London: HMSO.

Watson, R. and Weinberg, M. (1982). Interviews and the interactional construction of accounts of homosexual identity. *Social Analysis*, 11, 56-78.

Watson, R. (1997) Some general reflections on "categorization" and "sequence" in the analysis of conversation. In S. Hester and P. Eglin (Eds.) *Culture in action. Studies in Membership Categorization Analysis* (pp. 49-75). Washington: International Institute for Ethnomethodology and Conversation Analysis and University Press of America.

In: Family Caregiving for Older Disabled People
Editor: Isabella Paoletti, pp. 19-34
ISBN 1-59454-808-0

Chapter 2

ECONOMICALLY UN-RATIONAL FARM BUSINESS FAMILIES IN FINLAND

Saija Katila
Department of Business and Management
University of Kuopio, Kuopio, Finland

INTRODUCTION

There are great differences between countries regarding how welfare systems are designed and what the role of the informal support system is for the care of the elderly. Nevertheless, it is well-known that care for the elderly by members of the informal support system is characteristic of all countries in the world (Chappel, 1990) and care by family members is the most common alternative within the informal support system (Cicirelli, 1983; Kosberg, 1992). In Finland, as in other Nordic countries, the welfare system has developed into a universal welfare regime where the basic welfare benefits and services have been developed for all citizens, and in practice a large majority of the citizens also use these benefits and services. In other words, publicly provided care is a citizen's right, and should be available for any individual or family in need of these services. In the case of older disabled people, it is not the families but the government that is responsible for the care. The decision regarding the mix of informal and formal care is a choice that rests with the family.

It further seems to be a rather universal phenomenon that caring work done in homes is gender-segregated. Female members of the family are the major caregivers for elderly persons in most of the countries in the world (e.g. Gibson, 1984; Kosberg, 1992). Finland is no exception in this respect. The main caregivers in Finland in the private as well as the public sphere are women (Anttonen, 1997). It is, however, a less acknowledged fact that even if the welfare benefits and services are universal within a national context, groups differ regarding the mix of formal and informal care that they choose when taking care of their old and disabled family members. Furthermore, the question of how the priority is given to homecare over other options of care might be embedded in the moral order of an occupational community has received little attention. In this chapter, I will be looking at these issues in the case of one occupational community, namely farmers in Finland.

Farmers are an interesting group to study because farming in Finland (Suomen maatalous ja maaseutuelinkeinot 1999/2000), and also in Europe in general, is mainly organised into a familial unit. The basic organisational unit of agriculture in Finland is a family farm that is passed on from generation to generation.[1] In farming families, land, housing, machinery and the skills needed in farming work are transmitted from one generation to the next. Also social values, and taken-for-granted ways of behaving are transmitted through intergenerational networks with emotional rules to support them. On the basis of an ethnographic study, this chapter will demonstrate that the value of taking care of the antecedent generation is part of the system of values and norms comprising the moral order of Finnish farming families.

The starting point of this chapter is that the 'family' is not a discrete social form but rather a cultural creation, something we construct in our cultural communities. As individuals are part of families and families are part of larger communities, the larger community and society enter into our understanding of what a family is and what kind of rights and obligations individuals have within a family in the given context. Hence, whether you become a primary caregiver of your elderly family members is not solely an individual choice. Individuals seldom make 'individual' decisions, but rather decisions within the context set by various collectives. In a collective, the social context is to a significant extent perceived as a legitimate and integral part of one's existence. One has a sense of shared identity and commitment to live up to the moral order of the community (Etzioni, 1988, p. 4-5). As a member of a family you are forced to consider the social, moral, economic (see Etzioni, 1988; Granovetter, 1985) and emotional implications of the decisions concerning the home care of your elderly family members.

It could be argued that families have specific moral orders that emerge from their individual and cultural histories. A moral order refers to the norms and values of a particular community. Each action is publicly marked with respect or contempt. Actions, whatever their practical aim, are treated as displays of character in accordance with local understandings of acceptable and context-appropriate personae. In the moral psychology of personal being, one's actions count not for themselves, but for what they reveal about individual character in regard to the communities' moral order. The standing of a person depends in part on the degree to which she/he is capable of fulfilling commitments. It is important to understand that honour can be besmirched not only by one's own actions but also by the actions of a family member that dishonour the whole family (Harré, 1983, p. 245). A moral order defines what is valuable in a community, and worthy to strive for, and what are the basic principles according to which one is expected to behave (Ylijoki, 1998). A moral order does not, however, causally determine the actions of community members. It could rather be seen as a loose frame within which community members reflect their decisions and actions. Moral orders are ambivalent in nature – they can both support and restrict the actions of community members, depending on the context.

A family could be seen as a site where rights and obligations regarding care are formed (see Gubrium, 1987). Paoletti in the previous chapter illustrated in detail how such rights and obligations are finely ingrained in ordinary talk. Looking at family caregiving relationships

[1] Eighty-eight per cent of active farms are owned by private persons and twelve per cent by estates and family co-operatives (Suomen maatalous ja maaseutuelinkeinot 1999/2000).

from the point of view of a moral order, the role of emotions should not be dismissed. To enhance our understanding of how emotions influence families and their decision-making regarding the care of the old and disabled, it is important, however, to go beyond individual emotional expressions. Emotions are the personal displays of affected states like joy, love, sadness, shame or guilt. They are, however, only partly individual. They acquire their meaning from the cultural context - national, local and organisational (Ratner, 1989; Lutz and White, 1986, ref. in Fineman, 1997, p. 546; Fineman, 1993). They also transmit the collective subjectivity of groups of individuals and reveal cultural rules and touch upon issues that characterise humans in general (Ruth and Vilkko, 1996).

Rather than focusing on the role of an individual value emphasising the homecare of the elderly, this chapter suggests that it would be more fruitful to look at the value in relation to the system of values and norms comprising the moral order of the community in question. The Finnish yeoman moral order is composed of the values of continuity of the family farm, the value of taking care of the antecedent generation, the norm of unpaid family labour and the yeoman economic ethos consisting of hard work, saving and self-sufficiency (Katila 2000, 2002). The aim of the chapter is firstly, to assess the connection between the value of taking care of the antecedent generation and the other norms and values of the Finnish yeoman moral order. Secondly, the chapter describes how the moral order is gendered and how it influences the division of caring work on the farms. Thirdly, the chapter highlights how the gendering of the yeoman moral order might be changing, and fourthly what emotions play a key role in supporting the moral order.

The next section of the chapter outlines the methodological choices of the study. It will be followed by a narrative, from the ethnographic study, highlighting the role of the value of taking care of the antecedent generation in the everyday lives of the farming families. The first part of the narrative concerns the gendered division of labour and its connection to the value of continuity of the family farm. The second part discusses the value of taking care of the antecedent generation and its entanglement with the issue of continuity of the farm. The last part of the narrative focuses on the emotional nature of the yeoman moral order in Finland. The chapter will end with specific recommendations based on this study.

Study Design

Farmers are the most homogenous group in Finland with respect to social background and economic standing (Alestalo, 1985, p. 125-134). To be able to surface the norms and values of the yeoman moral order in Finland and the emotions supporting it, an ethnographic study (e.g. Van Maanen, 1088, 1995) of five farm business families was conducted. All the farming businesses under study had started new businesses outside the subsidised agricultural sector. They were micro enterprises that merely created self-employment. An attempt was made to maximise the variability between the cases (see Hamersley, 1992) according to how much the families used the farmer's skills and the farm's resources and how much they needed new skills and new resources. The cases vary from a farm where the entrepreneurs mainly continue farming-like activities by diversifying on the land (organic farming, strawberry production) to a farm where the new activities do not have anything to do with the farmer's skills and the farm's resources (veterinarian clinic, carpenter shop).

The pool of candidates for the study was first contacted by letter, which described the research questions and the method of the study. The letter implied that the candidates would be contacted later by phone. The rationality behind this procedure was to give the families ample time to decide whether they wanted to participate in the study. From the 14 families that received the letter, five invited the researcher into their home for a week.

The study draws upon two main sources of data: interview material and field notes. The data were collected by living for one full week with each of the five farm business families – observing the activities, participating in them and making interviews with different family members. During the study week the informants were followed throughout the days, paying attention to the material surroundings, like housing, machinery and tools where everyday life was conducted. Special emphasis was placed on the division of labour between the family members as well as on the entanglement of public and private spheres of life. Events were noted down during the course of the day, and they were extended into a full field diary each evening.

To be able to answer the research questions a biographical interview technique was chosen for the study. It was crucial in revealing the moral order and its supportive emotions, which framed the actions of the members of the farm business families. When people tell who they are, what they are striving for, and what is meaningful for them in their lives (Ruth and Kenyon, 1996), they also explain the generally accepted rules of the society in which they are living (Bruner, 1990). Reminiscing about life events triggers emotions that are relived and re-experienced (Cohen, 1993). Self-reflexive judgments are especially sensitive to emotions where the narrators' self-esteem and their beliefs about their abilities are concerned. In biographies, episodes of practical activity integrate moral and ethical motives (Polkinghorne, 1991). The interviews highlighted the subjective interpretations and reinterpretations, the individual meaning-giving process of life episodes, the experiences of growing up on the farm. In biography, a personal story merges with collective memory and makes visible the complicated inter-generational influence of the family (Thompson, 1993, p. 15). Biographies that are entangled with each other and refer to each other touch the life of the same group of individuals (Bertaux and Delcroix, 2000). During the study altogether eleven persons were interviewed. The interviews lasted an average of two hours and all of them were taped recorded and transcribed.

The data gathered was analysed thematically, but because it fragmented the lives of the informants, making it difficult to understand their situated behaviour, a narrative approach was adopted for the study. A narrative tells the story of human intentions and deeds and situates them in time and space. It further mixes the objective and the subjective aspects, thereby relating the world as people see it. Narrative knowledge could be seen as the main bearer of knowledge in our societies (Brunner, 1986). Using the biographies of different family members and the field notes collected during the participant observation period, narratives of each of the five families under study were constructed. What is conveyed to the reader is based upon the textual formats, the rhetorical figures, the choice of descriptive vocabulary and the selection of illustrative materials (Atkinson 1990, p. 2).

Because the narratives are too long to present here, only part of one narrative is presented to highlight the arguments made. For this chapter, I have chosen a case where the homecare of the disabled parents was the most intensive and long-standing. It must be pointed out, however, that the general arguments made in this chapter would remain the same regardless of which one of the five narratives were presented here. In the sections of the chapter where the extracts of the narrative are taken into closer inspection, reference will also be made to the findings of the other cases. Parts of the extracts are in italics to indicate a direct quotation from a transcribed interview with the actor in question. All the names used in this narrative are pseudonyms.

The narrative 'The Committed Ones' describes how the issue of care is embedded in the everyday running of the family and the farm in the lives of Juhani (40 years old), and his wife Tiina (32 years old) as well as Juhani's sister Mervi (41 years old) and brother Marko (42 years old.) The first section of the narrative discusses the childhood of the informants revealing the gendered division of labour and the gendered nature of the yeoman moral order.

THE COMMITTED ONES

Farming and Caring

Mervi, Juhani and Marko were born in the 1950s into a farming family. They lived in a small house with their parents, granny and Minni who was a mentally handicapped woman whom the "*municipality had given them*" (Tiina, interview 1). Minni took part in all farming and household work for her upkeep. Their family farm was a bit bigger than farms on average in Finland at the time. They had milking cows and they grew cereal crops and potatoes for their own use, and some for sale as well. When Mervi was a child, all family members had to do their share of the work on the farm, and the kids were no exception. And there was a lot of work: chopping wood, forking hay, carrying water and fire wood, tending cattle, milking cows, forking dung, cleaning, cooking, washing dishes and laundry. There was not much time for play.

Mervi was the only girl in the family with her own duties. On a daily basis she helped in the household chores and farming work. She also had great responsibility for the financial matters of the family after she was ten years of age. Mervi was very good at school and skipped one year. Thus, she finished middle school at the age of 14 in 1965. Her dreams of getting a further education were crushed the very same year - her mother was diagnosed with rheumatism and lost her ability to work. After her mother got ill she took full responsibility for the financial matters of the farm, like keeping the accounts. That was not, however, her main responsibility. Her task was to take care of her mom and dad, who were both disabled. Her dad had been incapable of movement as long as the kids could remember. *"I kept thinking that how can I keep sane, it was really hard on a young girl to care for her parents day in, and day out. Sometimes I did not see anybody of my own age except my two brothers for six months. I remember, it was really, really hard."* (Mervi, interview 1). Mervi's parents were mentally strong and they held on to the reins in the house. The work on the farm was organised as the parents saw fit. Their two sons had the duty to go to school, and after school their duty was to take care of the farm. The division of labour between the brothers evolved quite naturally. Marko took over the responsibility of animal husbandry that had earlier been the women's domain on the farm, and Juhani specialised in crop production. After finishing middle school Juhani was sent to farming school. He was assigned to continue the family farm. He had no objections, though, because he liked farming work and had no other plans. Marko finished high school and applied to the university but it did not work out. He returned to the family farm and kept working there. Mervi's duty was to stay at home and take care of her parents. Mervi understood the reasoning of her parents – they were afraid that they would not have anyone to take care of them if Mervi found someone and got married. Then they would be forced to leave the farm that was their home.

The extract nicely depicts the gendered division of labour on the farm in general, and the gendering of care in particular. The division of labour in the family was by no means atypical of Finnish farming families - on the contrary. It could be seen as a manifestation of the gendered nature of the Finnish yeoman moral order. Girls and boys growing up on a farm have differentiated rights and obligations. Girls are mainly expected to do household and caring work and tend the livestock. Boys, on the other hand, are expected to learn the occupation and they are entitled to continue the family farm. Men have the right to run the farm and they are socialised and trained accordingly (see also Abrahams, 1991; Kumpulainen, 1999; Silvasti, 2001; Sireni, 2000). It seems to be a common practice on European family farms that boys are actively encouraged to take over the farm whereas girls are actively encouraged to leave it. Girls are trained to run a farm only when they are the only children in the family, the only ones who could continue (e.g. Haugen, 1994; Whatmore, 1991).

But let us shift our focus from the issue of division of labour and continuity of the family farm to the issues of care on the family farm. In the next section of the narrative we can follow the lives and motivations of the family members during the period when the structure of thc family living on the farm changed and the caring work intensified.

Caring and Farming

The worst nightmares of the parents came true in 1978 when Mervi got married. She met her husband in August and married him in December and moved to his family farm. There she continued her caregiver vocation as she had before without any financial compensation. In her new home she started to care for her husband's old and sick mother who lived in the same household. Leaving home and her parents was not an easy choice for Mervi. For the first three years before her kids were born she travelled home every other day - 50 km by bus - to help her brothers take care of their mother, father and granny, who had fallen down the stairs. In the worst period there were three bed-ridden patients living in the house. Eventually they had to admit granny to a nursing home. When Mervi had her own kids she was no longer able to visit home that often, nor was she able to visit granny at the nursing home every week. Her inability to care for all the family members in need made her feel guilty. She felt that it was her fault that her granny died because she could not visit her often enough.

Mervi had the main responsibility of caring for her chronically ill parents for 13 years. While Mervi was the main caregiver of the parents, Juhani and Marko were able to put all their energy into modernising the farm according to the needs of the times. And they did a good job, too. The area under cultivation and number of milking cows increased. Mervi's marriage did, however, put an end to the positive growth and development of the farm. Mervi's marriage brought about a period of uncertainty and confusion but eventually Juhani decided to became the primary caregiver for their old and disabled parents. It was his vocation for the next 15 years. After getting over the first shock Juhani learned to care for his parents and took great pride in it. *"I think I have been successful... it is not agriculture... successful in the respect that I was able to take care of my parents at home until they died. I think it is quite an accomplishment. A man has to have something to make him feel good, and this is what makes me feel good. Many people would not have succeeded in taking care of two bed patients at home."* (Juhani, interview 2). By the time Juhani started caring for their parents on a daily basis, their mother's health had deteriorated and she no longer could walk and needed a wheel chair. Given the circumstances, caring work on the farm took precedence over farming. Juhani had to help his parents with dressing, washing, going to the toilet etc. He had to fit ploughing, harrowing, sowing and harvesting in into his 24-hour caring shift. Thus, it is no wonder that farm started to decline over the years. There just was not enough time do all the work that needed to be done.

Years passed and the life on the farm went on as always – work, work and more work. At some point Juhani started dreaming of having a wife and a family of his own. He had not met anybody in the village but that was no surprise because he did not have much time go out in the evenings. They lived a rather isolated life. The farm was five kilometres from the village centre and you could not see any other houses from their windows. Juhani was feeling quite lonely and sought contact with women by answering several pen-friend advertisements he found in a Christian paper. Eventually he got into contact with Tiina, who was eager to come and visit him on the farm. They met face-to-face three times and got married. A rather uncommon choice in Finland the 1980s, when young people were more likely to live together for some time before marrying. Tiina was the more active party in the marriage arrangement. She liked Juhani and saw no objections to their marriage. She came from a farming family and had lived in a household with many generations. Hence, she found her husband's commitment to the family farm and his parents a natural phenomenon. This was nothing out of the ordinary in her social circles.

The extract emphasises the commitment to the homecare of the old and disabled shared by the family members. They were ready to make considerable sacrifices in regard to their freedom and economic welfare to be able to take care of them. Even though the caring practices of the household could be seen as more intense than usual, it still represented the behaviour found in farming communities. Caring for the elderly and the disabled at home is specifically a rural tradition in Finland (Siiskonen, 1990) and it was a fact taken for granted in all the families under study. The value is connected to the intergenerational transfer of the farm as well as the tradition of *syytinki.* The basic idea of the *syytinki* is that the preceding generation can stay on the farm and be supported for the rest of their lives by receiving a share of what the farm produces. Making the agreement has more to do with the wish of the children to take over the farm than it has to do with physical deterioration on the part of the old farmer. It is worth noting, however, that the agreement does not include nursing services. From a legalistic point of view *syytinki* is clearly an economic agreement (Järvi, 1986) according to which the parents agree to move to a cottage separate from the farmhouse or to live in the same household with the child who agrees to take over the family farm.

Two out of the five families under study had made a *syytinki*-agreement[2]. It would, however, be a mistake to look at the agreement solely from an economic point of view because this would disregard the moral aspects of the intergenerational transfer of the farm. In all the cases under study, the families had taken care of their elderly parents living on the farm. Taking care of them demanded considerable sacrifices on behalf of the successor. These caring practices do not, however, rise out of Finnish legislation or the general caring culture of Finland. They emerge from the Finnish yeoman moral order. When taking over the farm, one simultaneously commits oneself to the yeoman moral order as well. However, this

[2] The number of the agreements has declined since the 1980s. The main reasons for the declining trend has been the improvement of pension security, the rise of lump sums paid for the parents turning over the farm, and the growing need for independence of the next generation.

commitment is not necessarily a conscious one. It is more a question of a life-long learning process through which the value of taking care of your old and disabled family members at home becomes internalised. The tacit moral agreement becomes visible the moment the parents get so weak that they no longer can cope on their own.

The extract further highlights the masculinisation of care in farming families. The study suggests that the lack of wives in the beginning of the farming career of the men has a tendency to shift the traditional caregiver roles in farming families. The men under study had taken over the caregiver role before their wives moved to the farm, and that role remained theirs after marriage. In four out of the five families under study a man was the main caregiver of the old and disabled parent(s). In the fifth case, the family lived on the wife's family farm where the nursing of the wife's chronically ill parents was shared by the spouses. It must be emphasised, though, that in all the families both the husband and wife shared the commitment to the value of taking care of the elderly at home. The shared understanding arises from the farming background of the spouses. It seems, however, that the difficulty in finding wives for farming men is a fairly common problem in the Finnish farming communities (Högbacka, 2003; Katila, 2000; Siiskonen, 1990; Silvasti, 2001; Sireni, 2002) but it a rather common problem in Europe in general. Women who have grown up in towns have no interest in moving to the countryside where the work is hard, pay is low and in many cases you have to live right by your in-laws, if not even in the same household. These circumstances are not very appealing to farming women either. They prefer to move to urban localities and enter the labour force outside the traditional agricultural sector (e.g. O'Hara, 1994; Whatmore, 1994).

The behaviour of Juhani and the other farming and caring men in my study could be characterised with the concepts of rationality of care (Haavind 1982; Ve, 1982) or rationality of responsibility. Rationality of responsibility refers to action that carries a sense of meaningfulness, moral commitment and legitimacy. It is not rule-bound behaviour but situational (Nätkin 1986, 157; Ve, 1982). A person who acts out the rationality of responsibility also thinks of the consequences of one's action from the perspective of others (Korvajärvi, 1986)[3]. Rationality of responsibility has usually been perceived as typical behaviour for women, as something that women learn through their socialisation process (Anttonen, 1997; Haavind, 1982). Caring work has been considered an example of rationality of responsibility that is typical for women whether it is done at home or in the public realm (for example Anttonen, 1997; Graham, 1983) and it has traditionally been women's domain on Finnish farms (Siiskonen, 1990, p. 76-78). The study indicates, however, that caring is not essentially a 'feminine' trait as some tend to claim. It is instead connected to the group norms that define whether one should take care of one's relatives or not, and if so, is it the duty of both genders or only the duty of the other. As Froland (1981) has pointed out, giving informal help is not innate but connected to cultural traditions of different groups as well as to learning taking place at home.

Living in a household with several generations is not an easy task in any circumstances, but it is substantially harder when there are old and disabled parents to care for. In the next section of the narrative we will focus on the emotional turmoil brought about by the caring responsibilities, and the entry of an "outsider" in the family.

---

[3] The concept of rationality of responsibility is very close to Caroll Gilligan's concept of 'ethics of care' (1982).

Emotions Run High

Tiina badly wanted to have a home and family of her own. She just did not quite grasp what it meant to move to a house where she was the only newcomer. She thought that she was the new lady of the house and could decorate it according to her taste. She started to move furniture around and got rid of some old furniture that Juhani's parents cherished. In no time, Tiina and her mother-in-law were at odds and there seemed to be no way out. Tiina stopped talking to her in-laws altogether and no longer visited their room. Juhani was really distressed about the situation " *My father asked her to forgive him, and my mother said she was sorry if she had hurt her feelings. But Tiina did not talk to them any more. I thought that it was a rather odd way to solve the problem. I do not blame Tiina, but I do not blame my parents, either. I had never come across a temperament like Tiina's. It was completely new for me that someone can just stop talking. They were very hard times for me.*" (Juhani, interview 2). If Tiina's actions were not to the liking of her in-laws, the caring practices of the household were difficult for Tiina to handle. "*When I was expecting my first baby I cried an awful lot. I really cried. Of course you are in a sensitive and vulnerable state, but still. Juhani's father had his bed put on a platform so that he could knock on the ceiling with his long stick whenever he needed Juhani. He knocked in the middle of the night and just any time.*" (Tiina, interview 2).

Tiina lasted on the farm for two years and decided that she, Juhani and their two kids should move to the village centre into a council flat. She told Juhani her decision, but Juhani refused to leave home and his old and disabled parents. Tiina did not accept it and threatened to take the kids and move back to western Finland if Juhani did not sign the lease. Juhani gave in and signed. "*I thought it over for several days. At the time, leaving this place felt really difficult. I considered it my home. I also was looking after my parents and I thought that I cannot take care of them while I'm living in the village. I kept thinking that they might not survive this move, and my father did not make it. He died in less than a year after I had moved and started running back and forth between the farm and the flat. I said that I had a feeling that my dad would die, if I left. But, of course, people must die when it is their time to go. The main reason why I hesitated with the move was that I felt that my dad was so dependent on me.*" (Juhani, interview 2).

Looking at family caregiving relationships from the point of view of a moral order, guilt and shame become relevant emotions in understanding the mix of care chosen. In this extract, as well as the in the previous ones, the issue of guilt is prevalent. According to Brody (1985), guilt is a major motivation to provide care. Rather than seeing guilt as an individual motivation to take care of someone, this study suggests that is would be more fruitful to look at it in connection with the moral order it is supporting.

Emotional displays are subject to rules and conventions. They are embedded in culturally specific moral orders and normative systems that allow for assessments of the correctness or impropriety of emotions within the group (Armon-Jones, 1986; Averill, 1985; Crawford et al. 1992; Harré, 1986; Harré and Parrot, 1996; Landman, 1996; Oatley, 1993). Thus, guilt and shame are both inherently connected to all moral orders (Eztioni, 1988; Harré, 1983). Guilt and shame are central to the nature of the organisational order, be it family or work organization. They are the sources of self-regulation that social organisations require to function. These emotions are nurtured in the processes of socialisation in a nation's culture and fine-tuned in a specific work organisation (Fineman, 1997, p. 551) and family.

Through the processes of identification and imitation with the parents and the grandparents living in Finnish yeoman households, children learn the values and norms of the yeoman moral order and also the appropriate emotions that go with it. The key emotions supporting the Finnish yeoman moral order are guilt and shame. A person who has internalised the value of taking care of your disabled and old family members accepts that disregarding the value is forbidden. By accepting that it is forbidden, one thereby accepts the authority of whomever or whatever forbids it. So the authority becomes the voice of conscience (Taylor, 1996). One is willing to work hard without any financial compensation just to live up to the expectations of the moral order. It could therefore be argued that taking care of your old and disabled family members on a family farm is also a matter of honour. Inability to do so will bring shame on you and your family, whereas the ability to do it will bring you respect. Thus, in this context, relying on institutional care is not considered an appropriate expression of individuality. When thinking of family, however, it is difficult to dismiss the emotion of love all together. Love refers in the broadest sense to the principle(s) by which people organise their relationships with one another (Averill, 1985, p. 191).

In the families under study, companionate love seemed to be very present in the intergenerational relationships. Companionate love consists of affection, commitment and intimacy (Hatfield and Rapson, 1993: 9). The main element of companionate love – long-term commitment, even a life-long commitment (Stenberg, 1988) is well manifested throughout the narrative. All the families under study were willing to make sacrifices to be able to take care of their old and disabled parents at home. For example, one of the informants gave up one of her part-time jobs to be able to care for her demented mother and father who had Parkinson's disease. The willingness to make sacrifices for the loved has been noted as one of the core elements of all love relationships (Averil, 1985: 9). No wonder, caring has also been called a labour of love (Graham, 1983). The study suggests that the ideal of love between children and parents, entangled with the ideal of love between the farm and the farmer, provide the individuals under study with a model and rationale for behaviour. Different commitments reflect different emotional contracts - with others and with self - and this determines the commitment's potency (Pfeffer, 1982 ref. Fineman, 1997: 551).

In an intergenerational farming household there are, however, many, even conflicting, love relationships, for example, between parents and children, grandparents and grandchildren, between spouses and between family members and the family farm. The different relationships may have conflicting commitments, and they are bound to change during the life-course of the family. For example, the commitment to your own parents may weaken when you marry and start your own family but it may strengthen again when your parents grow old. The extract further indicates that the commitments one has can potentially influence relationships that one has considered external to the relationship (see Beach and Tesser, 1988). In Juhani's case, the commitment to the homecare of his parents influenced among other things his marriage as well as the state of the farm on which their livelihood relied upon. Caregiving has many hidden costs for the caregivers and their families (see Oddone and Aguirre; Paoletti; Watson in this volume)

The narrative further highlights the potential conflicts and distress involved in caregiving relationships. Regardless of the fact that Tiina shared and understood Juhani's commitment to his family farm and the homecare of his parents, she could not handle everyday life in these circumstances. Families that are in the formation and child-rearing stages are the most hard pressed with respect to caregiving resources (Aldous 1994). Tiina seemed to be in a situation that is rather common in farming households comprising several generations. In such households serious conflicts and difficult human relations are well documented (e.g. Hutson, 1987; Katila, 2000; 2002; Rogers and Salamon, 1983; Silvasti, 2001). Coping with the conflicting demands that the different commitments impose on the members of the farming and caring families demands emotion management on a daily basis. Living close to each other requires you to be able to hold back your emotions and display them within socially accepted norms (Hochschild, 1983), thereby causing extra strain on family relations.

Discussion

The findings of the study are interesting in regard to two conflicting societal trends, namely the simultaneous intensification of working life and the declining possibilities of the state to provide universal care for the sick and the elderly. The increasing competition on global markets has forced companies across Europe to become more efficient. In their attempts to be more effective, companies have called for a more flexible work force. In this context, flexibility has come to mean intensification of work, readiness to work overtime and willingness to accept unorthodox employment. Those who are unable or unwilling to work under these circumstances, for example, because they want to take care of their children or elderly parents at home, have limited potential to remain employed. In the case of the agricultural sector demands for competitiveness and effectiveness has apparent in the goal-directed attempts of agricultural policy makers to challenge and alter the meanings of farming by building up a new identity for farmers as farm businessmen who are driven by profit maximisation and economic achievement. Declining subsidies and expectations of entrepreneurial behaviour have resulted in a substantial decline in the number of farms as well as in the intensification of farming and entrepreneuring on the remaining farms in Finland.

It seems that we have been able to improve the efficiency of the Finnish economy for the time being. But the situation is more contested when we look at these developments in relation to the needs of the growing population of the aged, and the declining possibilities of state to provide universal care for the sick and the elderly. It seems that in Finland, a new discourse that is in drastic contrast with the principle of universal care is emerging. There are increasing demands on families to provide the care for their sick and elderly family members; This suggests that there is a need to change the cultural preference of relying on societal care over family care. This tendency is also manifested in the new support systems being created to enable families to take more responsibility for the care of the old and disabled. It can be concluded that the demands of the growing older population are not in line with the demands imposed upon families by working life, especially in countries like Finland where both women and men fully participate in working life.

The farming population seems to differ from the general population in regard to the mix of informal and formal care for elderly family members. In Finnish farming families the cultural habit of taking care of the old and disabled at home still seems to be favoured. The developments taking place in the agricultural sector seem, however, to threaten the very practice and value. Changes in the agricultural sector are not only practical and economical but also value-laden. The emphasis on efficiency and entrepreneurship defines non-business activities as unimportant and unwanted. Thus, there is less and less time, and interest, for activities defined as "non-business", like the care of the old and disabled. The trend, coupled with the general individualisation of the society, may reduce the value of taking care of the old and disabled in farming communities in times where the needs of the older population are growing and the possibilities of state provided care are declining.

Although the farming population in Finland has been pressured to act more entrepreneurially, they still seem to hold on to their economically un-rational, non-entrepreneurial behaviour of taking care of the elderly at home. It seems that the entanglement of public and private spheres of life in the farm business families contribute to the preservation of a moral order that supports the survival and reproduction of the business as well as the family. The study suggests that we need to appreciate the meaningfulness of local, situated action in order to understand why what is rational action from the point of view of the farm business families may not be rational from another groups' perspective.

Conclusion

The chapter has focused on untangling the reasons why farming families in Finland seem to prioritise homecare over other options of care in a situation where publicly provided care is a citizen's right. The chapter suggested that the answer to this question lies in the moral order of the farming community. To be able to surface the norms and values of the yeoman moral order (Harré 1983) in Finland and the emotions supporting it, an ethnographic study of five farm business families was conducted.

The study points to the fact that the value of taking care of the antecedent generation is still recognised and observed in farming communities. In the Finnish farm business families, decisions to care for the elderly at home are based on internalised values and norms of the moral order. The husbands and wives in the farming families seemed to share a common interpretation of reality in this respect. The shared understanding relied on a shared template of prior expectation that was laid down by cultural habits of thought and practice. In this context, relying on institutional care was not considered an appropriate expression of individuality. It was considered to be outside the boundaries of the local moral order that prioritises family welfare over narrow self-interest. Breaking the value of taking care of the elderly at home gave rise to feelings of guilt and shame. The very caring practice did, however, constrain family relationships and business activities, and demanded considerable sacrifices on behalf of the family members.

The study further suggests that the gendered occupational identities and boundaries in farming families are historically constructed. Caring work has usually been part of the female domain in Finnish (farming) families. The chapter suggests, however, that the modernization of agriculture and the difficulty of farming men in finding wives tend to shift the care responsibility on the farms from women to men. Thus, it seems that the yeoman moral order is stronger than the gender order of the professional community.

Recommendations

Based on the study we recommend that

- the economic needs of caregivers must be met by providing them with sufficient economic support covering the loss of income due to caregiving responsibilities.
- the emotional needs of caregivers must be met by providing them with sufficient holidays where they can rest, do errands and maintain their social relationships.
- policy makers should consider the diverse needs of different occupational groups when making support systems aimed at the home care of the elderly.
- economic and social policies should be developed in concert to reveal how the changes in one sector of the society influence the other sectors of the society.

References

Abrahams, R. (1991). *A Place of Their Own. Family Farming in Eastern Finland.* Cambridge, UK: Cambridge University Press.

Alestalo, M. (1985). Yhteiskuntaluokat ja sosiaaliset kerrostumat toisen maailmansodan jälkeen. In M. Valkonen et.al. (eds.) *Suomalaiset. Yhteiskunnan rakenne teollistumisen aikana* (pp.101-200). Juva: WSOY.

Aldous, J. (1994). Someone to Watch Over Me: Family Responsibility and Their Realization Across Family Lives. In E. Kahana, D. E. Biegel, and M. L. Wyckle (Eds.), *Family Caregiving Across the Lifespan. Family Caregiver Applications Series, vol. 4*. London: Sage, 42-68.

Anttonen, A. (1997). *Feminismi ja sosiaalipolitiikka.* Tampere: Tampere University Press.

Armon-Jones, C. (1986). The Thesis of Constructionism. In R. Harré, (ed.), *The Social Construction of Emotions* (pp. 57-82) . Oxford: Basil Blackwell.

Atkinson, P. (1990) *The Ethnographic Imagination. Textual constructions of reality*. London: Routledge.

Averill, J. (1985). The Social Construction of Emotion: With Special Reference to Love. In K. Gergen, and K. Davis (eds.), *The Social Construction of the Person* (pp. 89-109). New York: Springer-Verlag.

Beach, S. R. and Tesser, A. (1988). Love in Marriage: A Cognitive Account. In R. Sternberg and M. Barnes (eds.) *The Psychology of Love* (pp. 330-355). London: Yale University Press.

Bertaux, D. and Delcroix, C. (2000). Case histories of families and social processes: enriching sociology. In P. Chamberlayne, J. Bornat and T. Wengraf (eds.) *The Turn to Biographical Methods in Social Sciences. Comparative issues and examples* (pp. 71-89) London, New York: Routledge.

Brody, E. M. (1985). Parent care as a normative family stress. *The Gerontologist*, 25, 19-25.

Bruner, J. S. (1990). *Acts of Meaning*. Cambridge, MA: Harvard University Press.

Bruner, J. (1986). *Actual Minds, Possible Worlds.* Cambridgem MA: Harvard University Press.

Chappel, N. L. (1990). Aging and social care. In R. H. Binstock and L. K. George (Eds.), *Aging and the social science*, 3 rd ed. (pp. 438-454). New York: Academic Press.

Cicirelli, V. G. (1983). Adult Children and Their Elderly Parents. In T. Brubaker (ed.), *Family Relations in Later Life* (pp. 31-46). Bervely Hills, CA: Sage.

Cohen, G. (1993). *Memory in the Real World.* Hillsdale, NJ: Lawrence Erlbaum Associates.

Crawford, J., Kippax, S., Onyx, J., Gault, U. and Benton, P. (1992). *Emotion and Gender. Constructing Meaning from Memory.* London: Sage.

Etzioni, A. (1988). *The Moral Dimension. Toward a New Economics.* London: The Free Press, Macmillan Publishers.

Fineman, S. (1993). *Emotion in Organizations.* London: Sage.

Fineman, S. (1997). Emotion and Organizing. In S. Glegg, C. Hardy, and W. Nord (Eds.) *Handbook of Organization Studies.* (pp. 553-564). London: Sage.

Froland C. (1981). *Helping Networks and the Human Services.* Sage Librarary of Social Research 128.

Gibson, M. J. (1984). Family support patterns, policies, and programs. In C. Busberg (Ed.) *Innovative aging programs abroad: Implications for the United States* (pp.159-195). Westport, CT: Greenwood.

Graham, H. (1983). Caring: a labour of love. In Finch, J. and Groves, D. (Eds.) *A Labour of Love: Women, Work and caring* (pp. 13-30). London: Routledge and Kegan Paul.

Granovetter, M. (1985). Economic Action and Social Structure: The Problem of Embeddedness. *American Journal of Sociology.* 91, 481-510.

Gubrium, J. F. (1987). Organizational Embeddedness and Family Life. In T. Brubaker (Ed.) *Aging, Health, and Family* (pp. 23-41). London: Sage.

Haavind, H. (1982). Makt og kjaerlighet I ektenskapet. In R. Haukaa et. al. *Kvinnoforksning: bidrag til samfunnsteori.* Oslo: Universitetsforlaget.

Hammersley, M. (1992) *What's Wrong with Ethnography*? London: Routledge.

Harré, Rom. (1983). *Personal Being.* Oxford, England: Basil Blackwell.

Harré, Rom. (1986). An outline of the Social Constructionist Viewpoint. In R. Harré (Ed.) *The Social Construction of Emotions* (pp. 2-14). Oxford, Basil Blackwell.

Harré, R. and Parrot, G. W. (1996). Overview. In R. Harré and G. W. Parrot (Eds.) *The Emotions. Social, Cultural and Biological Dimensions.* (pp. 1-38) London: Sage.

Hatfield, E. and Rapson, R. (1993). Love and Attachment Processes. In M. Lewis and J. Haviland (Eds.) *Handbook of emotions* (pp. 595-604). New York: The Guilford Press.

Haugen, M. (1994). Rural Women's status in family and property law: Lessons from Norway. In S. Whatmore, T. Marsden and P. Lowe (Eds.) *Gender and rurality. Critical Perspectives on Rural Change.* (pp. 87-101) Series VI. London: David Fulton Publishers.

Hutson, J. (1987). Fathers and Sons: Family Farms, Family Business and the Farming Industry. *Sociology*, 21, 2, 215-229.

Hochschild, A. (1983) *The Managed Heart. Commercialization of Human Feeling.* Berkley: University of California Press.

Höhbacka, R. (2003). *Naisten muuttuvat elämänmuodot maaseudulla.* Helsinki: Suomalaisen Kirjallisuuden Seura.

Järvi, E. (1986). *Syytinki ja maatiloilla tapahtuva sukupolvenvaihdos.* Maatalousyrittäjäin eläkelaitoksen julkaisuja 1/86.

Katila, S. (2000). *Moraalijärjestyksen rajaama tila: maanviljelijä-yrittäjäperheiden selviytymisstrategiat.* Helsinki School of Economics and Business Administration. Acta Universitatis Oeconomicae Helsingiensis A-174.

Katila, S. (2002). Emotions and the Moral Order of Farm Business Families in Finland. In Fletcher, D. (ed.) *Understanding the Small Family Business* (pp. 180-191) Small Business Series. London: Routledge.

Korvajärvi, P. (1986). Naisten yhteisö t - kahleita ja mahdollisuuksia. In Rantalaiho, L. (Ed.) *Miesten tiede, naisten puuhat* (pp. 181-209). Tampere: Vastapaino.

Kosberg, J. I. (1992). An International Perspective. In J. I. Kosberg (Ed.) *Family Care of the Elderly. Social and Cultural Changes* (pp.1-14). London: Sage.

Kumpulainen, M. (1999). *Maan ja talouden välissä. Viisi kertomusta suomalaisen maatilan luontosuhteen muutoksesta.* Joensuun yliopisto, Maantieteenlaitos, julkaisuja No 5.

Landman, J. (1996). Social Control of 'Negative Emotions': The Case of Regret. In R. Harré and G. W. Parrot (Eds.) *The Emotions. Social, Cultural and Biological Dimensions* (pp. 89-116). London

Lutz, C. A. and White, G. (1986). The anthropology of emotions. *Annual Review of Anthropology,* 15, 405-36.

Nätkin, R. (1986). Naiset, kontrolli ja hyvinvointivaltio. In Rantalaiho, L. (Ed.) *Miesten tiede, naisten puuhat* (pp. 181-209). Tampere: Vastapaino.

Oatley, K. (1993). Social Construction of Emotions. In M. Lewis and J. Haviland (Eds.) *Handbook of emotions* (pp. 341-352). New York: The Guilford Press.

O'Hara, P. (1994). Constructing the Future: Coperation and Resistance Among Farm Women in Ireland. In Whatmore, S. and Marsden, T. and Lowe, P. (Eds.) *Gender and Rurality. Critical Perspectives on Rural Change Series VI* (pp. 50-68). London: David Hulton Publishers.

Pfeffer, J. (1982). *Organizations and Organization Theory.* Marshfield, MA: Pitman.

Polkinghorne, D. (1991). Narrative and Self-Concept. *Journal of Narrative and Life History,* 2-3, 135-153.

Ratner, C. (1989). A Social Constructionist critique of the naturalistic theory of emotion. *The Journal of Mind and Behaviour* 10, (3), 211-30.

Rogers, S. C. and Salamon, S. (1983). Inheritance and Social Organization among Family Farmers. *American Ethnologist,* 10 (3), 529-549.

Ruth, J-E. and Kenyon, G. (1996). Biography in Adult Development and Ageing. In Birren, J. et. al (Eds.) *Ageing and Biography* (pp. 1-21) New York: Springer Publishing Company.

Ruth, J-E. and Vilkko, A. (1996). Emotion in the Construction of Autobiography. In C. Malatesta, C. Magai, and S. Mc Fadden (Eds.) *Handbook of Emotion, Adult Development and Ageing* (pp. 167-181). San Diego: Academic Press.

Siiskonen, P. (1990). *Emännän ja isännän roolin muutos maatalouden uudenaikaistuessa. Tutkimus maatilan emännän ja isännän muuttuvista rooleista työnjaon avulla tarkasteltuna.* Mikkeli: Helsingin yliopiston maaseudun tutkimus- ja koulutuskeskus.

Silvasti, T. (2001). Talonpojan elämä. *Tutkimus elämäntapaa jäsentävistä kulttuurisista malleista.* Suomalaisen kirjallisuuden seura: Helsinki

Sireni, M. (2000). Kunnon työtä ja oikeaa elämää kotiseudulla. Työn ja kotipaikkakunnan merkitys syrjäseudun nuorelle aikaiselle. *Alue ja Ympäristö* 29,1-16.

Sireni, M. (2002). Tilansa tekijät: tutkimus emännyydestä ja maatilasta naisen paikkana. Joensuun yliopiston yhteiskuntatieteellisiä julkaisuja, 56.

Sternberg, R. (1988). Triangulating Love. In Sternberg, R. and Barnes, M. (Eds.) *The Psychology of Love* (pp. 119-138). London: Yale University Press.

Suomen maatalous ja maaseutuelinkeinot 1999/2000. Maatalouden taloudellinen tutkimuslaitos, Finland, Publications 95.

Taylor, G. (1996). Guilt and Remorse. In R. Harré and G. W. Parrott *The Emotions. Social, Cultural and Biological Dimensions* (pp. 57-73). London: Sage.

Thompson, P. (1993). Family, Myth, Models, and Denials in the Shaping of Individual Life Paths. In Bertaux, Daniel and Thompson, Paul (Eds.) Between Generations. Family Models, Myths and Memories (pp. 13-38) *International Yearbook of Oral History and Life Stories* II.

Van Maanen, J. (1988). *Tales of the Field.* Chicago: The University of Chicago Press.

Van Maanen, J. (1995). *Representation in Ethnography.* London: Sage.

Ve, H. (1982). Makt, intresse och socialisation. *Kvinnovetenskapligt tidskrift,* 2, 23-32.

Whatmore, S. (1991). *Farming Women: Gender, Work and Family Enterprise.* London: Macmillan.

Whatmore, S. (1994). Theoretical Achievements and Challenges in European Rural Gender Studies. In M. van der Burg and M. Endeveld (Eds.) *Women on Family Farms. Gender Research, EC Policies and New Perspectives* (pp. 107-120). Wageningen: Circle for Rural European Studies / Dutch Network on Farm and Rural Women's Studies.

Ylijoki, O-H. (1998). *Akateemiset heimokulttuurit ja noviisien sosialisaatio.* Tampere: Vastapaino.

In: Family Caregiving for Older Disabled People
Editor: Isabella Paoletti, pp. 35-62
ISBN 1-59454-808-0

Chapter 3

A Pendular Movement between the Intergenerational Pact and the Exhaustion of Support Networks in Argentina

***María Julieta Oddone*[1] *and Mónica Beatriz Aguirre*[2]**
CONICET- FLACSO, Ayacucho 551 – Capital Federal
Universidad de Buenos Aires, Argentina

Introduction

The objective of this study is to reach an understanding of the problems that confront families burdened by the care of an elderly person with health problems. To this end, we approached key participants in "Caring for Those Who Care," a Buenos Aires City Government program. Basing our study on this organization, we interviewed family caregivers who have participated in the program. We worked with a sample of caregivers composed of spouses, sons and daughters, sons- and daughters-in-law, and grandchildren. The group of caregivers as well as the group of dependents includes participants of both genders; this permitted us to obtain a spread of cases ranging widely with regards to generation, to gender, and to familiar relationship; from these cases emerged the key issues in the caregiver´s situation to which we refer in this chapter.

The study focused on the City of Buenos Aires. The demographic structure of this capital city of the Republic of Argentina marks it as the country's most aged city, given that 22% (609,466) of its population is made up of people of 60 or more years of age.

Previous research conducted by this team (Oddone, 2001) indicates that 5% of the elderly population receives special care in a family setting. The Caring for Those Who Care data, which permits a general characterization of its attendees, indicate the following: that 88% of

---

[1] FLACSO, Facultad Latinoamericana de Ciencias Sociales y Consejo Nacional de Investigaciones Científicas y Técnicas (the Latin American Faculty of Social Sciences and the Nacional Council of Scientific and Technical Research). mjoddone@mail.retina.ar

[2] FLACSO, Facultad Latinoamericana de Ciencias Sociales. maguirre@mail.retina.ar

the caregivers are women, that 80% are over 50 years of age, that 60% spend more than 5 hours per day with the person in need of care, and that 72% carry out the caregiving duties on a daily basis[3].

In Argentina, and in particular in the city of Buenos Aires, various programs designed to help family caregivers have been implemented. These programs range from the formation of gerontological assistance to a program that proposes care for the family caregivers themselves. In between are found domestic internment, 24-hour attention centers, and retirement homes, among others. But the reach of these programs´ efficacy remains quite far from meeting demands, just as our interview subjects – who have been left alone in responding to the needs of their sick elderly and without hope of finding any help other than their own personal and family recourses -- prove. It seems to us that it is not the creation of new programs that is needed but rather their universality, seeing as the existing programs have had little chance to be assessed, given their limited reach. When the protective function of the state is reexamined, and the fact taken into account that the aging process is a phenomenon that modifies a society in its needs and demands, the problems of family caregivers will become solvable.

The Exhaustion of Family Support Networks

In everyday life, family units, in order to meet their needs, maintain networks of reciprocity and mutual help which are expressed through the exchange of tasks associated with the maintenance of members' well-being (Lomnitz, 1977). Both love and moral obligation play a role in these networks. Obviously, reciprocity is not always achieved in every interaction. Actors can expect a returned benefit mostly in the long term, sometimes even on the scale of the life cycle itself, across generations. The temporal dimension of these exchanges (their timing) that leads us to understand them as either short- or long-term constitutes a fundamental focal point for understanding family relationships with regard to aging. Effectively, in the short-term exchanges correspond to everyday situations; a typical example is that in which grandparents care for their grandchildren while their daughter works, and the daughter in turn assists her parents economically.

In the long-term generational-scale exchanges in which the help that parents give in their children's growth and development is returned by the children in the form of protection in the parents' old age are found. These exchanges are reciprocal and include the variable of time and are thus marked by normative values. In each act, the services exchanged are considered favors and the emotional availability of each person is tested. The exchange is valued as a link in and of itself and the very relationship is based upon the rationale – be it conscious or not of everyday or material needs, or of social values/norms that have been internalized as obligatory. In this sense, these exchanges form a part of the social capital which the old possess in our society. This form of organization is valid for all social sectors, though it changes the content of the exchange.

In his research conducted in France, P. Pitaud (1999) stresses that a large portion of the dependent elderly is involved in these exchange networks, and receives care from

[3] Data provided by Susana Aguas, Director of the Municipal Office for the Elderly of the City of Buenos Aires, year 2003.

predetermined sources in compensation for past assistance. This fact brings to mind a sort of symbolic debt.

In today's Argentine society, impacted by the crisis of the 1990s and the large-scale privatizations and devaluation, this social capital constitutes, in most cases, the only security for the elderly. It does not, however, escape a certain level of conflict. Within the circle of family relationships (especially those which link ancestors and descendents) the weight of moral obligation, reinforced by social expectation on the one hand and affection on the other, constitutes the reciprocity relationship (the proportions of these components in the determination of behavior is not easy to evaluate even in concrete cases). Disequilibrium is produced when these feelings are put to the test by material conditions – incomes, housing, health – that generate tensions within the systems (Oddone, 2002).

It is not only the factor of economic conditions that casts doubt on families' capacity to assume responsibilities which may overwhelm them. Nowadays certain social changes are arising which are affecting this capacity and will certainly come to affect it even more. In the first place, demographic changes – particularly the drop in fertility rates – have significant effects on the number of potential support providers. The correlative rise in life expectancy produces families of up to five generations, increasing the possibility of a greater number of aged dependents and, in consequence, the possibility that elderly persons must take charge of the caregiving of even older relatives[4] (Monk, 1997). Finally, if we bear in mind that females generally provide the family-member support, the greater participation of the woman in the labor market and the trend towards their greater social independence casts doubt on the continuity of a caregiving model headed by housewives.

> I have long believed we have the global capacity to support all the earth's people, but to do so will require a revolution in economic and political action which re-establishes human solidarity and reciprocity as central features of our social order. As has been argued these transformations are essentially moral; but failure to address them puts at risk not only the contact between young and old, but society itself". (Johnson, 1995, 262)

Just as Johnson stated, we believe that families preserve their capacity to sustain their members and in this sense continue to be the principal source of these members' wellbeing. But the changes that constantly challenge this capacity to the point of provoking true crisis at the group and individual level cannot be forgotten. For this reason, we think it necessary that public policy consider both aspects: the existence of these networks and the resilience of the families' classes to sustain themselves as well as the tensions to which they are subjected. The Caring for Those Who Care Program was conceived within these lines and for that reason we have chosen it as the entryway to access the caregiving families. Before presenting the result of our study, we will briefly describe recent developments in the support services system to family caregivers in Argentina.

---

[4] One issue which ought to be highlighted is that concerning caregivers of more than 60 years of age: the elderly who care for the elderly. This is obviously generally the case for spouses, but many caregiving daughters are also over 60 years old. The majority of out interviewees actually are aged over 60: Jorge W., 76, cares for his wife, 78; Hebe M., 72, cares for her husband, 82; Esther C., 70, cares for her husband of 85, María Isabel F.,

THE RETRACTION OF THE WELFARE STATE IN ARGENTINA

From the early 1940s to the late 1970s, a set of policies were developed, based on three legal principles: need, merit, and citizenship (Fraser, 1997). The aid policies – based on the first of these principles, need are meant for those who are unable to hold a job – above all, for the elderly and for children. Merit-based protection policies grant benefits according to the contributions of each person. Here we find employment policies, in which work takes on an important role as social integrator. Universal policies reach all people considered citizens, that is to say, any member of society. Through this set of public policies, the Welfare State fulfills its central role, guaranteeing protection.

In the last two decades, with the disappearance of this protective state, which has been the result of neoliberal adjustments, notable transformations have taken place in diverse dimensions (Vinocur and Halperín, 2004). Economically speaking, decentralization, privatization, greater concentration of wealth and inequity; socially speaking, impoverishment, vulnerability, and disaffiliation. All of these transformations restructure society, producing new characteristics in new configurations.

Confronted by the difficulties that the national state and its historical institutions have had in meeting the needs of the people, theorists have posited that various actors, by means of non-governmental organizations, will begin to re-knit the fabric of social networks. In this line of thought, belonging to such networks is a fundamental tool. It lends a sense of dignity to life because these networks suppose the existence of communicative processes carried out jointly with other actors, and give action a certain directionality. Things have not, however, turned out to work that way. Instead, what Wacquant (2001) calls organizational desertification has been observable.

In this new setting, the conditions for collective action are lost. Forms of participation are reduced to what is close at hand, given that, as has already been observed, institutions are shrinking. Close relationships are usually found in the family setting. The research of Bertaux (1996) demonstrates the importance of using the family as a unit of analysis and becoming acquainted with the transformations taking place within it. All family histories create a mirror wherein social history, great moments of change, and their various dimensions are reflected. Forging a family history makes people aware of the family unit importance in the formation and development of social activity and praxis. It is in this way that, gradually, generalized instability is reflected in family instability. The vulnerability of the family thus becomes evident in any emergency situation, in this case, the care of the oldest family members. As a counterpoint, the multiplication of cases of families with this type of need, reflects not only the aging of the population in general but also represents a situation of social risk to which institutions respond only very partially.

The exhaustion of family support networks is obvious in relation to the illness of the elderly. We must not continue burdening domestic groups with functions that are the general responsibility of society and the particular responsibility of institutions and state social programs. It is imminently important, then, that we find a position that will ensure that the planning of social policies will facilitate the complementation of informal family resources and more formal aid resources. To this end, it is necessary to rehabilitate and reconstruct the

65, cares for her 90-year-old mother; Lidia R., 60, cares for her mother, 84, and Teresita S., 66, cares for her mother, 91, and her aunt, 89.

Welfare State, with the goal of having it guarantee universal, high-quality services that assure citizens′ rights. Today these services are almost non-existent in the context of an emerging economy burdened by foreign debt.

As Neena Chappell (1996) argues, the new recognition of informal caregivers has highlighted the need for a thorough understanding of caregiving. However, "...without the expansion of formal community services, the tightening and steamlining of medical and hospital care can easily result in a greater burden on informal caregivers. This fact is not being considered seriously within the new vision [*of the health care system*]" (p. 149). Our point of view is that family caregivers remain the dominant source of assistance for elders and that there is very little actual concern in regards to the burden this assistance represents for them. So much so that we could make ours the words of Pitaud (1999), who, as we do, recognizes and values family support for the elderly as well as highlighting the social risk implicated by the burden and responsibility of caregiving: "I only hope that our government will not wait until the situation takes a turn for the worse before taking measures to aid dependent persons and their families!" (p.29). In the next section we will describe the method of data collection. Then in the analysis, reporting transcripts from the interviews, we describe the presence and character of support networks involved in the caring for older disabled family members. Moreover we highlight the position of the main caregiver (spouse, son/daughter, grandchildren, etc.), the tensions within the family, the financial implication of caregiving (the weight on the family budget) and the role of community resources. We conclude providing a set of recommendations based on our findings.

THE STUDY

Methodological Aspects

"Caring for Those Who Care," a Buenos Aires City Government program, included the organization of a course[5] for family caregivers to older disabled people. The course consisted of six weekly group meetings of two hours each.

The field work first centered on interviewing the key informants, professionals from the Center of Old Age of the Government of the City of Buenos Aires. These workers know the aged population and its central problems, and pointed us in the direction of individuals who would meet the definition of informal caregiver. The key informants enjoyed the trust of the group in question. Being assured of the seriousness, discretion, and utility of our work, they granted us the possibility of contacting the participant to the course.[6]

The material used in the field study was based on 15 freely-conducted in-depth interviews and on the information produced by the authors′ observations. This blend shows us the basics of the scenario in which the caregiver families go about their everyday lives. Of

5 The course coordinating team included a nurse, a social worker, and a psychologist. The course was divided into three sections:

I- General Information about gerontology.

II- Practices of the caregiver.

III- The connecting relationship. Responsibilities and limitations. The personal projects of the caregiver.

6 We especially thank the help offered by key informants Mariana Kesselman and Fabian Oliveira from the Buenos Aires City Government.

the 15 interview subjects, two were a married couple that cared for three elderly family members; another two were a mother and son that cared for two elderly family members. Two subjects were dropped from the analysis, in one case because the dependent was not a family member and in the other because the interviewee's answers did not correspond with the study´s objective. (his wife had begun to manifest some cognitive disorders but did not need special care yet) The sample ended up comprised of ten women and five men, each representing a different family relations to the dependent they cared for.

The main objective of the interviews was to distinguish the strategies that families have created to meet the needs of the elderly dependent as well as to detect the economic, emotional, and health costs which these strategies imply for the caregivers. We also evaluated the success or failure of these same strategies in terms of quality of life of both caregiver and dependent. To this end, we analyze the presence and character of support networks, family tensions, financial aspects, and the role of community resources.

The semi-structured in-depth interviews took place in the houses of the informants. Each interview covers a mixture of topics, according to the following list:

Family caregivers´ information: Sociodemographic and economic information (age, gender, etc.), Personal family situation (marriage, children, age of children, etc.), Work and earning situation. Family relation with the dependent person. Why did they take charge of the dependent? Does the dependent live with them?

Information about the dependent: Sociodemographic and economic information (age, gender, etc), Work and earning situation, Ownership of the living quarters, living quarters´ adequateness for the necessities of the dependent person, Sickness, Level of incapacity or dependency. Treatement, time, and attention required.

Composition and history of the family: Live-in and non live-in family members, family history and relationship networks.

Relationship of the dependent person: Quality of the caregiver-dependent relationship. Help of friends and family, help of institutions and economic questions.

- Free time.
- Changes in the quality of life of the caregiver (stress, depression, physical illness, etc.)
- Conflicts in family relationships (fatigue, tension, aggression, violence, abandonment, negligence, usurpation).
- Strategy implemented for the dependent person.
- Level of satisfaction with the implemented strategy.

Records of attitudes and expressions of the interviewees were reported in ethnographic notes, together with the descriptions of the physical space, the surroundings, and the quality of the caregiver-cared for relationship, according to what could be observed in the interviewees´ houses.

The duration of the interviews varied, according to the cases, between four and eight hours, divided among one or various sessions. They were done in the city of Buenos Aires during the months of October and November, 2003. With the consent of the subjects, the interviews were recorded on mini-cassette and transcribed. The topics were codified and categorized by the computer program Atlas Ti in a matrix of data obtained in the aforementioned manner making webs of thematic relationships. Analysis of the data was done by exemplifying characteristics (types) that arose from the interviewees′ narration, and these cases are those that appear in the text. In the next section we are going to illustrate the results of the analysis.

THE ANALYSIS

In the presentation of this study we have given priority to the actors' voices[7], though the richness of the face-to-face interviews is so great that it would be impossible to fully communicate its force. We have chosen to present interviewees' perspective articulated around thematic focuses. The most important elements of the testimonies are unfolded gradually in order to show the links between various themes. We cannot deny that in this method some of the interviews' substance is lost; however, we believe that this form of presentation transmits the lived experiences of the interviewees while at the same time permits us to treat in some depth the issues which we consider ought to be highlighted.

With regards to the various units into which we have grouped the content, we shall try to approach them separately so as to lend order to our presentation. These units, however, are so closely related that this separation sometimes becomes a bit artificial. Despite these provisos, we continue to believe that this is the best option and the most likely to promote a serious discussion of the cared for problems which in turn could yield the implementation of social policies targeted towards caregiving families. First, we address the ethics of care to prove the existence of the intergenerational pact. Second, we focus on the caregiving relation, its positive and negative aspects, regarded as punishments and rewards by the caregiver. Then we consider at length the costs of care. Here we take into account the consequences occasioned by caregiving such as lack of free time, health problems, economic costs, etc. We then describe the strategies that these families employed to cope with the situation and, finally, we examine the reasons for which the caregivers signed up for the class.

THE ETHICS OF CARE: WHAT SUSTAINS ITS FUNCTIONING?

We contacted our interview subjects during high-stress times for the networks to which they belong. The fact that they resorted to a support program to seek relief proves the existence of tension and stress.

One of the first issues we wanted to investigate is the reason for which the families took responsibility for the dependents. The moral values and feeling that sustain the commitment to care then began to appear:

> From a certain point of view, I feel fine. I feel that I'm finishing or fulfilling something that was done for me. One can only hope that the same thing happens with his own children. It's like a payback. That wouldn't be the exact word, because payback would be like giving

[7] We consider that the actors have an important weight in the authorship of the ethnographic text. (J. Clifford, 1998)

> something that they… it's more that it has to come naturally. Without a doubt, the word would be… it's a way of showing your affection for them. (Jorge K.)[8]

Jorge K. cannot find the exact word to express what he feels he is doing. It is not a payback of something concrete that his parents have given him, but rather something more. It is the fulfillment of a tacit agreement which seals intergenerational solidarity. The existence of this intergenerational pact becomes clearer when he says:

> At home we had my grandparents, my grandparents lived and died in our house. Because of that I feel like, for me, it´s familiar, the fact that it´s my turn now to care for them. (Jorge K.)

The same feeling of duty is reiterated in the words of María Isabel F. and Alicia B.:

> I feel that it's my obligation, it's my duty. That she cared for me when I was little and that I… (María Isabel F.)[9]
>
> It's what we're given in life. He (referring to her husband) is the son of Italians and he follows his duty 'til death. An only son… it's having a clean, clear conscience. To be able to say, well, that you looked after them while you could. (Alicia B.)[10]

Lidia R., in contrast, is less sure that she is complying with some duty. Her response show a process of elaborating the reasons that she feels she must stay by her mother's side.

> I don't know. I was sort of angry with my brothers but I also know I have no right to be angry. I don't know, I'm probably being selfish. I don't really understand it all. I like to supervise everything. I do, I really do. And then it all weighs me down…and I don't know why it has to be me. Why I think I am… it's because I'm the only woman. My brothers haven't said so, but I get the impression that my brothers think that I'm already retired and so it's up to me to go take care of my mom. Because it's my house. The house where my mom lives is mine. When my dad made his will, I got that house. It's a house I really love, truly. And, well, it's mine. And it's like, I get the impression that it's an obligation. And, hey, I'm already retired and so I have to go to take care of my mom. But look, it's not a hassle, when I do for her. I get worn out because, logically, I'm a human being and I can overdo it. But it's

---

[8] Jorge K., 48, single. He lives with his parents and a brother. He cares for his 82-year-old father who suffers neurological disorders which cause mobility problems. Family of Japanese origin. Jorge has several married brothers and sisters and has organized family aid so that when he has to be away for work or to be with his girlfriend, they take his place. He believes that his task is to "be there" controlling the situation.

[9] María Isabel F., 65, married, one married son, two grandchildren. He took the course so as to be able to care for his widowed mother, 90, who suffers cognitive disorders. María Isabel has always lived with her parents, though she is married. Three years ago she cared for her sick father until he passed away. At that time she counted on the help of her only sister and her niece. Currently, her sister is showing signs of Alzheimer's and her niece must care for her, and therefore she no longer has them to help care for her mother.

[10] Couple B., made up of Alicia, 55, and Salvador, 53. They have a son, a student, 19. They care for Alicia's mother, a widow, 89, for Salvador's mother, 75, and for his father, 78. The father suffers paraplegia and aphasia as the consequence of a stroke, for the last four years. When they got married, Salvador and Alicia built their house behind that of Salvador's parents and they have always lived together. When Alicia's mother was widowed, they brought her to live with them. Currently they are charged with the care of all three. They took the course because the situation had become intolerable.

not a hassle. I have a good relationship with my mom. We've never had problems. I've never had problems with my mom. Thank God. (Lidia R.)[11]

As we can see, the reasons Lidia R. alludes to are multiple, as much about gender — being the only woman — as economic — her parents' having put the house in her name — and work-related — her being retired. However, it seems that she feels most burdened from the need of control: if she does not supervise everything she can't feel calm. This doubtless has to do with duty.

It is noteworthy that, coming from the notion of the intergenerational pact, this emotional commitment appears with force and clarity in the case of parent-child relationships. The same obligation, however, does not occur with regards to the care of a spouse. This is what Hebe M., 72 years old, who cares for her 82-year-old husband, expresses:

Because there's no choice, I have no alternative. (Hebe M.)12

In the same situation, Esther C. declares:

…and so, it's up to me now to take care of him and I have to be aware that I have to be there, at his side. (Esther C.)13

The sense of being compelled to care, and the complex array of reasons bound to it were pointed out in various chapters, in particular by Paoletti, in chapter 1 and Katila, in chapter 2. In the next section we are going to discuss the caregiving relationship.

The Caregiving Relationship

The Power Within the Couple

In the case of wife-caregivers gender issues appear clearly linked to wives' "taking power" in the relationship. Esther C. expresses this:

-…Positive, though he tells me I'm like his cane, and I don't like it. The handle of the cane, that I have to be always with… that he leans on me. But it's positive that I've made my own decisions, which before I couldn't do.

-Was he very dominating?

-No, he was just a man of his time. He decides, he decided, and he will decide. It's his character. No, I don't know if it's his character, the role he has to have. Let's give it a more

---

[11] Lidia R., 60, separated, one son. She cares for her widowed mother, 83, who lives alone. She is retired but continues to work. She spends all weekends with her mother. Initially she came to take the course thinking mistakenly that it was about learning to be with older people. She took it anyway and it has helped her feel less dependent on her mother. She regrets than in spite of there being four brothers and sisters in her family they are not close, and suffer family tensions.

[12] Hebe M., 72, married, one married daughter, two grandchildren. Currently retired, she lives with her 82-year-old husband, also retired, for whom she must care due to his cognitive disorders. She took the course because she realized that even if the illness of her husband limits her, she is also limiting herself.

[13] Esther C., 70, married, four children, several grandchildren. She took the course three years ago foreseeing the future, given the age difference between herself and her husband, who is currently 85. At the moment of the interview his cognitive disorders had worsened.

> psychological image, then, the role. The role he has assigned himself. I'm more in the condescending role, and everything. (Esther C.)

Esther C's contradictions make clear that only in the interview itself does she begin to question what role each partner had in her marriage and probably also question if it was necessary to wait until her husband fell ill to begin to make decisions. In any case, her allusions to masculine and feminine roles refer to the traditional gender differentiation which, on the other hand, she seems to accept.

By contrast, Hebe M., who always worked and managed her money, experiences ambivalent feelings in terms of caring for her husband, but she nonetheless highlights as positive that he is now much more manageable. She says it this way:

> ...When he was still with it, he wasn't even remotely my companion, someone to go out with. He had his group, his friends, didn't give me the time of day. So now, of course, my payback is pretty big. Because sometimes he says to me, "Are you going to leave me alone?" And I go out to buy something at the store and come back. And sometimes I've just had it, and I say, "How many times did you leave me alone!" "Sure, but, you're being so mean!" And then afterwards it passes, but the anger is there. So sometimes it makes it harder for me. Because I remember certain things, when, well, I really needed him, when I got sick.(Hebe M.)[14]

And later on:

> The positive part is that he's much more manageable than before. More manageable for me is more comfortable. Because before he saw everything differently than me, thought of everything different. Then it was a lot more work. Now he's much more manageable. Dependent, because he depends on me. Not manageable because he likes to be, he has no choice. (Hebe M.)

It seems that in the marriage relationship the woman often takes her revenge, seizing the power in the relationship, and sees this as a benefit. This does not appear in other types of relationships; the intergenerational pact between parents and children differs from the marriage contract, the spousal duty is lived differently from the filial. This observation that arises from the data must be considered as a hypothesis to be tested in upcoming research.

As we have seen, the feelings that the function of caring awaken in the caregiver are multiple. But we shall focus first, as we have done so far, on those feelings which sustain the caregiving function in spite of how exhausting it generally proves. One of these feelings is related to the responsibility that constantly weighs on the caregiver as a result of the dependent´s vulnerability.

Constant Vigilance

Many caregivers manifest something similar to the "nursemaid's sleep"; they are never completely at ease but instead feel constantly vigilant, even in their sleep. But no one better

[14] See footnote number 10

than them to describe what they feel. Alejandro S., who along with his mother cares for his grandmother, tells us:

> It's lots of things together. I should spend more time looking for work, and I share this feeling with some friends of mine who take care of their loved ones. What they've found, just like what I'm finding, is that they're constantly in a state of vigilance. The first few nights my grandmother was in my house we all kept being jerked awake because of the constant cough she has which she can't stop. So it messes up your normal sleep. We just generally lived in a state of permanent vigilance. My mother more than I because she's more involved. But ít hits me too, transitively, because I see my mother, who's caring for my grandmother. The feeling we have is that no matter how much we do for her it isn't enough. Its because we lack means. She feels caregiver's fatigue. And I feel it, personally. (Alejandro S.) [15]

Salvador B. (husband of Alicia B.), who takes care of his paraplegic father, tells us that something similar happens with him:

> And uneasiness... as a psychologist said, about the bad nights, the hard nights… I don't sleep. I wake up a lot. He has these attacks. And he gets convulsions. My mom comes... I sleep in fits and starts. It's never sound sleep. My mom comes at night and when I hear anything, like if she calls me, Ah! … (Salvador B.)[16]

Another frequent consequence — whether made explicit by the caregivers or inferred from their behavior — of the anxiety provoked by the elderly person's vulnerability is an unnecessary and counterproductive overprotection which induces dependence. Lidia R., 60, who cares for her 84-year-old mother, clearly understands this when she tells us:

> Oh yeah, she moves fine. She does the shopping, everything. She even walks pretty fast. She can move great, thank God. Because of that the girls here always said: But if your mom is fine, why do you feel so obligated? Because I feel sort of … when, sometimes, I'm invited to do something on a Saturday and I still stay in. Until, the other day I was telling Mariana, until… generally, a little past one o'clock I leave and come back Sunday evening. All week we talk, every day we speak on the phone. If need be, two or three times a day, whatever. And I can't tell her until Saturday morning, at twelve o'clock noon, only then I tell her: Mom, you know I'm not going to be able to go… And Mom, happy in life, because my mom isn't irritating, at all. I don't know why. It's me who has some issue with my mom. I don't know why it's so hard for me. (Lidia R.)[17]

---

[15] Alejandro S., 38, single, and his mother, Teresita S., 66, widow. Alejandro lives with his mother and took the course so as to be able to help her care for his widowed grandmother, 91, and his great-aunt, also a widow, 89. Teresita has always lived close to her parents. In the last few years she has had to take charge of the care of her father and later of her own husband until they passed away. To cover costs she sold property. Seven months ago her only brother died. After this, the health of her mother, who suffered heart problems, worsened, and she became depressed. A sister of her mother, 89, a widow, has begun to manifest cognitive disorders which make it impossible for her to continue living alone. Teresita plans to bring this aunt to live with her so as to be able to care for her and sell her apartment to cover the costs, since the three women have very reduced pensions. Her strategy is, therefore, to sell property.

[16] See footnote number 8

[17] See footnote number 9.

A similar feeling, though certainly nuanced differently, tends to arise in the situation where the dependent—especially when it is a parent or loved one—is deteriorating (especially in cognitive function):

> I had a stage… because, well, there are a lot of things to it. One is seeing one's parents' deterioration which certainly isn't any fun. I don't think anyone would find it funny, the fact that… But you also take it as a part of that… that cycle we all go through. There comes a time when your mind raises those questions: what's going to happen here… and you sometimes try not to agonize over it, but… there is a sort of underlying anxiety there that, well, sometimes I can shake it off until later and sometimes it really hits me and, well, it's a matter of getting through it, and it passes. It passes because you have other distractions. If you didn't, you might get stuck on that, and that would be terrible. (Jorge K.)[18]

A similar sentiment appears in the words of Liliana P.:

> Emotionally, it takes me a long time. And I feel a lot of emotional pressure because my mother was always all-powerful. And suddenly she isn't all-powerful, she wants to keep being all-powerful. But there's also a fight. You have to fight to make her understand that there are things she can't do anymore and that you have to adapt to the way things are now. Apart from that it's as though the myth has fallen, the idol. Because all her life she was independent, she did everything according to her whim. She came and went. She raised all of us by herself. Without my dad's help, because he was fading. But she didn't ask anything of him, because she was all-powerful. (Liliana P.)[19]

Summarizing, we find that, among the feelings that sustain the caregiving function, the subjects note some that, in some way or another, cause anxiety for the caregiver. This anxiety generally derives from the precarious state of the dependent, who seems unprotected, weak, needy, and from the fact that a strong internal sense of duty mandates that the caregiver take the responsibility of ensuring the well-being of that sick dependent. As we stated before, this sense of duty can be conceptualized as the payment of a symbolic debt (P. Pitaud 1999) or as the fulfillment of an intergenerational pact (M. Johnson, 1995), but its existence is observed on all fronts.

We have also seen the distinctions in the relationships between parents and children and husband and wife. In respect to these differences, it must be said that while the former feel great anxiety as they witness the deterioration of their parents, the wives, in some cases, seem to experience a sort of revenge upon seeing their husbands undergo the process. This feeling results from the traditional gender roles that marked the man´s decision-making power in the couple, especially in this generation.

---

[18] See footnote number 6.

[19] . Liliana P., 37, married, one son. She took the course so as to collaborate with her sister who currently cares for her widowed mother, 77, who suffers cardiac problems and has begun to suffer cognitive disorders and depression. In the past the mother lived with one of their sisters, a drug addict, who made various attempts at suicide. All the brothers and sisters got together and decided to send the mother to live in another city with one of the daughters, since they considered that she needed a more tranquil environment.

The Lack of Gratitude

Especially when the dependent suffers from cognitive disorders, or is very dependent, the caregiver receives little or no sign of gratitude from the dependent person, which generates great resentment and makes the caregivers begin to question the reason for their sacrifice. Teresita S. dares to express this in all its harshness:

> I take care of her as if she were a queen, clean, impeccable. Now I have to buy her diapers. In her life, she has used diapers. Just think, she has no strength… and then: "Forget you have a mother," she tells me. How can I not… because my defenses are down. So then I leave and start to swear. Because I have this attitude of anger. Which I don't want. I can't help it… (Teresita S.)[20]

And then she later adds:

> Because she says: "Bring me the coffin so I can get inside…" all those things… you know what happens, I can't, I don't listen to her. Then yesterday I was furious because my friend asked me: "Teresita, why have you treated her badly?" And I said: "No, if I don't explode like that I'll have a heart attack." I have been taking two anxiety pills a day, that's how bad I felt. Because it overwhelms me. It overwhelmed me. This situation has overwhelmed me. No, at that moment it was too much, because I know I'm making an effort to give her a quality of life that she doesn't want to have. Sincerely, I'm speaking harshly. Excuse me for talking this way. Because, I tell you. I'd rather she closed her eyes and went peacefully. And I could say: "Dear, I owe you nothing, dear, we are at peace." (Teresita S.)

Teresita S. is, without a doubt, overwhelmed by her situation. Her anxiety is perceptible at every moment, throughout her story. As we can see, aside from the economic problems that caring for her mother have caused her, and to which we will refer later on, it is this lack of recognition on her mother's part that most upsets her. In this scenario, she tries to move her mother and, in doing so, becomes a torturer who wants to force her out of bed:

> Yesterday I take off her glasses and she says, "Ah! Why do you treat me this way?" I swear, that's what she does. And I tell her: "Because we've got to take your glasses off." But she has to see me like the bad guy in a movie. It's like that. Because I make her sit down… I may be a little hot-headed, but, yes, I'm always a disturbance, the one who forces her to sit. She yells like someone who's being… and besides, she does nothing to help me. She's a dead body… (Teresita S.)

Though without these dramatic extremes, María Isabel F. is going through similar situations with her 90-year-old mother, especially since the death of her father:

> Yes, 65 years of marriage. And she says that dad is calling her. That he sees her when she is alone. These are things that I have to get over, but it's hard. (María Isabel F.)[21]

In spite of her efforts to renew her mother's will to live, she cannot:

---

[20] See footnote number 13.

[21] See footnote 7.

> My family is very close. For Mother's Day, even, since my father was a person who likes to get the whole family together, we tried to get everyone to come and I was happy, and the response my mother gave me was: "Yes, but someone is missing." How do I solve that? There is no solution. My son was there, my niece, the great-grandchildren. She has four great-grandchildren, and they all came. We had a barbecue. Even my mother-in-law, from the geriatric home. We had a really nice get-together of 25 people. And I was happy because Dad would have wanted it and she says to me: "yes, but someone is missing." And, okay, well, I can't solve that. (María Isabel F.)

In the caregiver-dependent dyad, reciprocal victim-victimizer situations involving mutual mistreatment often arise. It is a vicious cycle in which relationship forms establishes in infancy are doubtless reproduced. As counterevidence, Lidia R. highlights the good relationship she has with her mother:

> As far as positive aspects go, it seems to me that the relationship is nicer. I can tell her I love you and before I couldn't. My son taught me to say I love you to someone. Because my son calls me on the phone: "I love you, Mom" ... and I learned to say it to my mom. And I like that. I've also probably grown up more, I'm older... the relationship is different. A good relationship with my mother. (Lidia R.) [22]

To summarize, the dependent frequently fails to recognize the caregivers´ efforts. This lack of recognition generates feelings that can range from sadness and powerlessness to anger and rage. In the caregiver-dependent relationship, reciprocal relationships of victimization are common, and this victimization, in turn, gives way to violent responses and possible somatic/pyschological illnesses in the caregivers (McDonald, L, 1996). In the next section, we refer more specifically to the burden — objective and subjective — that the dependents represent for the family members who have the primary responsibility of supporting them.

The Costs of Care

Throughout this chapter reference is made to the extremely high costs that all of these families are paying in order to care for an elderly relative; it seems opportune, then, to analyze this concept. Various studies have attempted to arrive at a definition. Montgomery, Gonyea and Hooyman (1985) introduce the term "burden," conceptualizing a subjective state associated with the grade of inconvenience or bother occasioned by caregiving. Their definition also includes objective consequences such as the restriction of free time or the health deterioration; in nothing these effects, the burden inherent in the act of caregiving ceases to be merely a concrete fact. Instead, it has a definite subjective effect, which is apparently related to the mishmash of negative feelings and perceptions that caregivers experience in regards to their function, that is to say, to the level of bother or inconvenience originated by the continual care of the dependent.

[22] See footnote 9.

From the stories of our interviewees arose various significant topics related to the costs or the burden of the caregivers, such as the abandonment of projects that we are going to present in the next section.

Abandonment of Projects

María Juliana T. and Jorge K. have given up their independence.

> I would have been able to do it easily and say, okay, all set... At the moment I had my home. Or, I left the house to live with my partner, everything. And just afterwards my mom lost her job and I went back. I went back because I was saying "I'll just invest some money in a rental, because I know my family has always helped me." It just didn't seem fair to me... But, well, we were talking about how I could have stopped and said, okay, all set, done. I don't know why I didn't. They're things that... I couldn't break that tie with my family, even though it's often hard for me, makes me groan. I can't break ties. (María Juliana T.)[23]

Jorge K. tells us something similar:

> Yes, maybe, at some point I've wanted to do certain things, which I needed some time to be able to do and it's been impossible to do them because I'm with my parents. That's an aspect which... I had the opportunity a few years ago to go and live with someone and I kept putting it off... I think that at the relationship level the subject was sort of off-limits. (Jorge K.)[24]

As it appear clear from those transcripts, there are no alternatives, different caring arrangement are not possible, not as much because they are not available, but they are not even thinkable. Another major cost of caregiving is having no time left for oneself, this is probably the most frequent complaint of caregivers.

Time Gone By

The costs to which all subjects without exception make reference are those which pertain to the lack of available time: with having life restricted and being unable to decide freely what they want to do. Hebe M., 72, who cares for her 82-year-old husband, with cognitive disorders, laments:

---

[23] María Juliana T., 27 years old, single. She took the course so as to solve a very complex family problem caused by the illness of her widowed grandmother, 75. Together with her mother and grandmother she is part of a typical verticalized family group. They have always lived all three together, the mother has worked as a domestic employee who slept at the site of her employment while María Juliana lived with her grandmother. When the grandmother began to have heart troubles María Juliana took care of her. But currently she works and studies and her grandmother suffers cognitive disorders which make it impossible for her to stay home alone. After much suffering they decided to send her to a geriatric home close to the house so they could visit her regularly. This is an enormous economic burden for them, and the three women have all felt the reduction in their quality of life.

[24] See footnote 6.

> Emotionally, I'm mad. My life is passing by. Am I going to end my life this way, caring for others, in this case for him? And I also see the deterioration. A really brutal kind. Sometimes he asks me, "what should I wear?" and I tell him "wear the same thing you wore yesterday, the pants and the polo shirt." And he comes in wearing pajamas. But not always. And I tell him, "No, that's to sleep in, Raúl, look closely." For example, sometimes I come home and tell him, briefly... "you didn't tell me where you went." And, a little while later, "why don't you tell me." I live on one floor... I either get mad myself or get mad at him. "I already told you a thousand times." "You didn't tell me anything!" My question is, how long will I be able to stand it? For example, I'd like to go on vacation. Alone, with my daughter, on an exchange with a group. And where would I leave him? He can't stay alone, there's no way. He wouldn't want to stay alone, either. It's a pretty heavy backpack, sometimes. (Hebe M.)[25]

Teresita S., to whose case we have dedicated much space, expresses it this way:

> I'm doing as much as I can. Then, God will decide. But I, right now, no, it's like I've stopped living. Because I used to go out to walk. Simple things. I took my rosary, prayed the rosary. Now I haven't gone to mass in three or four weeks. I don't have time and when the moment comes I don't feel like it. I had a little Virgin in the house, I prayed. But now I don't have the strength. I don't know if it's physical strength or mental strength I lack. But it's too much for me. See, when you've been taken over, you do what you have to do like a robot... So the bad part is that I'd like to see the sun and say, "what a beautiful sun!" Go out walking. The other day I put my sneakers on, walked four blocks, and came back. It's like my energy is exhausted. (Teresita S.)[26]

The lack of time for relaxation, the stress connected to caregiving, often translate in actual sickness and health problems for the caregiver, as it will be discussed in the next section.

Costs for the Health of the Caregiver

The health costs, physical as well as mental, are also very high, especially for primary caregivers, that is to say, for those who are most involved in the task. Alicia B. tells us that she began psychological treatment:

> And now I take psychological treatment. When he met me he said that I was bitter, but I used to be happy. I like to go out, but now I stay at home more and more. And I'm more and more exhausted. (Alicia B.)[27]

Liliana P. refers to the disorders suffered by her sister who cares for their mother in Córdoba:

> The other day I was talking with my brother-in-law and he was telling me that when there's some kind of or whatever, immediately my sister's health seems affected. She has

[25] See footnote 10.
[26] See footnote 13.
[27] See footnote 8.

> digestive problems, something like that. Nerves. Because she, when my mother gets really nervous or out of it… my sister starts feeling bad, and, yeah, she falls apart. She loses her voice. (Liliana P.) [28]

María Margarita B., 47, who cares for her mother, 78, also feels that her health has suffered:

> My health has been endangered, too. I've been getting checkups, because I feel something like exhaustion. But, no, luckily there's nothing. You can tell that it was tiredness, from coming and going. But no, it's under control now, for me, too. I realized in time that I needed to get under control, see someone… (María Margarita B.)[29]

Liliana P. also indicates having gone through spells of depression:

> Yes, even, when all of this had just recently come up and I began my class, two months, three months, it was really hard for me to go to class because it was hard to leave the house. I shut myself in… one of the symptoms that it said on the paper that they gave us the first day was about isolation and that sort of thing. And it was really hard for me to leave my house. I stayed shut in all day, in bed. I got up in the morning, gave the boy his breakfast. My husband took him to school, and I stayed there until three-thirty in the afternoon until I got off to run and pick him up from school and only then did I start doing anything at all. (Liliana P.)

Caregiving often represent an health hazard, it is also often a significant financial burden for the family involved. In the next section we are going to present some interviewees' accounts in relation to the effect of caregiving on the financial stability of the family.

Economic Costs

Without a doubt, under the category of "costs" experienced by the caregiver, the economic one is relevant. In effect, financial problems arise over and over in our interviewees' stories and are recurrently mentioned in this chapter:

> Yes, there have been economic problems. I've taken responsibility for that as well. Because, economically, there was nothing… like I couldn't give her money and I couldn't buy her medicine. It's not that she went without eating, but many of her needs could not be met… (Liliana P.)
>
> My father's medicines are expensive. We go without some things of our own to give them to them. (Salvador B.)[30]

---

[28] See footnote 17

[29] María Margarita B., 47, has a married son and a grandson. She lives with her partner. She works cleaning family homes. She cares for her mother, 78, a widow, who lives alone even though she suffers problems with her legs which limit her ability to walk to the point that she does not leave the house. The family group is composed of nine brothers and sisters of which only four take responsibility for their mother's care. María Margarita is the principal caregiver but counts on her brother's and a niece's contributions.

[30] See footnote 8.

> There are times when she needs to buy her medications, but her pension isn't enough. That's why I have economic problems, because I get paid by the hour, I don't have a salary. I may do some juggling, but my mom will not go without. (María Margarita B.)[31]
>
> We've had a lot of expenses, especially hiring people to be with her during the day and at night. (Alejandro S.)[32]
>
> The problem is money. I'm spending what I don't have. I take out loans and I have to pay them back. Money doesn't come into the house, it only goes out. The savings are gone. I don't know where to get money from. (Teresita S.)32

The economic cost of care passes the breaking point and frequently implies deterioration in the family economy which can be suffered by future generations of the involved families. Furthermore, when the caregivers are older people themselves, their savings may be negatively impacted, affecting their quality of life in their own old age. This is the case of Teresita S., to whom we refer in more detail upon discussing the topic of strategies implemented. Housing issues are often implicated in caring, they are mentioned in various chapters throughout the book and they are discussed in details by Watson, in chapter 8. In the next paragraph we present in particular the problems connected to different generations living in the same household.

Costs of Being a Verticalized Family

One couple among our interviewees constitutes a paradigmatic example of a verticalized family. Living in the same household seems to be a supplementary stressing factor. We will take the space here to tell their story because we believe that it shows a concentration of various key aspects of the family caregivers' problem.

Alicia B., 55, and Salvador B., 52, a married couple, are taking responsibility for the care of three of their respective parents, with whom they live, while at the same time supporting their only son, a 19-year-old student. This is a typical example of a verticalized family; Salvador is an only son and at the same time has had an only son; Alicia has only one brother. Between the two they care for the father of Salvador, who is 78, the mother of Salvador, 75, and Alicia's mother, 88. Furthermore, they are part of the so-called "sandwich generation," which must look after its parents while its children are themselves not yet independent. They are overcome by the weight of this responsibility and the demands of the people under their care. As we mentioned earlier in reference to the families with many elderly members who must be cared for and the few younger family members available to help, this couple has reached the limit of their possibilities.

In the unfolding of their story they have made decisions which now seem like mistakes, most importantly the decision to live with their parents. They explain it this way:

> It's all theirs. It's all in my dad's name, the land. So when we got married, we built our place behind theirs...it's not that we want leave them alone, because to start off with we

[31] See footnote 27.

32 See footnote 13.

> would have to have been apart. I didn't realize, because I lived there. The place is pretty, we did something nice, whatever, but... (Salvador B.)[33]
>
> ...my mother was widowed and she came to live with me. Since my parents-in-law already lived with us.... I don't know. And now that we've gotten started, we're not going to leave them. (Alicia B.)32

Four years ago, when Salvador's father got sick and became paraplegic, the problems started. Salvador feels that he must be at his father's side and Alicia blames him for not being able to tear himself away.

> Because we were already going crazy. Because the situation got worse. When he got sick my father-in-law was terrible. And my mother-in-law doesn't really know how to stay uninvolved, more like not at all. So it was chaos. At that point I more or less took the wheel, but the time came when we were totally destroyed. We fought a lot because he, every little thing... he wanted to be on top of every little thing. And I didn't. We went through hell. (Alicia B.)

Throughout the entire interview Alicia does not stop explaining that it's not caring for her relatives that bothers her, but rather living with them. She would have rather had them live in another house and had to go there to care for them, to be able to enjoy some intimacy with her husband and son.

> For me, taking care of them doesn't bother me at all. Even helping them economically, if I have to buy their medications, because they aren't bad people, bad parents. The only thing that kills me is living all together. If we lived separately I'd go to them. Because, sometimes, I've taken his aunt to the doctor. You can tell that I'm inclined to do that. So what bothers me isn't the... what bothers me more than anything is the living together. (Alicia B.)

To summarize, the "costs" refer to the level of inconvenience produced by the caregivers´ efforts, as measured by objective indicators such as restriction of free time, deterioration of health, abandonment of personal projects, or economic pressure derived from caregiving costs. "Cost" implies the objective and subjective encumbrance that the caregivers´ task brings. In order to lighten the load of costs, the caregiver tries out various organizational strategies. Those strategies implemented by our subjects are discussed in the next section.

Strategies for the Organization of Care

One aspect of our research that has especially interested us is the strategy that these families employed to cope with this situation. And we encountered a wide variety of different solutions. In effect, in some cases the families were able to somehow organize themselves and this way kept the situation under control, while in others, the organization seemed chaotic and irresolute.

---

[33] See footnote 8.

The Home Office

Jorge K., who is a real estate agent by profession, opted to work at home in order to "be there," as he puts it, and keep control over household events. He is single, and this permits him to be with his parents for the most time possible. On the weekends, as well as on days when he must travel for work, one of his brothers or sisters takes his place. He is confident that he can count on one of them whenever he might need to. He himself declares that the strategy that he has found is satisfactory, but also implies the sacrifice of some aspects of personal life.

> I'm usually around in the morning. My office is my house. I do everything by phone, and so... maybe I go by the office in the afternoon, or, like today, I'm doing things downtown because we're diversifying. Besides, I have to travel every once in a while, and at those times another family member steps in. (Jorge K.)[34]

As we can see, Jorge K. seems to be the organizer of a family support network in which members can trade places, sometimes being the primary, secondary, or tertiary caregiver, as becomes necessary.

Internment in a Retirement Home Close to the Family Home

María Juliana T., 27, tells us that she and her mother had to take the decision to intern her grandmother when the situation became unmanageable, given that both must work. She says:

> ...Before, it was under control, she made her own food, did some things, and lately she's stopped doing anything. If she doesn't have her food served to her she doesn't eat, or get hungry, or remember to eat. There were three people in our house taking care of her, and we couldn't manage. She wouldn't take her medicines, she wouldn't eat. And, well, given all that we had to opt to put her in a home one block from the house, so we're always over there visiting her... (María Juliana T.)[35]

This is another case of a verticalized family, of three generations of women, granddaughter, mother, and grandmother, who have always lived together. The internment decision had a very high cost for the family group, emotionally and economically. The grandmother´s retirement funds cover only half the cost of the geriatric ward and the rest must come out of the other two women's salaries.

> ...This home costs 470 pesos (160 US dollars) for a person like my grandmother who is mobile. My mother can't pay that amount, so she told them that what she can pay, with a lot of effort, is 400, and they left it at 400. But just now, today before coming here, we were doing all our bills, and we said, we won´t make it! (María Juliana T.)

[34] See footnote 6.
[35] See footnote 21.

This case also illustrates another of the aspects of the caregiving problematic which we initially mentioned: the changes in the situation of the woman. María Juliana T. works and does postgraduate studies and is not inclined to sacrifice these projects in order to stay at home and care for her grandmother.

> I´m trying to see things objectively because when I didn't, I suffered a lot. I cried a lot. And I said no. I think it was unfair for me. (María Juliana T.)

Though she thinks they made the right choice, she has not stopped suffering for having made it. Often, caregiving imply moving house for the cared for. This is a choice that is often difficult for both parts.

Move to Another City with a Daughter

Liliana P. has a large family: there are seven brothers and sisters. The difficulty that arose was reaching an agreement regarding what was best for their mother. But they did it, and decided that she would go to live with one of the daughters, in Córdoba, where the surroundings are calmer. The other children collaborate economically, when they can, from Buenos Aires. This way they took her out of an extreme situation linked to a suicidal drug-addict daughter who was negatively affecting the family network.

> ...somehow, we all got together. When we had to take her to Córdoba even the furthest gone of us was there. Since it was very difficult to take her, even the furthest gone... we used to take her to Córdoba, or send her on a bus, and it was tremendously traumatic because it was my sister Silvia and me and my brothers and sisters had taken themselves out of it. They gave us the money, but it was "you do it." Or, more like, you be the bad guy. The other one still used to come to my house to console my mother before she left. This time he didn't. This time we broke down and said: it's like this and it has to be like this and this is what we're going to do. And we all sort of took that stance. (Liliana P.)[36]

Family conflicts are often generated in relation to the allocation of caring responsibilities as in this case; in the next section we discuss as the property of one's house can be at risk because of the costs of caregiving.

Selling the House and Using up One's Personal Wealth

Teresita S.'s is another typical case. She is a widow of 62 years who takes care of her 91-year-old mother. In the past, she cared for her husband and father until they passed away. Her only brother passed away seven moths ago. She is now alone, and desperate. Little by little she has been using up her savings so as to be able to meet the costs of her mother's care and now she finds herself having to sell her possessions. She tells us:

[36] See footnote 17.

> Here the problem is basically money. I am spending what I don't have. I've taken out loans, I have to repay that money… the problem is that there is no money coming into the house, it´s only going out. So all my savings are used up, everything has been used up and I find myself in a really tough situation at a time when I have to make any number of decisions… I'm killing myself. I'm giving… I don't want to be tragic, but I am sacrificing myself. And I don't want to sacrifice myself, sincerely… I've had to pawn jewels to be able to stay afloat. Because my economic situation is very bad… (Teresita S.)[37]

But Teresita S. does not only take care of her mother, but also of an 89-year-old aunt, who suffers early Alzheimer's symptoms which makes her unable to continue to live alone. This aunt has donated her apartment and Teresita plans to sell it and bring the aunt to live with her, to make ends meet. She explains this to us:

> Imagine now that I have to bring over my aunt, it's a mess. My aunt is in the early stages of Alzheimer's. I have to sell her apartment to be able to survive myself. Because she gave it to me. But until I sell it… I'm going through… I've had some terrible moments when my father, when my husband died I was left with debts, I sold the house, I paid it all… but now this is the worst moment of my life, emotionally and psychically speaking… the only thing I want is to lie in bed with the heating pad and not think. Because when I wake up in the morning my head is chaos. I don't know how to fix all this… (Teresita S.)

In Teresita S's story we observe a middle-class family with a good economic history whose wealth has shrunk during the last few years to afford the care of the oldest family members. The strategy has remained the same, to sell property in order to pay debts. This is another highlighted aspect of the caregiving problem: the possibility of inheriting wealth from the previous generation becomes less and less, since that wealth must be used for their care in old age.

In this section, we presented the strategies that the subjects implemented to resolve the problems of every day life. Some may be considered sucessful because they have allowed the caregiver to control the situation; others, on the other hand, have driven the families toward situations of even more vulnerability. Attending the course "Caring for Those Who Care" was considered by the participants an additional strategy, but we think it is worthwhile to examine the class in a separate section.

Why the Course?

In this section, we will reveal the interviewees´ opinions about the course—how they came across it and the impact it has made in their lives. We will point out how attending classes was a strategy that some caregivers adopted in the hope of alleviating the burden they felt in their caregiving role.

---

[37] See footnote 13.

Different Kinds of Motivations

Among the myriad of interesting responses our subjects gave us during interviews, the reasons for which they approached Caring for Those Who Care and their success in the program surprised us. We found a wide variety of answers, from those who did it in the moment of maximum family tension to those who turned to the program anticipating future troubles and even those who sought to collaborate with a fellow family caregiver; there were even some who mistakenly approached the course thinking its subject matter was something different and who stayed because it interested them anyway. The following interviewees related these different motivations. At the most dramatic extreme, Salvador B. and Alicia B., as we saw before, say:

> Because we were already going crazy… we went through hell. (Alicia B.) [38]

The course was greatly helpful to them:

> It was very useful for us in the sense of getting away a little bit. Because we were all very close to the problem. What's more, we started leaving the house a little more. Because staying that way, with my father-in-law, paraplegic, it was like we were all paraplegic. We used to go out walking, the two of us, and we stopped. We started staying inside all the time. (Alicia B.)

Esther C., by contrast, began the course so as to prepare herself for possible future situations:

> What's going on now is that at this moment I am taking charge. When I took the course for caregivers I was sort of foreseeing the future. He's (*referring to her husband*) 85 years old. It's a 15-year difference. I could already see that I would have to take care of him and of myself. Not just take care of him, but of me, too, keep myself up. (Esther C)[39]

Liliana P., for her part, saw in the course the possibility of supporting her sister, who cares for her mother in Córdoba:

> I took the course because, at that time, I could not take charge of her myself, have her living with me and all that… She went to live at my sister's house in Córdoba and the situation is a little complicated. She started with cognitive problems, she still doesn't have a certain diagnosis of her illness… so it seemed to me to be a way to contribute something to my sister, who was there, to take the class and pass it along to her, because where she is this sort of course doesn't exist, and I'd pass along all the information. (Liliana P.)[40]

Alejandro S. also thought that participating in the course would permit him to help his mother care for his grandmother and great-aunt:

> And why did I do the course, well, up until a year ago there was the possibility of her coming to live with us and now she is going to have to. So I wanted to be prepared. Because

[38] See footnote 8.
[39] See footnote 11.
[40] See footnote 17.

the course generates a structure, information and assistance from the social workers. There was a nurse in the course, and also psychological assistance. The course helped me a lot, and it keeps helping me. My worry was how to open my head up to be able to help these older people and, in case of not being able to assist them full-time, how to give ideas to my mother or whoever was right there, to tell them: look, we have people to turn to. (Alejandro S.)[41]

Others did the course because they felt bad for the people they cared for, as is the case for María Isabel F., 65, who cares for her 90-year-old mother. She tells us:

> Because I felt bad. I felt like I was being aggressive with Mom. Because Mom has a problem which is like an arteriosclerosis of old age. So she says things that hurt me. And I respond badly and then make myself feel worse. So because of all that I took the course, and they told me that my mom's problem was first, and I had to understand that, but it was hard. She's medicated, they took her to another doctor and medicated her. For a month and a half she's doing well with the forgetting and all. But yesterday we started with the robberies. Because she keeps thinking she's being robbed. So since I'm the only one in the house it's hard for me to hear that. For example, we fought yesterday and today she's like a puppy and I feel bad. And now she's been saying that everything hurts, so they'll pamper her. Before I came I gave her some tea with aspirin and told her to go to sleep... but yes, it's hard for me. It's really hard on me, that's why I took the course. *(María Isabel F.)* [42]

Jorge K. also felt conflicted about his role as caregiver and wanted to receive help:

> Strictly speaking, I did the course because my sister recommended it to me. The course's rationale is consistent with a certain unease one sometimes feels. It's that about caring for those who care, like the term says. We needed to take another look at what was happening to us. Sometimes one gets worked up over certain things. And sometimes the trigger is, of course, those we care for. And it's not their fault that they are the way they are. It's part of our life. *(Jorge K.)*[43]

In actual fact the course had a positive impact on the participants' life as it is illustrated in the next section.

How the Course Helped Caregivers

Regarding whether the course gave him skills which help him better carry out his duties, he has the following opinion:

> To say that it wears me out... it would be a lie to say it didn't. But I think those are moments, and they pass later. I think that, exactly, after the course, the way I get made has changed a little bit. I think I started to take some time, started to delegate some things a little bit. I've got a ways to go yet, but... *(Jorge K.)*

---

[41] See footnote 13 .

[42] See footnote 7.

[43] See footnote 6.

We have observed that one of the principal aids that the course gives to the caregivers is something very simple: it gives them permission to take distance and delegate their duties to others, even temporarily. We believe that the "mandate" that in large part sustains the situation generates a sense of responsibility that make caregivers nervous when they are absent. Jorge K. again illustrates what "being there" means:

> I believe that what I do, more than anything, is just be there. Sometimes that term seems a little passive, but the fact of being there implies that my mom is calmer. I tell you this because, sometimes, I find myself in situations like: we have to bathe him. Usually my mom goes with him when he bathes. But, my mom has some problems, so I ask her to bathe him when someone else is there, just in case. I might hand her a towel, or help with the chair… the fact is that, well, while someone else is there everything that could be dangerous has to be done. I think that's my job, the simplest one at least. There's also taking him to the hospital, of course, staying with him, talking to the doctors, going to buy medicine. I do take charge of that, which no one else does. It's generally me. (Jorge K.)

This needs to ensure that nothing bad happen therefore generates a permanent nervousness, a sense of anxiety, sometimes produced by the overprotection of the dependent, which over time leads to exhaustion. The course enables the caregiver to take some distance and delegate his tasks to others, which brings relief. The sequence would be like this:

Anxiety
↓
Overprotection
↓
Exhaustion
↓
COURSE
↓
Permission to take distance
↓
Relief

María Juliana T., 27, who has her grandmother in a geriatric home, tells us that the course helped her to set limits, to know how far she had to take her dedication to the dependent.

> -Because I wanted to be capable, to do my best. I wanted, well, there are things that I believe that because of my age I might not know, might not have enough experience. And also a little restraint. Maybe sometimes I said: okay, I'm young, I'm intolerant, and, well, how much do I have to put up with, and what things are really okay? To what extent I have to set limits. And, well, these days I'm the one who sets the limits.
>
> -Did you learn that in the course or is that your character?
>
> -Well, in the course it was like they told me: Okay, it's all right for you to set limits. Or at least that's the message I got. It's okay, setting limits. Even if she's like a kid, and all, because

> she isn't a baby. Sometimes you say: no, because she's older and she has severe cognitive disorders she's acting like a little kid. Yes, she might be acting like a little kid, but you have to set limits for little kids. And my mom can't. My mom can't set limits. So she suffers and now she's suffering, seeing her mother in the geriatric home: no, it shouldn't be like this. And, well, so that's the restraint that I have to have, on both counts. (María Juliana T.)[44]

To summarize, the interviewees′ responses indicate that one of the courses′ main effects was the possibility of establishing limits on their dedication, by coming up with alternative strategies for alleviating family and personal strain.

To take a distance from the caregiving situation physically, but above all psychologically, was the most important positive effect of the course.

CONCLUSION

In this chapter, we have discussed the key themes that play roles in family care of the elderly with health problems. Using these as a basis, we examined the existence of networks of solidarity and the intergenerational pact as the fundamental basic ethic that forms and sustains the caregivers′ personal mandate. Families that take care of their elderly relatives and, consequently, experience stressful situations remain strong by invoking moral and ethical values. These values are maintained due to a strong psychological sense of duty in the caregiver. This sense of duty derives from the tacit pact that clinches solidarity between generations, which we call the intergenerational pact. There is a difference in the caregiving-ethic between the feeling of obligation that a parent-child relationship elicits (intergenerational pact) and the obligation that derives from a marriage contract. In the latter case, changes in the exercise of power are observed, given that women seem to take advantage of their spouses′ dependent situation. This observation should be taken up as a hypothesis in future research.

Of the multiple feelings – positive and negative – that arise in the caregiving situation, the responsibility that encumbers the caregiver due to the dependent person′s vulnerability generates a situation of permanent unease, even while sleeping the "nursemaid′s sleep." It has been observed that overprotection of the elderly person augments dependence, creating a vicious cycle. In the caregiver-dependent dyad, reciprocal relationships of victimization commonly arise that generate situations of mutual abuse and sickness. Family caregivers refer to the "high costs" incurred by supporting their sick elderly. Among the most important ones that arose in this project are: the abandonment of personal projects, lack of independence, lack of free time, lack of future personal time, the caregivers′ loss of physical and psychological health, and massive economic payments that endanger the future of the family caregivers.

Caregivers have come up with various strategies in an attempt to deal with the uncertainties of daily life. Some of these strategies we consider successful because they manage to control the situation; others, on the other hand, have not been able to resolve the crisis. Among the proposed strategies, attendance in the course "Caring for Those Who Care" has been found to offer caregivers information and facilitate a conscientious understanding of

[44] See footnote 21.

the situation. This knowledge helps the caregivers to distance themselves and set limits, and thus modifies the emotional burden of caregiving.

Recommendations

Be attentive to the demands for help that caregiving families and their elderly present, with the purpose of contributing to the job they are undertaking. These demands focus fundamentally in:

1. economic help (monthly subsidy, loans, etc);
2. complimentary services of domestic help (gerontolocial caregiver, nurse, domestic hospitalization, etc);
3. institutional care for the elderly during some period of time or season.
    - Make known, through various means of communication, the different programs that exist to help family caregivers and end their isolation.
    - Develop stable, uniform means and procedures of socio-healthcare coordination and complementation, given that a plan for caregivers integrates health questions as well as social ones.
    - Develop and broaden a diversified aggregate of social services, with the idea of being able to furnish each case with adequate resources. Keep in mind that some families may need one or more services at the same time or in alternate form.
    - Strengthen technical-professional services with the purpose of being able to guide the caregivers in utilizing and reaping their benefits of services at the level they require. Create the position of "Case Administrator." This could be a formal or voluntary job.
    - Stimulate development of the complementation of social policies, given that currently, in practice, the informal caregiver is "punished" by the fact that in-home help services are not offered.
    - Favor the possibility of making professional life compatible with the care of a dependent by means of legislation that would facilitate obtaining special licenses (remunerated or unremunerated).
    - Encourage volunteering by facilitating a greater presence of such work in the field of the caring for the elderly and in helping the caregiving families. Technical and economic help should be given to them.
    - Offer technical help in regards to adapting living quarters. This includes everything from the orientation to the execution of the modifications.
    - Promote research in different regions whose results would permit the adjustment of policies and programs destined for caregiving families, keeping in mind their socio-cultural differences.

References

Bertaux, D. (1996) Historias de casos de familias como método para la investigación de la pobreza. *Revista de Sociedad, Cultura y Política,* 1, 10-21 Buenos Aires.

Chappell, N. (1996) The Sociological Meaning of Caregiving and Social Support: Issues for Older People, the Family and Community. In V. Minichiello, N. Chappell, H. Kendig and A. Walker (Eds.), *Sociology of Aging. International Perspectives.* (pp. 148-151) Melbourne: ISA, Research Committee on Aging.

Clifford, J. (1998) Sobre la autoridad etnográfica. En C. Reynoso (Comp.), *El surgimiento de la Antropología Posmoderna.* (pp. 141-170) Barcelona: Gedisa.

Fraser, N. (1997) *Iustitia Interrupta. Reflexiones críticas desde la posición postsocialista.* Bogotá: Universidad de los Andes-Siglo del Hombre Editores.

Instituto Nacional de Estadísticas y Censos (INDEC) (2003) La población argentina envejece. *Aquí se cuenta. Revista informativa del censo 2001,* 6, 1-4. En http://www.indec.mecon.gov.ar/webcenso/aquisecuenta/aquisecuenta.asp

Johnson, M. (1995) Interdependency and the Generational Compact. *Ageing and Society*, 15, 243-265.

Lomnitz, L. (1977) *Como sobreviven los marginados*. México: Editorial Siglo XXI.

McDonald, L. (1996) Abuse and Neglect of Elders. In J. Birren (ed.) *Encyclopedia of Gerontology*. (Vol.1, pp. 1-10). Los Angeles: Academic Press.

Monk, A. (1997) *Actualización en Gerontología.* Buenos Aires: Asociación Gerontológica Argentina.

Montgomery, R., Gonyea J. and Hooyman N. (1985). Caregiving and the experience of subjective and objective burden. *Family Relations. Journal of Applied Family and Child Studies, 34, 19-26.*

Oddone, M. J. (2001) Actitudes, percepciones y expectativas de las personas de mayor edad. Buenos Aires: FLACSO/STEAS. Versión electrónica en http://www.flacso.org.ar/posgrados/cursos/ig/publicaciones.jsp

Oddone, M. J. (2002) Ageing and Society. In S.D. Gorkhale and N. Pandit (Eds.), *Ageing in Search of its Identity.* (pp. 262-271). Pune: IFA, Community Aid and Sponsorship Programme and Aameyra Publishers.

Pitaud, P. (1999) La dependencia y su price en charge (responsabilidad) en Francia: Análisis crítico de un nuevo dispositivo. In R. Moragas Moragas (Ed.), *El reto de la dependencia al envejecer.* (pp. 17-30) Barcelona: Herder.

Vinocur, P. y Halperín, L. (2004) Pobreza y Políticas Sociales en Argentina de los años 90. Santiago de Chile: CEPAL. Versión *electrónica en http://www.eclac.org/*

Wacquant, L. (2001) *Parias Urbanos. Marginalidad en la ciudad a comienzos del milenio.* Buenos Aires: Manantial.

In: Family Caregiving for Older Disabled People
Editor: Isabella Paoletti, pp. 63-83
ISBN 1-59454-808-0

Chapter 4

A STUDY OF THE CAREGIVING ROLE OF THE SANDWICH GENERATION IN HONG KONG*

Richard Cheung Lam*
Department of Sociology,
Hong Kong Shue Yan College, North Point, Hong Kong

INTRODUCTION

The present day aging population is a worldwide phenomenon that is primarily caused by an increase in life expectancy and the resulting growth in the number and percentage of the elderly population. Hong Kong is no exception to this global trend of population aging. In 1971, 7.4% of the Hong Kong population was aged 60 and above. The percentage increased at an alarming rate, to 14.8% in 2001, and it is estimated that it will be 15.2% in 2006, 20.8% in 2016, and 31.8% in 2026 (Hong Kong Census and Statistics Department, 2002). The number of people aged 60 and above is forecast to increase from 1,004,400 in 2001 to about 2,435,400 in 2026 — an increase of 142% (HKCSD, 2002). The rapid increase in the numbers of the aged is having a tremendous impact on the distribution of social resources, including social security, pensions, health care, housing and the labor market. This phenomenon has increased public awareness of the need to review the issues related to its impact, especially the caregiving to the elderly (Bengtson and Putney, 2000; Chi, 1999; Liu, Cheng and McGhee, 2001; Mok, 1994).

In facing the provision of caregiving to the elderly, two major dilemmas need to be solved. The first one is the issue of who should provide the care to the elderly; should this be the responsibility of the family or the government? The second dilemma is the question of what kinds of care are to be provided (Bengtson and Putney, 2000). In a traditional Chinese society, the values of Confucian filial piety provide the basis to define culturally the inter-generational relationship and what kinds of caregiving are to be provided. These values outweigh all other ethical imperatives and some of the component ideas are even shared by

* Assistant Professor, Telephone: (852) 21048235. Fax: (852) 28068044. Email: rclam@hksyc.edu

other cultures (Ho, 1996). Confucian values assume that care for the elderly is the responsibility of the adult children, and therefore, basically the family's responsibility (Bengtson and Putney, 2000; Chow, 2001; Pak, 1996). In addition, Confucius defined filial piety in terms of nine acts and Mencius described eight features of filial piety or care for parents (Lin 1992). "In the Chinese context, filial piety is prominent in the classics arising from Confucian philosophy that has prevailed for two and a half millennia." (Kwan, et al., 2003, p.16). However, in Hong Kong, because of the change of family structure and the perception and practice of traditional Chinese values, filial piety, as described by Confucius or Mencius, does not appear to be the consensual norm (Cheung, et al., 1994). Since the traditional filial piety basis for supporting the elderly is largely modified or changed, the provision of caregiving will be at risk. In this case, the role of formal sources of support will probably need to be strengthened. This will lead to a tremendous increase in the Government's burden and resources when providing caregiving to the elderly.

In studying caregiving, the sandwich generation has been under-represented in research on caregiving and filial responsibility (Kwok, 2000). The sandwich generation has to take care of their elderly and their own children at the same time. This implies that they may face much greater potential difficulties than other non sandwich-generation adult children in handling this situation. In response to this grey area of our understanding and the change of filial piety values, this research focuses on how the present-day Hong Kong sandwich generation perceives and performs its caregiving roles towards the elderly, and the constraints it faces in performing those roles.

PERSPECTIVES ON CAREGIVING

The Confucian Filial Piety

Confucianism, Chinese ethical religion, has dominated Chinese thought for over two thousand years. The goal of Confucians is to achieve harmony with the world and nature. Based on this goal, Confucius established a set of rules which were intended to maintain the harmony and proper relationships between rulers and ministers, fathers and sons, husbands and wives, between brothers and between friends. In the father and son dimension, the Confucian concept of filial piety contains important rules and guidelines governing intergenerational relationship. Confucius defined nine acts involved when adult children practice filial piety toward the elderly. They include: providing care; not being rebellious; showing love, respect, and support; displaying courtesy; continuing the family line; promoting fraternity among siblings; advising parents; concealing parents' blunders; and displaying sorrow for parents' illness and death (Lin, 1992). In the Confucian school, Mencius described eight features of filial piety. They include: supporting; respecting; taking care; minding; showing courtesy; pleasing; abiding by righteousness; and reproducing (Lin, 1992). These nine acts and eight features describe and define proper behavior and attitudes for adult children to have towards the elderly.

The practice of Chinese filial piety in the traditional society has its moral and economic background. "In pre-industrial economics both land and businesses, which served as the family's source of sustenance, were owned by the oldest generation and passed down to the younger generation only at death. Hence, it was not the oldest generation that was dependent upon the younger generation, but rather the younger generation that was dependent on the older generation for housing and income. What care may have been provided to parents was, therefore, not necessarily based on a sense of moral obligation, but instead stemmed from economic necessity" (Montgomery, 2000, p.1019). However, the introduction of an industrial economy has substantially changed the economic necessity behind the moral obligation. First, when the traditional extended and interdependent family moves to the city, the adult children begin working for other employers rather than having their father as their employer. The economic independence and financial power of the sons frequently enables them to achieve a dominant position in the family. Consequently, the adult children will usually move out to form their own nuclear families. Thus, the economic independence and the formation of nuclear families have affected the new generation's perception and performance acts of filial piety.

Second, the responsibilities of the family are diminishing in modern society; the family no longer functions as the provider of education, health care, and vocational training for its members. These functions have now been largely taken over by the Government and other institutions. Moreover, the family is no longer the only source of moral training. More and more schools, nurseries, clubs, and the state are molding the worldview of the Chinese. Modern education tends to produce a generation which rationally values achievement and also makes decisions on rational grounds. In addition, economic independence has also fostered rational and independent thinking and behavior (Ng, 1991, pp. 178–181). Consequently, the introduction of an industrial economy, the subsequent change of family structure and the rise of rational and independent thinking have substantially modified or changed how the new generation perceives and practices the values of Confucian filial piety.

The contemporary society of Mainland China still has the characteristics of high filial piety, such as legal sanction on filial responsibility and gerontocracy. In contrast, Hong Kong which is dominated by an 'East meets West' culture, shows myriad differences from Mainland China cities because of historical factors that differentially shape their structure and culture (Kwan, et al., 2003, p.20). The perception and performance of filial piety is to a great extent different across societies where Chinese culture is still prevailing. Research on the perception of traditional Chinese filial piety has clearly indicated that filial piety is on the decline or under transformation (Chow, 2001; Ho, 1996; Lui, et al., 1997; Ng, 1991). Others found that one modern manifestation of filial piety would include greeting parents, respecting parents, caring for parents, pleasing parents, financially assisting parents, and obeying parents (Kwan, et al., 2003, p.1). It is significant to study the extent to which this traditional Confucian value has been changed or transformed in Hong Kong. This has an implication that the responsibilities of taking care of the elderly need to be rearranged to provide a balance between family and state support. In studying the practice of filial piety, many dimensions of filial piety could be included, such as respecting, pleasing and caring for the elderly. However, this chapter focuses on the dimension of informal caring for the elderly.

Reasons for Caring

In explaining why adult children provide caregiving to their elderly, perspectives on caregiving can be useful. According to sociobiological theory, the fundamental goal of the organism is not mere survival of its offspring, but to 'inclusive fitness,' to pass on the maximum number of genes to the next generation (Hamilton, 1964). Based on this principle, human beings helping each other can be best understood in terms of the human evolutionary past — close relatives help each other, even at risk of their lives and against a 'selfish' purpose, in order to increase the chances that their genes will survive in their relatives (Forsyth, 1987). Consequently, helping is much more common among close relatives than among strangers and in dense, rather dispersed communities (Barash, 1982), and intrafamilial helping of all types is desirable — the old helping the young as well as the young helping the old (Schulz, 1990). The strength of the theory seems to explain why adult children provide care to their offspring, but doesn't explain the provision of care to their elderly, especially in the case of limited resources that should be allocated to the young rather than the old in order to maintain the survival of the genes (Schulz, 1990).

In sociological analysis, it is values that provide the moral rationale and motivation, and the role of social norms such as the norm of reciprocity or social responsibility that governs caregiving behavior. The reciprocity norm emphasizes the social exchange that paying back what one receives when young, while social responsibility stresses that helping others in need is a social obligation (Schulz, 1990). In fact, there is an implicit social contract within families that has traditionally emphasized the reciprocal obligations between generations. Parents support children in return for their assistance in old age. This is typically a social, not a legal, contract (Treas and Wang, 1993, p.87). In Confucianism, filial piety provides the core element of morality, and in the case of Hong Kong, Confucianism, familism, and the norm of reciprocity in general are three ideological sources bolstering filial piety (Kwan, et al., 2003, p.15).

The above studies have clearly indicated that the provision of caregiving is not necessarily based on a moral sense of filial piety but also stems from a socio-economic structure. In the face of these changes in the family structure and in the perception and practice of traditional Chinese values, this research aims to study how the present day Hong Kong sandwich generation perceives and practices filial piety. Based on this research goal, three research questions will be examined. First, how does the modern sandwich generation perceive the values of Confucian filial piety and to what extent have they internalized the values. Second, to what extent have the Confucian values affected the informal caregiving behavior of the sandwich generation in contemporary Hong Kong society. The third research question is to identify the structural constraints that may affect the performance of the caregiving roles of the sandwich generation.

In this section, the literature review on filial piety has shown that the traditional Chinese filial piety is the primary moral obligation that governs the Chinese adult children in performing and perceiving the caregiving roles. However, in the case of Hong Kong, filial piety has been modified and changed. This research aims to examine how the present-day sandwich generation perceive and practice the caregiving roles and the difficulties they encounter. In the next section, The method of data collection and data analysis will be described. Then the section 'Findings' outlines the general distribution of the respondent's demographics and examines the associations between perception of filial piety and actual caregiving performance, and explores the difficulties that respondents encounter. The findings are then discussed before conclusion and recommendations.

METHOD

Quantitative data was collected from a random sample of 503 respondents in the CATI survey and qualitative data from 20 in-depth follow-up interviews. This study used computer-aided telephone interviews (CATI) (see Appendix 1). This method has become increasingly popular in Hong Kong community surveys because the well-developed local telecommunication networks (it is estimated that every household has at least one telephone line). It is regarded by previous researchers to be less embarrassing for respondents when answering sensitive questions and encourages them to be more forthcoming (Tang and Chung, 1997). For each of the telephone interviews, the trained interviewers completed a structured forty item questionnaire in an average of twelve minutes. The questionnaire involved five main categories of respondent's information: personal characteristics; beliefs and perception of filial piety; actual caregiving performance; and difficulties and problems encountered. The collected data was subject to SPSS quantitative analysis.

In addition, 20 in-depth interviews were conducted as follow-up research. Because the follow-up research could not re-call the sample collected by CATI, the respondents were different from those participating in the CATI and a snowball sampling method was adopted. A semi-structured questionnaire was developed with a checklist of variables mainly concerning information on the rationale behind the sandwich generation performing its caregiving roles. Consequently, with the random sample of the sandwich generation and the follow-up interviews, the findings of this research have a highly generalized capacity and can be used as a crucial reference point for the government when formulating social policies regarding the elderly. In the next section the result of the survey and of the qualitative study will be illustrated.

FINDINGS

The Sandwich Generation and their Perception of Caregiving Roles

Socio-Demographics of Respondents

In this section, the findings will be classified into three parts. Firstly, selected socio-demographics of respondents are described and these variables are assumed to influence respondent's perception and performance of caregiving roles. This part will also involve the presentation of six domains of respondent's perception on caregiving. Secondly, the caregiving performance of the respondent will be depicted, and followed with an investigation on the association between the respondent's perception and performance of the caregiving role. In the third part, socio-demographic variables and selected structural variables are used to cross-tab with respondent's caregiving performance. These cross-tabulations can assist in examining the rationale and factors that influencing respondent's caregiving performance.

The findings of the respondents' general socio-demographics shown in Table 1 include the respondent's gender, relationship with their elderly, age of respondent, age of elderly and family income. In the gender distribution, the majority of respondents were female 62.2%, and the rest 37.8% were male. (This distribution implied that the female performed caregiving more than the male. However, the distribution might not reflect this phenomenon because the rates of refusal to be interviewed for male and female were not available). The second distribution of the variables indicated that 34.2% of the respondent's identity of its care-receiver was son, 38.2% was daughter, 23.9% was daughter-in-law and 3.7% was other relation. This distribution of the identities indicated that the major care provision rested on the son and daughter of the elderly. As for the daughter-in-law, it occupied the second majority category 23.9%. The other relation was only 3.7% (It is a Chinese traditional merit for Chinese daughter-in-law to help her husband take care of her husband's parents. That is why the daughter-in-law also had a high percentage 23.9%). The majority age group of respondents was between 35–54. It occupied 80% of the total respondents. The rest 20% was either below 34 or above 55. While the majority age group of the elderly was between 65-84. It occupied over 73% of the total care-receivers. The rest 26.6% was either below 65 or above 85. Almost half of respondent's family income per month lied between HK$ 10,000 – 30,000 per month and the other half lied below HK$ 10,000 or above HK$ 30,000. These variables are expected to have an influence on the perception and performance of caregiving roles and will be cross-tabulated with other variables later.

Table 1. Demographic Characteristics of Study Sample

Variable	Percent	Number of respondents
Gender of Respondent		
Male	37.8	(190)
Female	62.2	(313)
Relationship between Respondent and Elderly (The identity of the respondent to the care receiver)		
Son	34.2	(167)
Daughter	38.2	(187)
Daughter-in-law	23.9	(117)
Other Relation	3.7	(18)
Age of Respondent		
Below 34	14.5	(71)
35–44	46.8	(230)
45–54	33.2	(163)
Above 55	5.5	(27)
Age of Elderly		
Below 65	14.7	(73)
65–74	34.9	(173)
75–84	38.4	(190)
Above 85	11.9	(59)

Table 1. (Continued)

Variable	Percent	Number of respondents
Family Income per month		
Below HK $10,000	18.2	(72)
HK$ 10,000–20,000	36.1	(143)
HK$ 20,000–30,000	20.5	(81)
Above HK$ 30,000	25.3	(100)

PERCEPTION OF CAREGIVING ROLES

In this research, six questions were used to measure the different aspects of how the sandwich generation perceived the values of Confucian filial piety (the questions were based on a modification of Kwok's (2000) research). These include: the adult child has the responsibility for taking care of his/her parents (child's responsibility); the adult child should not only provide the resources for care but also, should the need arise, be concerned about his/her parents (care and concern); the adult child should take care of his/her parents — even without any reward (care without reward); the adult child should sacrifice time, money and energy in taking care of his/her parents (sacrifice); performing the caregiving roles is an expression of filial piety (filial piety); and if there is the opportunity to be free from any caring-responsibility requirements for their parents, adult children should still be willing to take care of them (choose to take care) anyway. The findings of these measurements are shown in Table 2.

Table 2. Various domains of perceptions on caregiving

	Child's responsibility (Percentage and Frequency)	Care and concern	Care without reward	Sacrifice	Filial piety	Choose to take care
Strongly agree/ certainly willing	45.3 (224)	47.4 (236)	42.7 (208)	28.3 (136)	34.1 (166)	77.9 (381)
Agree/ perhaps willing	46.5 (230)	46 (229)	50.5 (246)	44.2 (212)	43.3 (211)	11 (54)
Neutral	7.3 (36)	5.2 (26)	4.7 (23)	15.8 (78)	8.4 (41)	2 (10)
Disagree/ perhaps unwilling	1 (5)	1.4 (7)	2.1 (10)	11.3 (54)	12.1 (59)	3.1 (15)
Strongly disagree/ certainly unwilling	0 (0)	0 (0)	0 (0)	0.4 (2)	2.1 (10)	5.9 (29)
Total	100 (495)	100 (498)	100 (487)	100 (480)	100 (487)	100 (489)

In the three main domains, child's responsibility', 'care and concern' and 'care without reward', over 92% of the respondents (sandwich generation) strongly agree or agree how they perceive the caregiving roles of the adult child. However, in contrast to these three domains, the 'sacrifice' domain registers less recognition with 73% of respondents saying they strongly agree or agree. The comparison of the distribution among these four domains implies that the filial piety obligation has its material limits. Respondents agree on the filial piety values, however, when requiring sacrificing their money and time, their willingness to perform caregiving dropped almost 20%. The 'filial piety' domain, regarding the taking care of their elderly to be an expression of filial piety, has a relatively low percentage, 77%. However, the 'choose to take care' domain, regarding the respondents' willingness to take care of their elderly when they have the opportunity of being free from the caring of their elderly, was a higher to 89% including 'certainly willing' and 'perhaps willing'. (All these percentages on the various domains are significant at the 0.001 level)

The higher percentage of the respondents' willingness to care even if they had an opportunity to avoid this responsibility indicates that some other values lead respondents to take care of their elderly even if there are no such values as filial piety, or the respondents are willing to take care of their elderly but do not regard these caregiving roles as a sign of filial piety. For instance, respondents may regard the provision of care to their elderly as a justified action since the adult children had been taken care of by their elderly and they should do something in return. Treas and Wong (1993, p.87) regard that as the implicit social contract within families. These findings indicate that the majority of the respondents treat caring for their elderly as an expression of filial piety. They regard this caring as the responsibility of the adult child and most important of all is that even without any pressure being applied to perform the role or without the social norms constraints they are still willing to do this. In other words, most respondents are willing to take care of their elderly and internalize the values affecting their behavior towards their elderly. However, the relative low percentage of 73% in the domain of "sacrifice" indicates that there are limits to the filial obligation.

The six questions were further subjected to a reliability test that has an acceptable Alpha value of 0.63 for measuring an abstract construct. The scores of the six questions were added together to form an index – 'The Strength of Filial Piety Values'. The index shows a similar distribution to the distribution of the questions shown in Table 2, and will be used to conduct regression analysis with the caregiving performance in the next section.

THE ACTUAL CAREGIVING PERFORMANCE OF THE SANDWICH GENERATION

With respect to how respondents perform the caregiving roles to their elderly, five questions were used to measure different domains of caring. The domains were: 'emotional care'; 'economic care'; 'information care' – i.e. knowledge and information care; 'daily care'; and 'nursing care'. The distinction between the different domains of caring was primarily based on the respondent's subjective definition. In the case of respondents feeling doubt about the distinction, the telephone interviewer quoted examples to illustrate the content of each domain, for instance, 'visiting or making a phone call' as an example of emotional care; 'giving money' in economic care; 'filling in an application form or selecting the appropriate doctor' in information care; 'cooking or shopping' in daily care; and 'bathing or toileting' in nursing care. The findings are shown in Table 3.

The respondents' caregiving performance in the emotional and economic domains is quite consistent with their perceived conception of filial piety — 86% and 79%, respectively — if 'frequently' and 'sometimes' are added together. In the domains of information and daily care, it is quite diverse from the previous two — 57% and 30%, respectively. Around 80% of the respondents never performed nursing care for their elderly.

In the last section, the findings on how the respondents perceive their caregiving roles indicated that most respondents had internalized the values of filial piety as their intrinsic values in influencing how they performed the caregiving roles (see Table 2). Consequently, it was assumed that the respondents would perform in all the care domains. However, the distribution in Table 3 indicates that the traditional values seem to affect only the first two domains of the performance — emotional and economic — both have a similar high percentage.

Table 3. Various Domains of Care

	Emotional care (percentage and frequency)	Economic care	Information care	Daily care	Nursing care
Frequently	53.3 (266)	48 (240)	26.3 (131)	12.3 (62)	4.6 (23)
Sometimes	32.7 (163)	30.8 (154)	30.3 (151)	17.5 (88)	7.2 (36)
Seldom	7.2 (36)	8.4 (42)	13.5 (67)	14.9 (75)	9 (45)
Never	6.8 (34)	12.8 (64)	29.9 (149)	55.3 (278)	79.3 (398)
Total	100 (499)	100 (500)	100 (498)	100 (503)	100 (502)

The performance became diverse in information, daily and nursing care domains. The diverse distribution indicates that their actual performance in caregiving did not match with how they perceived filial piety. The findings of the follow-up in-depth interviews can partly explain this phenomenon, as it will be illustrated in the next section

Interesting Inconsistencies in the Data

In the information care domain, the older generation usually obtained knowledge and information from their friends, neighbors and television, rather than from their adult child. In the Chinese traditional conception of the elderly, the elderly have relatively more life experience knowledge and are considered to be wiser than the young, and should be respected by the young. The generation gap and the self-respect of the elderly causes them to be reluctant to ask the younger generation especially a third generation child for knowledge and information.

With respect to the daily care domain, if the elderly could take care of themselves, the sandwich generation seldom or never performed this role. In addition, the sandwich generation will usually ask the elder offspring (the third generation children) to provide certain daily care such as shopping to the elderly. It is role differentiation that the sandwich generation as the main bread-earners needs to concentrate on providing the financial support the family. While if the elderly could not manage to take care of themselves and needed nursing care, the findings show that around 80% of respondents had never performed such a role. Three main factors can contribute to an explanation of this phenomenon. First, nursing care is usually beyond the sandwich generation's knowledge and, in fact, such care should probably be provided by a nursing professional. Second, the high percentage of those showing 'never perform nursing care' was partly due to the respondents' traditional Chinese belief that the respondents should highly respect their elderly and would feel embarrassed about having any physical contact with their elderly. In addition, the findings of follow-up interviews show that once the elderly could not take care of themselves, the respondents probably recruited a maid or a nursing professional to perform the daily care or nursing care respectively (provided that their family income enabled them to do so).

The five questions measuring the different domains of caregiving performance can also be subjected to reliability and factor analysis. The result of the analyses shows that the first factor included 'nursing care' and 'daily care'. The second factor included 'emotional care', 'information care' and 'economic care'. Based on the content of these six questions, the first factor could be regarded as the construct to measure 'physical care' that involved the substantial physical action in the domains of 'nursing care' and 'daily care'. These two questions formed an index as 'The Intensity of Physical Care Performance'. The second factor could be regarded as the construct to measure 'symbolic care' that involved the symbolic expression of care in 'emotional care', 'information care' and 'economic care'. These three questions also formed an index --- 'The Intensity of Symbolic Care Performance'. The two analyses indicated that there was ambiguity and a low reliability for the two caregiving performance constructs. This implied that there might be some other factors affecting the actual performance of caregiving. Hence, the performance of various care domains did not have had a high internal consistency in the two constructs. Consequently, the analysis of these two constructs should be handled with particular care.

To examine the relation between filial piety values and the actual caregiving performance, the correlation between the values and various care domains, and the values and the recoded cares (physical and symbolic cares) are shown in Table 4.

Based on traditional sociological analysis, it is assumed that a person's value system will provide the rationale for their social actions. Hence, it is expected that the stronger a person internalizes the caregiving values, the more domains and intensity of caregiving that person would perform. However, the regression analysis did not match this expectation and assumption. The strength of filial piety values is positively correlated with the intensity of emotional, economic, information and symbolic cares, but negatively with daily, nursing and physical cares. In addition, they are weakly correlated. Other research also found a similar result that "the high filial responsibility does not translate to high practice in filial piety" (Kwan, et al., 2003, p.7). The findings of the consistently high percentage perception of filial piety and caregiving as an internalized belief compared with the inconsistency in their actual performance in the caregiving roles indicates that the sandwich generation has some constraints which causes them to have difficulties in performing in all care domains.

Table 4. The strength of filial piety values by various domains of care

	The Strength of filial piety values (Gamma)
Emotional care	0.19*
Economic care	0.14*
Information care	0.145*
Daily care	-0.05
Nursing care	-0.12*
Symbolic care (index)	0.17*
Physical care (index)	-0.03

Note: * $\rho < 0.05$

FACTORS AFFECTING THE CAREGIVING PERFORMANCE

To investigate the discrepancy between the perception and the performance of the respondents in the caregiving roles, seven variables were selected to examine how they affected the respondents' perception and performance. The seven variables were: gender and age of the respondents (Gender; Age R); living arrangements (Living Arrangements); respondents' family income (Family Income); respondents' relationship with the care-receiver (Relation); age of the care-receiver (Age O); and the ability of the elderly to take care of themselves (Care of Themselves), see Table 5. (Some of the variables involved are nominal and others are ordinal or interval; for the sake of simplicity in interpretation, all measures of associations (except two) take Cramer's V to show the strength of their associations)

The cross-tabulation showed that the respondents' gender affected only economic care; the association also showed that males were generally more willing to provide economic care than females. It seems to relate to the traditional value that males need to take care of the financial support of the family.

The variable, respondents' age, did not have a significant association with any care domains. This result implied that a respondent's age did not affect how a respondent performed in various care domains.

Table 5. Demographic variables by various domains of care

	Gender	Age R	Living arrangements	Family income	Relation	Age O	Care of themselves
Emotional care	0.11	0.04	0.16 **	0.08	0.12 *	0.08	0.01
Economic care	0.15 **	0.06	0.11	0.16 ***	0.12 *	0.07	0.05
Information care	0.06	0.06	0.17 **	0.11	0.08	0.1	0.11
Daily care	0.05	0.07	0.42 ***	0.09	0.1	0.14 ***	0.16 **
Nursing care	0.05	0.06	0.08	0.09	0.06	0.09	0.22 ***
Symbolic care (index)	0.11	0.1	0.1	0.17 ***	0.08	0.13 *	0.13* (G=-0.24)*
Physical Care (index)	0.11	0.07	0.3 ***	0.09	0.1	0.12 *	0.26*** (G=-0.3)**

Note: * $\rho < 0.05$; ** $\rho < 0.01$; *** $\rho < 0.001$
Figures inside the box are the value of Cramer's V
Figures in brackets denote the value of Gamma G

The Living Arrangements

The variable of 'living arrangements' had a very significant association with four out of seven domains of care, including emotional, information, daily and physical cares. In the domain of daily care, it achieved the highest association index value (Cramer's V) of 0.42 in the cross-tabulation. The result of a very significant association with four domains of care obviously indicates that 'living arrangements' had a strong impact on how the respondents performed their caregiving roles.

It is well known that family support given to the elderly is often affected by the living arrangements of the elderly. However, some social scientists (Kim, 1996; Koyano and Okamura, 1996) have argued that the strength of the family support to the elderly cannot be based simply on the frequency of contact or co-residence within the family. Rather, the strength lies in the ties of obligation and affection, bound in custom and the social process. It is because frequent contacts or co-residence may lead to lower levels of satisfaction among family members and of commitment to the obligation. Maintaining a good relationship among family members is a problem. Ensuring the elderly have someone to take care of them is another matter. Changes in living arrangements are likely to be associated with changes in the level of care and assistance received by the elderly. These changes are supported by the findings of this research and the follow-up interviews.

The Family Income

The variable of 'family income' had a reasonably significant association with only one domain — economic care. It is understandable that different family income levels would affect the respondents' ability to provide economic care. In addition, there is a negative and very significant association between 'family income' and 'symbolic care'. Since the symbolic care includes the economic domain it follows that different income levels would affect the respondent's ability to provide symbolic care.

Other Variables

The variable 'respondents' relation with the care-receiver' had a fairly significant association with two care domains — emotional and economic cares. Both the cross-tabulations and the findings of the in-depth interviews indicated that the closer the relationship (for instance, son is closer than son-in-law and daughter is closer than daughter-in-law) between the respondents and the elderly, the more likely the respondents would care more for the emotions of the elderly and provide more economic care to the elderly.

The variable 'age of the elderly' had a very significant association with the daily, symbolic, and physical care domains. This association was similar for the variable 'Care of themselves' that also had a very significant association with daily, nursing, symbolic and physical cares. Although the variable 'Care of themselves' had a significant association with four out of seven care domains, it was not significantly associated with emotional, economic and information domains. These two significant associations reflected the reality of the respondents' actual performance in the caregiving roles. If the elderly could not manage to take care of themselves, it was logical that they required certain care domains, especially the nursing and daily care domains. In addition, there was a relatively stronger, negative and significant association between 'care of themselves' and both symbolic and physical care domains. The negative association indicated that when the elderly could not take care of themselves, the respondent would perform more symbolic and physical care. These four significant associations with 'Care of themselves' can explain partly why most respondents had internalized the caregiving values, yet did not perform in all care domains, see Table 2 and 3. There is a very simple explanation for this, because those they cared for did not need it, as it will be illustrated in the next section.

The Great Majority of Older People are Healthy and Independent

The high percentage of respondents that did not perform physical care only reflected the 92% of the elderly that could take care of themselves, see Table 6 below. It is very important to highlight the fact that the great majority of older people conduct independent lives.

Table 6. The ability of the elderly to take care of themselves

		Frequency	Percent	Valid Percent	Cumulative Percent
Valid	Certainly Yes	231	45.9	46.2	46.2
	Yes	190	37.8	38	84.2
	Fair	41	8.2	8.2	92.4
	Not and Certainly not	38	7.6	7.6	100.0
	Total	500	99.4	100.0	
Missing	System	3	0.6		
Total		503			

Therefore, it appears that it is not the case that those respondents internalizing the caregiving values refused to perform certain domains of care, especially physical care. Rather, it was that the elderly could take care of themselves. This should be spelled out clearly: a large proportion of the elderly population is healthy and active, consequently the respondents did not need to perform in these domain cares. If the above explanation of the inconsistency between the internalized caregiving values and the actual caregiving performance could be assumed, the value of Gamma for the association between 'care of themselves' and 'physical care' would be very high, i.e. if the elderly have difficulties in taking care of themselves, the adult child (sandwich generation) would perform more physical care. However, the obtained value of Gamma was only -0.3, see Table 5. It is relatively low to support the above explanation. The findings of the follow-up interviews can partly explain this low value. The findings of the interviews showed that if the elderly could not take care of themselves, the respondents usually employed a maid to perform the daily care or a nursing professional to perform the nursing care. (This is a very practical proposition in the Hong Kong context. The government imposed minimum wage for a full time maid imported from the Philippines or Indonesia is around HK$ 3,500 in Hong Kong. While a full time clerk or worker commands a salary at least two to three times more than that amount). Therefore, if the elderly could not take care of themselves, the respondents provided only a small amount of physical care as the remainder was performed by a paid service.

On the whole, the ability of the elderly to take care of themselves plays an important role in affecting how the respondents performed in the various care domains. If the elderly cannot take care of themselves, they would require the respondents to carry out more intensive care and, larger number of domains. At the same time, the cross-tabulation also indicated that if the elderly could not live with the respondents, there would be potential difficulties for the respondents in providing certain care domains to the elderly. The cross-tabulations in this section have indicated that the 'living arrangements', 'family income' and 'care of themselves' had significant impacts on both the physical and symbolic care performances. These impacts seemed stronger than the effect of their internalized values in affecting their caregiving performance. Moreover, the distinction between physical care and symbolic care, together with the consideration of the ability of the elderly to take care of themselves, can largely explain why those respondents who had internalized filial piety values did not perform in all care domains, and the strength of their internalized values reflected little on the various domains and intensity of their caregiving performance.

DISCUSSION

Based on the analysis of the above findings, three main factors affecting the caregiving performance can be identified. The first factor is the strength of the caregiving and filial piety values that can be regarded as the primary factor in affecting the respondents' caregiving performance. The findings of this research indicate that the majority of the respondents had internalized caregiving and filial piety values, see Table 2. The values provided the basic rationale for performing in the various care domains.

The second factor is the structural constraints, such as the living arrangements and the family income. This factor constituted a potential difficulty when performing various domains of care. For instance, whether or not the respondents lived with their elderly substantially affected the performance in all care domains, especially in the physical care performance.

The third factor is the ability of the care-receivers to take care of themselves. If the elderly could take care of themselves in all care domains, the sandwich generation would not perform in certain domains, in particular, the physical care performance. In this research, about 92% of the respondents' elderly could, to a great extent, take care of themselves, see Table 6. This implied that the majority of the respondents' elderly did not require much physical care such as daily care and nursing care. Consequently, the respondents would seldom perform in these care domains. The remaining 8% of the respondents' elderly that could not take care of themselves needed to receive care in the largest number of domains, especially physical care. However, the association between the ability of the elderly to take care of themselves and the physical care performance did not have a particularly high association — only –0.3 of Gamma, see Table 5. The findings of the 20 in-depth interviews have partly explained this phenomenon, that when the elderly could not take care of themselves, the respondents would usually (provided that the family income could support it) recruit a maid to provide daily care or a nursing professional to provide nursing care. On the whole, the analysis of the third factor indicated that the ability of the elderly to take care of themselves to a great extent could determine the specific domains and intensity of caregiving provided by the sandwich generation.

Based on the above analysis of the research findings, it is strongly recommended that an analysis of the caregiving performance should incorporate the three main factors simultaneously or else the analysis will provide a confused picture of the caregiving performance. For instance, if the explanation of caregiving performance is simply based on the first factor — the internalized caregiving values — then the consistently high percentage expressing filial piety and caregiving as their internalized belief compared with the inconsistency of their actual caregiving performance will be observed. If the third factor (the ability of the elderly to take care of themselves) is incorporated when analyzing the caregiving performance, it can partially explain the following inconsistency. Whether or not the care-receiver needs or accepts all domains of care determines, to a great extent, the respondent's caregiving performance, even though the respondent has internalized caregiving values and is ready to perform in all care domains.

To explain the caregiving performance fully, the second factor (structural constraints) also needs to be incorporated into the analysis of caregiving performance. For instance, having internalized caregiving values and the care-receivers' needs for the respondents to perform in all care domains, the second factor — constraints such as the living arrangements

— would also affect the respondents' performance both for physical and symbolic cares. Therefore, the three factors need to be incorporated simultaneously when explaining the caregiving performance of the sandwich generation.

In addition, there are three significant findings worthy of discussion or further research:

Firstly, the respondents show a very diverse response to the question that performing caregiving roles is an expression of filial piety, see Table 2. This implies that many respondents either do not regard practicing filial piety means one has to personally perform the caregiving role or that performing the caregiving role is not an expression of filial piety. However, the other question about the respondents' willingness to care even if they had an opportunity to avoid this responsibility shows a high percentage of 'certainly willing' (see Table 2). These two distributions clearly indicate that except for filial piety there are some other values affecting how the respondents perceive the caregiving roles (Chow, 2001; Ho, 1996; Lui, et al., 1997; Ng, 1991). The findings of Chow's recent research also show that " … people in Hong Kong have a different interpretation of how the values of filial piety should be practiced in today's world than what was perceived traditionally" (Chow, 2001, p. 134). Kwan has argued that "Confucianism, familism, and the norm of reciprocity in general are three ideological sources bolstering filial piety" (Kwan, et al, 2003, p.15). Further research is required to identify these values or beliefs.

Furthermore, a loose intergenerational relationship can hardly produce quality caregiving across generation. "Caregiving based on filial piety is greater in quality and is more helpful. On the other hand, caregiving would be less stressful to the caregiver who is high in filial piety. Filial piety is therefore a healthy cushion to caregiving offspring. The benefit of caregiving based on filial piety may draw on the affection of caregiver. Care with love would be more helpful" (Kwan, et al., 2003, p.15). The findings of empirical studies also support the idea that the values embodied in filial piety support warmth, love, harmony, and close family ties, all of which facilitate intergenerational relationship. Further, filial piety correlates with some positive aspects of personality that makes adult children feel more obligated to support their elderly parents and more responsible for caring for them, and reduces parent-child conflicts (Yeh, 2003, p.67). Hence, in order to facilitate a quality and harmonious intergenerational relationship the government should assert the status of Chinese filial piety values and educate people on the values when they are young.

Secondly, the ability of the elderly to take care of themselves has played an important role in affecting what care domains and the intensity of care the respondents need to provide. If the elderly cannot manage to take care of themselves, the respondents may become frustrated by the need to perform caregiving. Many care domains (especially the nursing care) are beyond the ordinary respondents' knowledge and capacity to perform and, in reality, require a nursing professional. However, as the elderly grow older, this situation will occur more frequently and it is beyond the respondents' ability to control. The findings of follow-up interviews indicated that the relatively higher-family-income respondents would recruit a maid to perform daily care and a nursing professional to perform nursing care. However, many families with low family income could not afford this recruitment. This imposes a great burden on the sandwich generation to perform simultaneously the caregiving roles for both their older and their younger generation. Therefore, it is suggested that the government should provide nursing care, or a service or a center for those elderly who cannot manage to take care of themselves, to ease this unsolvable burden imposed on the sandwich generation. Currently, Nursing Homes and Care and Attention Homes can provide a varying degree of medical and nursing care to the elderly people. In addition, the services of the Social Centers for the Elderly, the Multi-Service Center for the Elderly and Day Care Centers for the Elderly can ease the burden on the sandwich generation (Ngan, et al., 1996; Ngan and Cheung, 1999). However, as the numbers in the elderly population are increasing steadily, the provision of health, medical and nursing care from Government or non-Government organizations should be increased accordingly.

Thirdly, the variable of 'living arrangements' has shown a significant association with many care domains. It is understood that if the respondents cannot live with their elderly, they can hardly perform in many care domains, especially providing emotional support and care when the elderly is ill (Lam, et al., 1998). In addition, the sandwich generation will experience inconveniences in performing in some other care domains, such as daily care. Although living together may bring conflict or dissatisfaction between both the sandwich generation and its elderly parties, it is important to note that the elderly, to a great extent, do require some one to take care of them (Andrews and Phillips, 1998). Kwan and his colleagues (2003) also suggested that "promoting co-residence between parents and children would be a first step to induce filial piety practice among the younger generation" (p.7). Therefore, it is suggested that the government should offer certain social policies, such as a tax reduction, to encourage respondents to live with and take care of their elderly.

Conclusion

This research has examined how the Hong Kong sandwich generation perceives and performs its informal caregiving towards its elderly and the structural constraints that affect its caregiving performance. The findings of this research show that most respondents had internalized caregiving values and regarding caregiving as an expression of filial piety, see Table 2. The findings also indicated that most of the respondents did not perform physical care and were quite diverse in performing symbolic care, see Table 3. These two findings showed a confused picture, that although they had internalized caregiving values, the respondents did not perform in all domains of care accordingly. The findings on the structural constraints partly explain this phenomenon. Structural constraints, such as living arrangements and family income played a more important role in limiting the caregiving performance of the sandwich generation than did caregiving and filial piety values.

Recommendations

- To explain the caregiving performance of Chinese adult children, one should examine the extent they have internalized filial piety values, the ability of care-receivers to take care of themselves, and the structural constraints, such as living arrangements and family income that could affect caregiving performance.
- To improve the quality and quantity of informal caregiving by adult children, filial piety values should be emphasized. The values can provide a healthy cushion for some stressful and demanding caregiving, and support warmth, love and harmony in intergenerational relationship.

- Government should provide regular trainings, especially nursing care, to adult children in performing physical care.
- In light of an aging population, the government should accordingly increase the number and services of elderly health centers to reach those families that have elderly members and yet can not fulfill the caregiving roles.
- Government should develop social policies that could provide convenience to adult children to live together with elderly members in the family, so that adult children manage to perform various care domains with ease.

REFERENCES

Andrews, G. and Phillips, D.R. (1998). Markets and Private Residential Homes: Promoting Efficiency or Chaos? *Generations Review*, 8, 4, 9-11.

Barash, D. P. (1982). *Sociobiology and behavior* (2nd ed.). New York: Guilford Press.

Bengtson, Vern L. and Putney, Norella M. (2000). Who will care for tomorrow's elderly?: Consequences of population aging east and west. In Vern L. Bengtson, (et al) (Eds.), *Aging in East and West: Families, States, and the Elderly (*pp. 263-285). New York: Springer Pub. Co..

Cheung, Chau-kiu, Lee, Jik-joen and Chan, Cheung-ming (1994). Explicating Filial Piety in Relation to Family Cohesion. *Journal of Personality and Social Behaviour*, 22, 3, 565-580.

Chi, I. (Ed.) (1999). *A Study of the Chinese Elderly Issues*. Hong Kong: Hon Chung China.

Chow, Nelson W. S. (2001). The practice of filial piety among the Chinese in Hong Kong. In Iris Chi, Neena L. Chappell and James Lubben (Eds.), *Elderly Chinese in Pacific Rim Countries: Social Support and Integration* (pp. 125-136). Hong Kong: Hong Kong University Press.

Forsyth, D. R. (1987). *Social Psychology*. Belmont, CA: Brooks/ Cole.

Hamilton, W. D. (1964). The Genetical Evolution of Social Behavior, I and II. *Journal of Theoretical Biology*, 7, 1-52.

Ho, Y. F. (1996). Filial Piety and its Psychological Consequences. In Michael Harris Bond (Ed.), *The Handbook of Chinese Psychology* (pp. 155-165). Hong Kong: Oxford University Press.

Hong Kong Census and Statistics Department (2002). *Hong Kong Population Projections 2002-2031*. Hong Kong: Demographic Statistics Section, Census and Statistics Dept.

Kim, Dongbae (1996). Effect of Retirement Housing on Filial Responsibilities in Korea. In *Hong Kong Journal of Gerontology: Total Care of the Elderly — a Multidisciplinary Approach*. Vol. 10 supplement. Proceedings of 5th Asia/ Oceania Regional Congress of Gerontology (pp. 118-121).

Koyano, Wataru and Okamura, Kiyoko (1996). Filial Piety and Co-residence in the Japanese Context. In *Hong Kong Journal of Gerontology: Total Care of the Elderly — a Multidisciplinary Approach*. Vol. 10 supplement. Proceedings of 5th Asia/ Oceania Regional Congress of Gerontology (pp.122-125).

Kwan, Alex Yui-huen, Cheung, Jacky Chau-kiu and Ng, Sik Hung (2003). *Revisit of the Filial Piety Concept Among the Young, the Adult, and the Old in Beijing, Guangzhou,*

Hong Kong, Nanjing, Shanghai, Xiamen, and Xian: Research Report. Hong Kong: Dept. of Applied Social Studies, City University of Hong Kong.

Kwok, Hong Kin (2000). A Comparative Study of the Middle Class and Working Class Sandwich Generations, the Stress They Encounter and Their Coping Strategies in Contemporary Hong Kong Society. (Ph.D. Thesis) Hong Kong: The Chinese University of Hong Kong.

Lam, T.P. et al. (1998). Community Attitudes towards Living Arrangements between the Elderly and their Adult Children in Hong Kong. *Journal of Cross-Cultural Gerontology*, 13, 3, 215-228.

Lin, An-hong (1992). *Study of Filial Piety in Confucian Thought.* Taipei, Taiwan: Wen Jin.

Liu, Ben C. P., Cheng, Y. H. and McGhee, S. M. (2001). Health and Care Utilization Patterns of the Community-dwelling Elderly Persons in Hong Kong. In Iris Chi, Neena L. Chappell and James Lubben (Eds.), *Elderly Chinese in Pacific Rim Countries: Social Support and Integration* (pp. 241-256). Hong Kong: Hong Kong University Press.

Liu, William T., Yu, Elena S.H., Gong, S.S., and Kean, Y. (1997). *Filial Piety and Caregiving Burden in Shanghai, People's Republic of China.* Hong Kong: Faculty of Social Science, Lingnan University.

Mok, Henry T.K. (1994). Elderly in Need of Care and Financial Support. In Donald H. McMaillen and S.M. Man (Eds.), *The Other Hong Kong Report.* Hong Kong: The Chinese University Press.

Montgomery, Rhonda J. V. (2000). Filial Responsibility. In Rhonda J.V. Montgomery (Eds.), *Encyclopedia of Sociology* (pp.1018-1024). New York: Macmillan Reference.

Ng, Gan-theow (1991). *Religion, Culture, and Modernity: some Missiological Implications of the Process of Secularization in East Asia.* Ann Arbor, Mich.: University Microfilms International.

Ngan, M.H., Leung, M.F., Kwan, Y.H., Yeung, W.T. and Chong, M.L. (1996). *A Study of the Long-term Care Needs, Patterns and Impact of the Elderly in Hong Kong.* Hong Kong: Dept. of Applied Social Studies, City University of Hong Kong.

Ngan, Man-hung and Cheung, Chau-kin (1999). *A Study on the Effectiveness of the Home Care and Support Services for Frail Elderly People and their Caregivers.* Hong Kong: Haven of Hope Christian Service.

Pak, Jae Kam (1996). The Ideal of Filial Piety in Modern Times. In *Hong Kong Journal of Gerontology: Total Care of the Elderly — a Multidisciplinary Approach.* Vol. 10 supplement. Proceedings of 5th Asia/ Oceania Regional Congress of Gerontology (pp. 130-132).

Schulz, Richard (1990). Theoretical Perspectives on Caregiving, Concepts, Variables, and Methods. In David E. Biegel and Arthur Blum (Eds.), *Aging and Caregiving : Theory, Research, and Policy* (pp. 27-52). Newbury Park, CA : Sage.

Tang, C. and Chung, T. (1997). Psychosexual Adjustment Following Sterilization: A Prospective Controlled Study on Chinese Women. *Journal of Psychosomatic Research,* 42, 187-196.

Treas, Judith and Wang, Wei (1993). Of Deeds and Contracts: Filial Piety Perceived in Contemporary Shanghai. In Vern L. Bengtson and W. Andrew Achenbaum (Eds.), *The Changing Contract across Generations* (pp.87-98). New York: A.de Gruyter.

Yeh, Kuang-Hui (2003). The Beneficial and Harmful Effects of Filial Piety: an Integrative Analysis. In Kuo-Shu Yang, et al. (Eds.), *Progress in Asian Social Psychology: Conceptual and Empirical Contributions* (pp. 67-82). Westport, Conn.: Praeger.

APPENDIX 1

A brief description of selection process of the random sample is as follows:

1) enter all telephone numbers of the latest household telephone directory into a computer to form a telephone number database.
2) use computer to select randomly about 12,000 telephone numbers from this database and put them into another computer system and ready for the telephone interviewers to select randomly. (based on the result of similar CATI survey, to generate 500 successful cases of interview requires 10,000 to 15,000 random telephone numbers).
3) the last two digits of these selected telephone numbers are replaced by random digits. (this procedure can ensure that some telephone numbers not including in the latest household telephone directory will have a chance to be selected)
4) selection process after successful initial contact

a) select sandwich generation family, if not --- stop.
b) Select sandwich generation respondent, if not available --- stop.
c) Select the sandwich generation respondent who currently provides caregiving, if not --- stop (this selection criterion can ensure the respondent is currently performing some caregiving to its elderly, or else it is pointless to collect information of sandwich generation who does not perform caregiving).
d) A brief statistics of the telephone calls are shown in Table A.

Table A. A selected statistics of the telephone interview (the total telephone numbers dialed as the percentage base)

Frequency	Percentage	Remarks
503	4.8%	Successful completed case
1,912	18.4%	No one answer
52	0.5%	Telephone recording
1,416	13.6%	Household refused to be interviewed
612	5.9%	Cannot get through
555	5.3%	Respondent refuse to be interviewed
65	0.6%	Partly completed interview
458	4.4%	Fax number
98	0.9%	Language barrier
2,408	23.2%	No appropriate respondent

*Total telephone number dialed: 10,390 (in three consecutive days)

*The average interview duration: 00: 11: 52

*An earlier version of this chapter was presented at the XVth ISA World Congress of Sociology 2002 in Brisbane, Australia. The author wishes to thank David Ip, HK Kwok, Tony Roberts and Paul Stables for their critical comments and suggestions. The author is also indebted to the East Asian Development Network (EADN) for the funding of this research.

In: Family Caregiving for Older Disabled People
Editor: Isabella Paoletti, pp. 85-102
ISBN 1-59454-808-0

Chapter 5

CAREGIVERS, HELPERS, AND FAMILY: FAMILY CAREGIVING RESEARCH IN A CANADIAN CONTEXT

Joanie Sims-Gould*[*] *and Anne Martin-Matthews
School of Social Work and Family Studies
The University of British Columbia, Vancouver, BC

INTRODUCTION

To date, social scientists studying families have focused almost exclusively on studying family roles, not on family relationships or family responsibilities; there has been particular paucity in the examination of family responsibilities as relative and interconnected to one another (Matthews, 2002). This statement can be extended to research on family caregiving.

This chapter will further the current understanding of family caregiving through the examination of the context for research of family caregiving in Canada; and, through the analysis of Canadian longitudinal data examining the responsibilities and relationships of various family members involved in family caregiving to an older adult. Within our analysis, we make a distinction between those that are primary caregivers and those that are "helpers" or secondary caregivers and present their differential responsibilities within family caregiving. We also develop the argument for extending family caregiving research beyond the examination of the dyad (between primary caregiver and care recipient) to an exploration of networks of multiple individuals with multiple responsibilities.

* Email: simsg@interchange.ubc.ca, amm@interchange.ubc.ca

The Canadian Context: Population Aging, Healthcare and Family Caregiving

The Changes in the Structure of the Population

Canada's population[2] is still considered young in comparison with many countries in the industrialized world. Nevertheless, with increases in life expectancy and the aging of what is commonly known as the "baby boom generation," the proportion of the population over the age of 65 will increase even further, to approximately 25 percent by the year 2031. This trend will begin to accelerate around 2011, when the oldest baby boomers, born in 1946, reach age 65.

In an attempt to reflect the heterogeneity of old age, researchers and policy makers often distinguish between the "young old" (often those between 65 and 80 years of age) and the "old old" (usually those aged 80 or 85 and older). This "old old" population has been the fastest growing age group in Canada over the past decade. The numbers of Canadians over the age of 80 "soared by 41 percent" between 1991 and 2001, and by 2011 will include an estimated 1.3 million people. Not only are numbers of people reaching age 65 increasing, but also individuals arc living longer in old age. At age 65, women in Canada can expect to live another 20 years and men another 16 years (Chappell, Gee, MacDonald and Stones, 2003). Increased longevity has also meant a substantial increase in the duration of family ties across generations. It is now common for parents and children to share 50 or 60 years together. When persons born in 1910 reached their fiftieth birthday in 1960, only 16 percent of them had at least one of their parents still alive. By comparison, when persons born in 1930 reached their fiftieth birthday in 1980, 49 percent of them had at least one of their parents still alive. Projections suggest that when persons born in 1960 reach their fiftieth birthday in 2010, fully 60 percent of them will have at least one of their parents still alive to celebrate the event with them (Gee, 1990). The implications of these demographic trends for the roles of family members as caregivers and helpers are apparent.

In fact, many people over the age of 65 also have at least one child who is also over the age of 65. An examination of the Canadian demographic trends particularly with respect to population aging points very clearly to families spending more years together; this is turn potentially contributes to more years of family caregiving across generations. As family ties become more enduring, more Canadians find themselves involved in family care of an older relative.

Population aging is not the only feature of Canadian life that is contributing to a changing context and increased opportunity or likelihood for family caregiving. Health and social policies, and changes to them, have an impact on aging individuals and families. For example, in comparison with families in many countries of the world, Canadian families benefit enormously from our national medical insurance program (Martin-Matthews, 1999; Martin-Matthews, 2000). Although health-care policy is changing, currently it still functions to reduce the economic and social burden to families when their members, old or young, become ill. How long this continues to be true remains to be seen.

---

[2] 13 percent of Canada's total population of 31 million people is over the age of 65 years (Statistics Canada, 2003).

Health-Care Reforms

Throughout the 1990s, Canada was engaged in a thorough review of its federally and provincially funded social programs. Health-care programs and policies, under provincial jurisdiction, were of particular concern. Initially, health-care reforms were expected to benefit the elderly and those who care for them by channeling funds away from hospitals and institutions and to more preventative and community-based programs (Béland and Shapiro, 1994).

However, as the federal government tackled its deficit by reducing transfer payments to provinces for health, postsecondary education, and welfare, health-care provision has changed significantly in Canada. Although there are variations amongst the provinces, most have opted for caps on payments to individual physicians, along with the removal of certain products (for example, specific medications) and procedures (such as cataract surgery) from the list of insured services (Romanow, 2002).

The implications for elderly Canadians and their families are complex and as yet unclear since health care is still very much in the midst of restructuring (Chappell et al., 2003). Nevertheless, these changes in Canadian health-care policy and delivery stand to have substantial impact on Canada's elderly and those who care for them (Martin-Matthews, 1999). Several years ago Carolyn Rosenthal, a Canadian gerontologist, observed "...governments expect families to provide more care than ever to frail elderly who, increasingly, will remain in the community where...services and programs will increasingly be under-funded or absent... Such an assumption is clearly dangerous for everyone. Older people may be left without adequate sources of support. Or, women may leave paid employment, thereby damaging their own present and future economic situations" (1997: 18). These predictions have proven all too true. In a current review of the process of health reform in Canada, the researchers conclude that "the vision of health reform... has allowed for a shifting of the burden of care in old age from the public purse onto individuals and families even though this was not part of the rhetoric or the vision of health reform" (Chappell et al., 2003:432–33) Recent financial cutting to the support system to family caregiving is not a Canadian problem only, as it is pointed out in other chapters in this book, for example Pyysiäinen, in chapter 6 says that recently public care of the elderly has been drastically reduced in Finland where there was a long standing tradition of state intervention in elder care.

Research on Family Caregiving: The Focus on the Dyadic Relationship

While much of the responsibility of care of older adults has been shifted from the public purse to individuals and families, very little research has been conducted on the presence and responsibilities of family in family caregiving. To date the bulk of caregiving research has focused on the dyadic relationship between primary caregiver (most often a wife or adult daughter) and care recipient (Brody, 1995; MacRae, 1998; Peek and Zsembik, 1997). According to Pyke and Bengtson (1996: 380) "the intent of such [caregiving] research has been to describe commonalities in the caregiving process. The result has been a homogeneous portrait of caregiving provided by highly committed female individuals who are motivated by attachment and norms of filial obligation". With a focus on the primary caregiver, little research has been conducted on the contributions of other caregivers or "helpers" within the context of family caregiving. According to Marshall, Matthews and Rosenthal (1993: 39) the "protean nature of living in a family is not [currently] captured in the research literature".

The focus on primary caregiver dyads has restricted and limited our knowledge both of caregiving as a family system and of the best ways to support caregivers (Boaz and Hu, 1997; Keating, Otfinowski, Wenger, Fast and Derksen, 2003; Marshall, Matthews and Rosenthal, 1993; Peek and Zsembik, 1997). According to Keating et al. (2003) "there has been little systemic analysis of the ways in which groups of people with social or kin ties to older adults organize themselves to provide care". Similarly, Pyke and Bengtson (1996:380) assert that: "caregiving in the context of the larger family system, permitting the examination of secondary caregivers…has rarely been studied".

Keating et al. (2003) and Fast, Keating, Otfinowski and Derksen (2004) argue that a perspective on family caregiving, where caregiving is examined as a series of interconnected relationships, is the solution. Similarly, Haines and Henderson (2002: 235) contend that with Canadian health care reforms placing greater emphasis on family care of older adults it is essential to understand family systems, including other less understood ties and responsibilities, like those of helpers.

In the research literature, the activities that caregivers undertake in a variety of tasks are well known. Little is known, however, as to who, or if, anyone else participates in family caregiving through the provision of care and whether these contributions are viewed as supplementary or complimentary to the contributions of the primary caregiver (Cantor, 1979).

THE AIM OF THIS STUDY

As a step in advancing the current understanding of family caregiving our research explored the presence and contributions of "helpers" in caregiving. Our study focused on the development of a picture of helpers in family caregiving where the nature or character of help, who is delivering it and the enduring nature of help were examined.

To study helpers in caregiving, using data from The Canadian Aging Research Network's (CARNET) survey of employed Canadians, we examined two exploratory research questions:

- Who is a helper?
- How do helpers help?

In the next section the method of data collection and data analysis will be illustrated.

THE STUDY

Data for this investigation were drawn from the Canadian Aging and Research Network (CARNET) Work and Family Study. The study, conducted in 1991-1992, 1994 and 1995 involved the distribution of surveys to 9,693 employees in eight Canadian organizations. The organizations do not represent a random cross-section of Canadian employees, but efforts were made to select organizations representing different employment sectors, including government agencies, financial services, manufacturing, health services and educational institutions. Our analysis of the CARNET dataset specifically relied on longitudinal data collected from 250 individuals over 5 years at three points in time.

PROCEDURE

Personal meetings were conducted with employers to describe and explain the purpose of the study. Once an organization had agreed to participate, all employees over the age of 35 years were mailed an information letter describing the study and a questionnaire comprised of standardized scales from previous research, as well as items developed specifically for this study. Within each organization participants over the age of 35 were over-sampled to increase the likelihood of identifying people currently providing assistance to a relative aged 65 or older (Gignac, Kelloway and Gottelieb, 1996).

The questionnaire was self-administered and took approximately 35 to 45 minutes to complete. A reminder notice was then mailed one week later to all respondents who had not returned a questionnaire. Across all participating organizations, a total of 5, 496 usable surveys were returned, yielding an overall response rate of 57 per cent in the first wave of the study. Approximately 13% respondents identified themselves by providing contact information for further follow-up.

The second stage of the research, conducted two-three years after the first stage ended, involved a follow-up interview of the 13% who had provided contact information; this was done to identify individuals still involved in providing care to an older adult. This stage of the research identified 250 respondents who met the sample criteria of providing care to at least one relative and helping with one activity of daily living (feeding, bathing, dressing, etc.) or two instrumental activities of daily living (home maintenance, transportation, shopping, etc.).

The third and final wave of the CARNET study involved the distribution and completion of questionnaires to the 250 individuals: 108 men and 142 women completed the survey questionnaire. These respondent caregivers reported on various aspects of providing help to up to three elderly family members; they also provided information on caregiving contributions for up to three 'helpers". This third phase of the research was conducted in order to examine the patterns of formal service use and the frequency, type and duration of help provided by both respondent caregivers and helpers in family caregiving in a sample of employed Canadians. This third stage, once linked with the findings from Phase I and Phase II also provides detailed information at three points in time over five years on the 250 respondents and their families.

MEASURES

To develop an understanding of the contributions of helpers involved in family caregiving we relied on data from research questions that asked about the nature of help provided to both the respondent caregiver and their older relative.

In order to answer the research question 'who is a helper?' survey participants had been asked: "Are you the person most responsible for providing care to your older relative?"; "If no, then who is?"; and, "Who else has helped this relative?". These questions enabled us to determine if the respondent caregiver was the primary caregiver, and if so, who helped them and who helped their relative (the helpers). If the respondent caregiver was not the primary caregiver, these questions were used to determine who was the primary caregiver and thereby identify their helpers and as those providing help to their older relatives.

The second research question, 'how do helpers help' was answered through the analysis of responses to such questions as: "In the last six months has anyone assisted *you* in helping your elderly relatives/friend in any of the following ways: household chores, childcare, financial assistance, home/yard maintenance or repair, moral/emotional support or other?" . "Within the past six months, how often *has this person* (helper one, helper two, helper three) helped your older relative/friend with bathing, dressing, feeding, toileting or taking medication?".

The first set of questions enabled the researchers to examine patterns of indirect help to the older relative/friend (the help provided to the respondent caregiver who then in turn provided help to the older relative). The second set of questions enabled us to measure direct help (help from the respondent caregiver to the older relative and help from the helper to the older relatively).

At each phase of the study, the respondent caregivers were asked whether others helped them in the provision of care to their elderly relative(s). These data, with repeat measures at three points in time, permitted the examination of changing patterns of help received by these caregivers over time.

The linked quantitative data over time as well as written responses to long answer questions allowed for the development of descriptive vignettes. In addition to the development and analysis of vignette's the statistical software package SPSS was used to generate frequency data that contributed to a description of helpers in caregiving.

SAMPLE

Respondents in this study (N=250) averaged 43.3 years of age (SD = 7.10). Eighty four percent of respondent caregivers were married or living common-law. The sample was largely upper middle class with a median household income between $70,000 - $79,000. Eighty four percent of the sample had children (Mean = 0.8; SD = 0.85).

Caregivers reported working an average of 44.2 hours per week of paid employment (SD = 11.3). Their job positions varied with 36.7% of caregivers reporting supervisory/professional positions, 28.0% reporting clerical work, 15.9% sales/service occupations, 5.2% health-related jobs, 5.2% teaching, 3.2% manufacturing jobs, and 5.8% other occupations. In the next section we are going to present the findings from this study

ANALYSIS

A Methodological Finding

To begin to understand the role of helpers in family caregiving it is first important to understand the conceptual orientations that have dominated family caregiving research. To date much of family caregiving research has focused on understanding the caregiving dyad; research with an emphasis on caregiver stress has predominated this literature. Findings from studies on stress and burden have contributed to an understanding of relationships between stressful events and outcomes, although this research has largely been focused on the dyadic relationship between a care receiving elder and a family member who is the 'primary caregiver'. It has typically, although not exclusively, examined stress as measured at one point in time. According to George (1993: 357) family caregiving and stress research have paid "insufficient attention to social structure...and social contexts that are related to the occurrence and consequences of life events".

The Dyadic Focus

The following vignette, constructed using CARNET data from all phases of the study provides an example of the popular dyadic focus often utilized in family caregiving research.

> Mary, a 40 year-old divorced nursing attendant helps to provide care for her 74 year-old mother Lois on a very regular basis. Although Lois is in good physical and emotional health, Mary provides approximately ten hours of care each week, helping Lois to maintain an independent life in her own home. Mary assists her mother several times a week with dressing, medication, bathing, using the toilet, transportation, shopping, and household chores. Once a month, Mary helps Lois with completing forms, managing money and finances. When asked if "over the past month have you felt nervous or stressed" Mary answered " sometimes". While Mary helps her mother 10 hours a week, in addition to her 28 hour a week job, she feels that children have "a little" obligation to care for their older parents. In addition to work and caregiving responsibilities Mary also balances the needs of parenting her 14 year-old son Jeremy.

This vignette provides an example of how a number of variables specific to Mary and her mother Lois are utilized to depict family caregiving with a dyadic lens. This illustration provides some insight into what life for Mary and for Lois looks like and enables the reader to make assumptions about perceived levels of caregiver stress based on Mary's response to the stress question.

However, an alternative theoretical framework, one that expands the focus from the dyad to a network provides a rather different picture. Kahn and Antonucci's (1981) model of social networks, termed "convoys of social support" provides an example of this orientation where the idea of a single caregiver (a dyad) is rejected and instead suggest a stable network of care defined as a "convoy". In contrast to theories that characterize caregiving as a dyad, the convoy model with its attention to social ties and social relations, conceptualizes caregiving based on the constituting relationships between multiple individuals. According to Antonucci and Aykiyama (1995: 356) "individuals move through their lifetimes surrounded by people who are close and important to them and who have a critical influence on their life and well-being." The convoy model provides a framework for mapping and investigating the critical influence of individuals within networks of family caregiving. An understanding of the critical influence of network members moves the conceptualization of caregiving from a dyadic relationship to a system comprised of multiple players with multiple roles.

The Network Model

Using the same family care situation as described previously, and drawing on additional data from the CARNET surveys, the following vignette provides a network perspective.

> Mary, a 40 year-old divorced nursing attendant, provides regular care for her 74 year-old mother Lois. Lois lives independently in her own home and is in good physical and emotional health. Mary identifies herself as the primary caregiver to her mother Lois, and provides approximately ten hours of care each week. Mary assists Lois several times a week with dressing, medication, bathing, using the toilet, transportation, shopping, and household chores. Once a month, Mary helps Lois with completing forms, managing money and finances. In addition to a 14 year-old son Jeremy, Mary has two brothers, four sisters and a number of other family members many of whom also help provide assistance to both Mary and Lois. Mary receives help from her siblings with moral support as well as help with home and yard maintenance. In addition to the ten hours a week of care provided by Mary to Lois, Mary's sister and Lois's niece help to provide care for Lois. Mary's sister provides general care on a monthly basis and household care once a week. Lois's niece helps once a week with the provision of personal care, general care, household care as well as daily help with emotional support. When asked if "over the past month have you felt nervous or stressed" Mary answered " sometimes". While Mary helps her mother 10 hours a week, in addition to her 28 hour a week job, she feels that children have "a little" obligation to care for their older parents.

In this second depiction, one is able to see the complex interplay of family members with the widened network focus. In doing this, there is an improvement in understanding the richness of the caregiving experience; even the answer to the stress question has more context than in the dyadic vignette. Not only is there more information provided with a network focus, a sense of the complexity of individuals working together, to help in family caregiving is generated. A further research focus, which contributes to the advancement of understanding family caregiving beyond the dyad, involves the analysis of the passage of time.

The Passage of Time

The convoy model developed by Kahn and Antonucci, in addition to providing a network framework for understanding family caregiving, also introduces the importance of the passage of time or lifecourse of family caregiving. Kahn and Antonucci (1981) metaphorically describe an individual's movement through the life cycle as being "surrounded by a set of other people to whom he or she is related by the giving or receiving of social support" (Kahn and Antonucci, 1981: 393). According to Elder (1998) the convoy model reflects the notion of linked lives, or what Burton (1996: 200) describes as "interlocking pathways that individuals and families follow through an age-differentiated life span". The convoy model of support implicates both the continuous and reciprocal nature of exchanges within the context of a family caregiving relationship over time (Antonucci, 1990). The third vignette, based on additional data from the same CARNET data set and the same family as previously described, widens the research lens one step further to include the passage of time.

> When interviewed in 1990, Mary, a 40 year-old divorced nursing attendant and mother of 14 year-old Jeremy, provided care for her 74 year-old mother Lois on a very regular basis. Although Lois was in good physical and emotional health, Mary provided approximately ten hours of care each week, helping Lois to maintain an independent life in her own home. Mary assisted Lois several times a week with dressing, medication, bathing, using the toilet, transportation, shopping, and household chores. Once a month, Mary helped Lois with completing forms, managing money and finances. When asked if "over the past month have you felt nervous or stressed" Mary answered sometimes. In addition to the ten hours a week of care provided by Mary to Lois, Mary's sister and Lois's niece helped to provide care for Lois. Mary's sister provided general care on a monthly basis and household care once a week. Lois's niece helped once a week with the provision of personal care, general care, household care as well as daily help with emotional support. In 1995, when interviewed Mary's mother Lois had died one year earlier, but indicated that the family continued to provide support in the same manner until her death with support from Homecare. However, Mary did indicate that over time, the stress of caregiving took its toll on the entire family network. Mary stated in her 1995 interview: "while providing care for my mother before she died a year ago the assistance we received from the Home care nurses was exceptional. But until after Mom died I didn't realize how continually stressed I was nor how it had affected my son and my brothers' and sisters' families. I believe the caregivers need both emotional and in some cases financial assistance. I was asked to leave my new job as a Secretary because of stress and lost time when Mom was dying...it's amazing how well you think you're coping until the pressure is over and you realize you were just 'making it'."

In this third illustration, a widening of the research lens to include multiple family members and changing circumstances over time provides a more dynamic portrayal of family caregiving. Mary enhances the understanding of this family's experience of stress and burden through retrospective observations with respect to the entire family's level of stress.

The presentation of these three vignettes illustrates that there is much to be learned about family caregiving beyond the dyad. With a widening of the research lens in mind, we know turn to an analysis of the research questions of who is a helper, how helpers help and the enduring nature of help.

HELPERS IN FAMILY CAREGIVING

Who is a Helper?

Our first research question, 'who is a helper?' is a more complex question that it appears. The question must be tackled in two steps, first making a determination on who is the primary caregiver, and then who the helper(s) are; for example in the case of the dataset used in this analysis, the respondent caregiver is not necessarily the primary caregiver.

Respondents in this study were an average age of 43 years (sd 7.1) and the majority (85%) indicated having at least one child and another (15%) indicated having grandchildren. As shown in Table One, of the 250 individuals surveyed 54% indicated being the primary caregiver, while 46% indicated not being the primary caregiver (but were the respondent caregiver). The primary/respondent caregivers (primary caregivers) differed from the respondent/not primary caregivers (secondary caregivers) in the frequency distribution of reporting one helper, two helpers, or three helpers. In the case of the primary caregiver, where 82% indicated receiving help, the frequency of having one helper was 54%, two helpers 26% and three helpers 20%. In the secondary caregiver group, where 92% indicated having help, the frequency of having one helper was 30%, two helpers 32% and three helpers 38%. In both the primary caregiver category and the secondary caregiver category mothers were the person most often being cared for, while the identification of helpers varied.

Primary caregivers most often reported sisters as being their number one helper, while secondary caregivers most often reported their spouse as their number one helper. Of notable difference between the two, a higher percentage of primary caregivers were women while a higher percentage of secondary caregivers indicated being men. This points heavily to the gendered nature of family caregiving where women are most often primary caregivers, and in this study, if they are not the primary caregiver they are identified as being the number one secondary caregiver. Marital status also differed slightly between groups with secondary caregivers reporting being married more frequently than primary caregivers.

Primary caregivers, as shown Table One, differ from secondary caregivers in both their personal characteristics and in the type of assistance they extend to their older family members. The following vignette, which describes the care situation of another participant caregiver in the CARNET studies, gives a descriptive example of why it is important to make this distinction when conducting caregiving research as well as illustrating the richness of information obtained in doing so.

> Patricia, an accountant, is a 42 year-old divorced mother to twelve year-old Amy, does not consider herself as being the "most" responsible for the care of her aging parents (Maureen and Ted). Her sister Andrea is the primary support person. Maureen and Ted are in overall good physical and emotional health and live in their own apartment. Patricia does not live in the same community as her parents. Patricia assists from a distance with emotional and moral support, travelling to the town where her parents live when required. Patricia provides support whenever she can to her one sister (Andrea) who lives in the same city as Maureen and Ted. Patricia helps mostly with emotional support and financial support. Andrea, the primary caregiver, helps Maureen and Ted weekly with personal care, and financial support as well as daily assistance with emotional support. Maureen and Ted also receive help from Laurie (Patricia's other sister) and Candace (Patricia's cousin). Laurie helps weekly with general care, household care, emotional support and financial support. Candace on a monthly basis helps with personal care, household care as well as weekly assistance with emotional support. When asked about her sister's caregiving responsibilities, Patricia states the following: "for the primary support person, my sister in this case [Andrea], the time commitment is phenomenal. Also her patience and understanding has been challenged. Her work background has saved hours of research time but a personal cost to her and her family. She has put in untold hours of emotional support…The other of us "girls" live out of town but

have spent time reassuring parents and sister that we support all the decisions and directions suggested. Our goals are all the same, to have Mom and Dad settled and as happy and stress free as possible".

Table 1. Respondent Caregiver Characteristics

	Respondent Caregiver Primary Caregiver N=135		Respondent Caregiver Not Primary Caregiver N=114	
	N	%	N	%
Gender				
Male	51	37.8	57	49.6
Female	84	62.2	58	50.4
Marital Status				
Married	107	79.9	98	85.2
Common-law	9	6.7	3	2.6
Separated	4	3.0	4	3.5
Divorced	8	6.0	3	2.6
Widowed	0	0	2	1.7
Single/Never Married	6	4.5	5	4.3
Only Person Providing Help*				
No	103	81.7	96	92.3
Yes	23	18.3	8	7.7
Number of Helpers*				
One	56	54.0	29	30.0
Two	27	26.0	31	32.0
Three	21	20.0	36	38.0
Identification of Helper One**				
Respondents Spouse	23	22.1	31	32.3
Respondents Sister	30	28.8	21	21.9
Respondents Brother	22	21.2	16	16.7
Relatives Spouse	6	5.8	5	5.2
Identification of Helper Two**				
Respondents Spouse	3	6.3	5	7.5
Respondents Sister	5	10.4	15	22.4
Respondents Brother	12	25.0	8	11.9
Respondents Sister-in-law	6	12.5	15	22.4
Identification of Helper Three**				
Respondents Spouse	3	14.3	5	13.9
Respondents Sister	3	14.3	3	8.3
Respondents Brother	3	14.3	7	19.4
Respondents Brother-in-law	2	9.5	5	13.9
Identification of Person Receiving Most Care				
Spouse				
Mother	3	2.2	0	0
Father	79	58.5	55	49.1
Mother-in-law	15	11.1	7	6.3
Father-in-law	12	8.9	21	18.8
Grandmother/Grandfather	1	0.7	3	2.7
Aunt/Uncle	4	2.9	7	6.3
Parents/Parents-in-law	4	3.0	9	8.1
Friend/Neighbour	13	9.6	6	5.4
Other Family	3	2.2	3	2.7
	1	0.7	1	0.9

*In this table "help" is the assistance given directly to the older person receiving care.

** Top four listed.

By examining a case where the respondent caregiver is not the primary caregiver (rather a secondary caregiver), but by also including the primary caregiver in the respondent's answers (as in this vignette), we get a much fuller picture of what is actually happening as compared to limiting ourselves to studying the dyadic relationship between solely the respondent caregiver and older adult(s). If we had considered only the respondent caregiver, it would have appeared like little was happening in the context of this family caregiving situation, clearly this is not the case.

In this vignette we see the unique perspective of a family member who is not a primary caregiver reporting on the activities of other family members even though this family member is not the individual 'most responsible' for caregiving. This approach contrasts with most studies on caregiving that focus solely on primary caregiver responses. This vignette gives the perspective of helper or secondary caregivers, those participants in family caregiving networks who rarely have a 'voice' in caregiving research.

The Helpers' Caring Tasks

Our second question, 'how do helpers help?' is also a multi-faceted research question. To determine the ways in which 'helpers' help, it is essential to first consider whether 'help' or tasks are provided directly (help to the older family member) or indirectly (by way of help given to the primary caregiver who then assists the older adult). For example, do helpers participate in providing instrumental support or in providing affective relations to the primary caregiver who then in turn performed the bulk of instrumental tasks? As another component of understanding how helpers help we also felt it important to note the 'character of caregiving relationship exchange'. According to Abel and Nelson (1990:4) the character or nature of a caregiving exchange can encompass "instrumental tasks and/or affective relations".

Table 2. Frequency of Type of Help Provided to Respondent Caregivers From "Helper" Caregivers

Type of Help Provided to Respondent Caregiver from Helper Caregiver	Primary Caregiver N=135		Secondary Caregiver N=114	
	N	%	N	%
Household Chores	37	44.6	34	48.6
Childcare	1	1.2	3	4.3
Financial Assistance	5	6.0	11	15.7
Home-Yard Maintenance	36	43.4	31	44.3
Moral Support	62	74.7	52	74.3
Other: e.g., transportation, running errands, meal preparation, socializing.	14	16.9	15	21.4

Table Two highlights the responsibilities of helpers in caregiving to those who are primary caregivers and those who are secondary caregivers. Moral support (75%), household chores (45%) and home-yard maintenance (43%) are the types of help most often provided to primary caregivers. Similarly, moral support (74%), household chores (49%) and home-yard maintenance (44%) are the types of help most often provided to secondary caregivers. Results show that help to the respondent caregiver (primary or secondary) is predominantly affective in nature.

Table Three documents help given to the older adult by helper one, helper two and helper three. It is shown that helper one, two and three most often help with general care, emotional support, followed by household care. The type of help given by helpers to the older adult is instrumental in nature followed by affective assistance. The results in Table three also illustrates that those who report having three helpers have an increase in assistance with emotional support (affective support). In this way help from helpers both supplements and compliments care given by primary caregivers.

Table 3. Frequency and Type of Help Provided By"Helper" Caregivers to Older Relative/Friend

Help Provided	Helper #1 N=199		Helper #2 N=113		Helper #3 N=56	
	N	%	N	%	N	%
Personal Care	76	38.2	43	38.1	18	32.1
General Care*	174	87.4	94	83.9	43	76.8
Household Care	143	72.6	77	68.7	30	53.6
Emotional Support	172	87.3	90	80.2	50	90.9
Financial Support	100	50.8	43	38.4	17	30.4

* General Care is defined as: transportation, shopping and/or errands.

To illustrate this point, the following vignette, taken from verbatim and survey data from the third stage of the CARNET studies reflects the complexity of the social structure of family caregiving, the nature of help provided (affective/instrumental) and the balance of both direct and indirect help.

> Maria is an elementary school teacher, 40 years old, married and with two children ages six and three. Both her parents are still living. She has one brother and one sister. She provides help/care to her widowed mother-in-law, Gloria age 75, who lives in her own home/apartment. Her mother-in-law's physical health is described as excellent, but her emotional health as "fair". Instrumental activities performed by Maria include help with transportation and meal preparation (three years ago Maria was helping weekly with meal preparation, transportation, shopping and running errands, but now she helps two to three times a week with the same tasks as well as helping several times a week with emotional support). Although Maria provides more help than does anyone else to her mother-in-law, others also provide assistance to both Gloria and to Maria. Maria receives help with household chores and also moral support from her husband Willem and friends. This assistance helps Maria in that it "frees her up" to provide assistance/care to Gloria. Gloria receives help from Maria's husband Willem, Maria's sister-in-law Carrie, and Gloria's friend Gertrude. While

> Maria is the primary caregiver for her mother-in-law Gloria she is also concerned about the well-being and future of her own parents who are in there 80's and live outside Canada. Maria states: "I am just beginning to undertake arranging for my parents to come to Canada if and when necessary for health reasons. This has taken a fair bit of time already, and I've made a little headway. Having one "elder" in town takes time, but when your own parents are far away, it raises many issues and problems that are not easy to solve. I'm not sure what will happen if either of my parents becomes seriously ill or hospitalized. I think my sister and I will have to take time off work and leave our families to take care of them...work and family responsibilities obviously come into the picture when making the difficult decisions that lay ahead".

This vignette describes a family caregiving scenario with a relatively low level of caregiving need and responsibility. However, even within the context of this rather straightforward family caregiving scenario the complexity of direct and indirect care is clearly demonstrated. Maria while balancing the needs of a young family helps to sustain her mother-in-law living on her own with both direct and indirect help. The vignette, with attention to describing indirect/direct care and affective/instrumental support highlights both the differentiation and the intertwining of family caregiving responsibilities.

The Longitudinal Perspective

An interesting component of this vignette, related to the significance of a widened focus in studying family caregiving, is the reference to the passage of time. In this vignette, Maria has concerns regarding the balance of help, as articulated in her verbatim account of current and anticipated care roles. She is concerned that the potential and probable changing needs her own parents will require ongoing adjustment and re-organization of work and family lives. This raises an additional perspective on the family: that while research captures a current perspective on their caregiving situation, it may be, and is likely, anticipated to change. This raises an important aspect of family caregiving – it is dynamic. The further broadening of caregiving research from a dyadic focus, to a network focus, to a network that includes reference or attention to the passage of time, serves to improve our understanding of family caregiving.

Table 4. Help Received Over Time by Respondent Caregiver

	Help Received		No Help Received	
	N	%	N	%
Time One	96	56.1	75	43.9
Time Two	105	42.0	145	58.0
Time Three	199	86.5	31	13.5

Table Four summarizes, at three points in time over five years (Phase I, Phase II, Phase III), the frequency of the respondent caregiver receiving help from a helper for the care of the older relative to whom they provide the most care (NB. The data is for same older relative at all three points in time). Results show that the frequency of reporting a helper increases from Phase I to Phase III with a slight dip at Phase II. Approximately 56% of respondents indicate receiving help in Phase I, 42.0% at Phase II and 86.5% in Phase III. This last table points to the enduring nature of help within family caregiving.

DISCUSSION

When research on family caregiving is broadened to include multiple individuals with varied responsibilities, as in our study of 'helpers', we see family caregiving as a complex network of individuals. This 'illumination of complexity' has two main effects. First, it allows us to begin to describe and examine what Marshall, Matthews and Rosenthal (1993: 39) call the "protean nature of living in a family". The "protean nature" being the messiness, complexity and intricacies that are characteristic of family life and dynamics that can't necessarily be summarized by looking at the interactions between two individuals. Second, it enables us to begin to ask and answer new questions about family caregiving beyond caregiving dyads. For example, in our study of helpers, with a widened focus, we can begin to tease out some of the dimensions of helping and caregiving, such as the distinction between respondent caregivers and primary caregivers and the intersection(s) with direct and indirect help.

In addition to considering the perspectives of secondary caregivers and primary caregivers, we focused on the intersection of these two groups in terms of their receipt of direct and indirect assistance in caregiving. Direct assistance was conceptualized as being help or care given directly to the older person receiving care. Indirect assistance was the help given to the respondent caregiver (whether the primary caregiver or secondary caregiver). The nature or type of assistance given was also considered. As shown in our results, direct and indirect help to the caregiver and help to the older adult are quite different. Respondent caregivers most often receive assistance in the form of moral support and aid with household chores while 'helpers' most often assist their older relative/friend with transportation, shopping and errands, followed by emotional support. Indirect help is most often affective in nature while direct helps tend to be instrumental. While some helpers provide instrumental support to the respondent caregiver it is less frequent than the affective help. Helpers in caregiving emotionally support caregivers offering encouragement and validation, which in turn enables or supports the provision of care to the older relative. 'Help' therefore both compliments and supplements care to the respondent caregiver and to the older relative.

As shown in our results, in Phase III a more respondents indicate having a helper than in Phase I or Phase II. As family caregiving extends through time a number of possible and probable changes occur that serve to increase the likelihood of helpers being involved, some of which might include: changing health status of the older relative, changing work/family responsibilities of the respondent caregiver, and/or increased competency and delegation of family responsibilities by the respondent caregiver.

Conclusion

Our expanded focus on helpers and respondent caregivers who are not primary caregivers illustrates the complex and dynamic nature of family's involved in family caregiving. According to Fast et al. (2004: 17) "research that uses the care network as the unit of analysis will provide a more comprehensive understanding of the capacity and needs of the family/friend sector".

Our research attempted to explore the complex interplay of responsibilities and relationships within the family caregiving context with attendant emphasis on the presence of 'helpers' in family caregiving. A comprehensive understanding of the families involved in family caregiving provides the foundation for improvements in academic gerontological caregiving research and education. Gottlieb (1992: 307) contends that a better understanding of caregiving serves to contribute to the "ways in which we conceive and measure social support". In the Canadian context, where we are seeking to gain an enhanced understanding of the issues facing families as our population ages and health care is restructured, a heightened awareness of the complexity of family caregiving will contribute to improved methods of operationalizing and measuring caregiving as a research concept. In the end, these refinements have the potential to led to improvements in service, program, policy and research for caregivers, care recipients and their families (Guberman and Maheu, 2002; Marshall, Matthews, and Rosenthal, 1993; Martin-Matthews and Campbell, 1995; Peek and Zsembik, 1997).

Recommendations For Future Research

Considerations for future research on family caregiving networks will benefit from including:

- The influence of the passage or element of time on caregiving networks. Specifically, how networks fluctuate and change over time with respect to the responsibilities and relationships between primary caregivers, helpers and the older person(s) receiving care.
- The perspective(s) of multiple family members within the same family caregiving network. The inclusion of multiple perspectives will assist in the development of an understanding of family caregiving, one that represents multiple voices and perspectives on the provision of care within the same family. Ultimately these developments will serve to influence research and policy frameworks where the complexity and multiplicity of family caregiving responsibilities and relationships beyond the caregiver/care recipient dyad are taken into consideration.

REFERENCES

Abel, E. K. and Nelson, M. K. (1990). Circle of care: An introductory essay. In Abel, E. K. and Nelson, M. K. (Eds.), *Circles of Care: Work and Identity in Women's Lives*, (4 – 34). New York: State University of New York Press.

Antonucci, T. C. (1990). Social supports and social relationships. In R. H. Binstock and L. K. George (Eds.), *Handbook of Aging and the Social Sciences, 3rd Edition*, (205-227). San Diego: Academic Press.

Antonucci T. C., and Akiyama, H. (1995). Convoys of social relations: Family and friendships within a life span context. In Bleiszner, R. and Bedford, V. H. (Eds.), *Handbook of Aging and the Family*, (355-371). Westport: Greenwood Press.

Béland, F. and E. Shapiro. 1994. "Ten Provinces in Search of a Long Term Care Policy." In V. W. Marshall and B. D. McPherson, eds., *Aging: Canadian Perspectives.* Peterborough, (pp. 245-267). Ontario: Broadview.

Boaz, R. F. and Hu, J. (1997). Determining the amount of help used by disabled elderly persons at home: The role of coping resources. *Journal of Gerontology: Social Sciences* 52B(6), S317 – S324.

Brody, E. M. (1995). Prospects for family caregiving. In Kane, R., and Penrod, J. D. (Eds.), *Family caregiving in an aging society*, (pp. 15 - 28). Thousand Oaks: Sage Publications.

Burton, L. (1996). Age norms, the timing of family role transitions, and intergenerational caregiving among aging African American women. *The* Gerontologist, 36 (2), 199- 208.

Cantor, M. H. (1979). Neighbors and friends. *Research on Aging*, 1(4), 434 – 463.

Chappell, N.L., E. M. Gee, L. McDonald and M. Stones (eds.). 2003. *Aging in Contemporary Canada.* Toronto: Prentice Hall.

Elder, G. H. Jr. (1998). The life course as developmental theory. *Child Development*, 69, 1 – 12.

Fast, J., Keating, N., Otfinowski, P. and Derksen, L. (2004). Characteristics of family/friend care networks of frail seniors. *Canadian Journal on Aging*, 23(1) 5 – 19.

Gee, Ellen M. (1990). Demographic Change and Intergenerational Relations in Canadian Families: Findings and Social Policy Implications. *Canadian Public Policy,* 16: 191–99.

George, L. K. (1993). Sociological perspectives on life transitions. *Annual Review of Sociology*, 19, 353 – 373.

Gignac, M., Kelloway, K. E., and Gottlieb, B. H. (1996). The impact of caregiving on employment: a mediational model of work-family conflict. *Canadian Journal on Aging*, 15(4), 525 – 542.

Gottlieb, B. H. (1992). Social support: A relationship process, not a commodity. *Canadian Journal on Aging*, 11(4), 306 – 310.

Guberman, N. and Maheu, P. (2002). Conceptions of family caregivers: Implications for professional practice. *Canadian Journal on Aging*, 21(1), 27 – 37.

Haines, V. A. and Henderson, L. J. (2002). Targeting social support: A network assessment of the Convoy Model of Social Support. *Canadian Journal on Aging*, 21(2), 243 – 256.

Kahn, R. L. and Antonucci, T. C. (1981). Convoys of social support: a life-course approach. In March, J. G., Kiesler, S. B., Morgan, J. N., and Oppenheimer, V. K. (Eds.), *Aging: Social Change*, (pp. 383 – 405). New York: Academic Press.

Keating, N. C., Otfinowski, P., Wenger, C., Fast, J. E. and Derksen, L. (2003). Understanding the caring capacity of informal networks of frail seniors: A case for care networks. *Ageing and Society*, 23, 115-127.

MacRae, H. (1998). Managing feelings: caregiving as emotion work. *Research on Aging*, 20(1), 137- 160.

Marshall, V. W., Matthews, S. H., Rosenthal, C. J. (1993). Elusiveness of family life: a challenge for the sociology of aging. In Maddox G. L., and Powell Lawton M. (Eds.). *Annual Review of Gerontology and Geriatrics: Focus on Kinship, Aging, and Social Change*, (pp. 39 – 72). New York: Springer.

Martin-Matthews, A. (1999). "Widowhood: Dominant renditions, changing demography and variable meaning". In S. M. Neysmith (ed.), *Critical Issues for Future Social Work Practice with Aging Persons*, (pp. 27 – 69). New York: Columbia University Press.

Martin-Matthews, A. (2000). Intergenerational caregiving: how apocalyptic and dominant demographies frame the questions and shape the answers. In Gee, E. and Guttman (Eds). *The Overselling Population of Aging: Apocalyptic Demography, Intergenerational Challenges, and Social Policy*, (pp.64 – 79). Don Mills: Oxford University Press.

Martin-Matthews, A. and Campbell, L. D. (1995). Gender roles, employment and informal care. In Arber, S. and Ginn, J. (Eds). *Connecting Gender and Ageing: A Sociological Approach*, (pp. 129-144). Buckingham: Open University Press.

Matthews, S. (2002). *Sisters and Brothers/Daughters and Sons: Meeting the Needs of Old Parents*. Bloomington: Unlimited Publishing.

Peek, C. W. and Zsembik, B.A. (1997). The changing caregiving networks of older adults. *Research on Aging*, 19(3), 333 – 362.

Pyke, K. D. and Bengtson, V. L. (1996). Caring more or less: Individualistic and collectivist systems. *Journal of Marriage and Family*, 58(2), 379 – 383.

Romanow, R. (2002). *Building on Values: The Future of Health Care in Canada*. Government of Canada. <http://finalreport.healthcarecommission.ca/ >

Rosenthal, C. (1997). "Family Care in Canada in the Context of Social and Demographic Change." *Ageing International,* 24/1: 13–31.

Statistics Canada. (1997). Measuring the Age of Retirement. *The Daily,* June 6. *http://www.statcan.ca/Daily/English/970611/d970611.htm#ART1*

Statistics Canada. (2003). Population by sex and age group. <http://www.statcan.ca/ english/Pgdb/demo31d.htm>

In: Family Caregiving for Older Disabled People
Editor: Isabella Paoletti, pp. 103-126
ISBN 1-59454-808-0

Chapter 6

NEGOTIATIONS AND ROOM FOR MANOEUVRE IN CARING FOR AN ELDERLY PARENT

Jaana Pyysiäinen
University of Helsinki,
Helsinki, Finland

INTRODUCTION

The general aim of the study was to examine how the commitments of caring for an elderly parent come into being and develop. Caring was thus seen as a process, which forms in the course of time as the condition of the elderly parent and the situations in the life of the carer change. The focus of the study was on *how* things happen in the care arrangement, not *what* happens. The latter has been the more customary way to treat the subject of caring for an elderly relative.

The position of the daughter who cares for her elderly parent could be best described with the concept of *room for maneuver*. The daughter is neither totally free to choose her position in the care arrangement, nor is she completely restricted by the pressures from her social environment. The commitments of caring are created by individuals, but they tend to become a part of the social structure in the sense that they restrict and facilitate future decisions and action. The individual has thus a certain degree of freedom to define his or her position in the care arrangement. This limited freedom is what is meant here with the concept of room for manoeuvre. This concept is used by Janet Finch and Jennifer Mason (1993) in the same sense of limited freedom as they discuss negotiations about different kinds of family commitments. However they use the concept only in passing. The concept of room for manoeuvre is the focus of this study as it seems to characterize realistically the position of the daughter who cares for her elderly parent. The main question centres on how much room for manoeuvre the daughter has within the care arrangement.

The limited freedom – or room for maneuver – to choose ones position in the care arrangement is what makes daughters (in some cases also sons) such an interesting group among the carers of an elderly person. The context of this study is Finland. In Finland children are the second largest group of carers of an elderly person right after spouses (Vaarama, Hakkarainen, Voutilainen and Päivärinta, 2000). In the Finnish context it has been noted that spouses have no freedom of choice when the need for care of a husband or a wife arises (Gothóni, 1991). The spouse is an evident carer whereas children should have at least a hypothetical possibility to decide whether or not to become a carer.

I will begin by introducing some points that have been brought out by previous studies that have considered the caring relationship between the elderly parent and their children (mostly the daughters), but before that a few words about the Finnish context of the care for the elderly.

In Finland it has been customary to see the society as being responsible for the care of the elderly (e.g. Koskela, Kunnas, Salanko-Vuorela, Vaarama, Vanamo, 1991). In the Finnish culture, there has been an emphasis on elderly people maintaining their own independence from their adult children. Studies looking at the attitudes of older people towards their care show that the elderly do not want to be a burden to their family; instead they expect to receive care at the public expense.

During the 1990s, public care of the elderly in Finland has been drastically reduced. The aim was to reduce specifically the institutional care and to increase the professional, non-institutional care such as home help and district nursing. There are now fewer elderly people in institutional care, but the elderly do not receive any more professional care to their homes. In fact, the relative coverage of the professional home-care (home help and district nursing) for the elderly was also reduced by more than 40% from 1988 to 1998 (Vaarama, Hakkarainen, Voutilainen and Päivärinta, 2000). This means that during the last fifteen years the responsibility for the care of the elderly in Finland has shifted more and more from social institutions to the relatives. Overall, relatives now provide approximately 70% of the elderly care (Vaarama and Kautto, 1998).

Factors Affecting the Choice of Becoming a Carer

In most literature concerning family caregiving, affection and reciprocity have been seen as important and often also self-evident factors that define the caring relationship between family members (Qureshi and Walker, 1989). People are willing to become carers for persons with whom they have become close in a long-lasting relationship. Factors that affect the willingness to help are gratitude, love, sense of duty, responsibility and reciprocity (Gothóni, 1991). According to Hazel Qureshi and Alan Walker (1989), however, factors like affection, responsibility and reciprocity are not necessarily involved in a caring relationship between a daughter (or son) and her elderly parent. In their data they also encountered children whose relationship to the elderly parent they cared for had always been one-sided or even hostile. They may have experienced violence or molestation in their childhood. These children could not be seen as caring for their elderly parents because of a feeling of owing something to the parent, nor were they motivated by affection towards the parent. (See Baillie, in chapter 7 for an extended discussion of the issue of caregiving when relationships are poor.)

In a large, quantitative Finnish study about family caregiving for the elderly (Gothóni, 1991) many of the respondents could not specify which factors had made them become carers. A typical answer was that "the responsibility of caring has fallen on me quite naturally". The carers announced that their motive for caring was simply the fact that their relative needed help. Also Attias-Donfut and Wolff (2000) state that the logic of family relationships is simple: the one who needs help also receives it. In the study of Qureshi and Walker (1989) the respondents regarded the caring for an elderly relative as natural. The researchers explain the naturalness by normative expectations towards relatives. According to them there is a normative hierarchy about the most suitable carer for an elderly family member. The hierarchy is: spouse, relative living in the same household, daughter, daughter-in-law, son, other relative or neighbour. These normative expectations work via outside pressure and also an inner feeling of guilt if one cannot fulfill these expectations.

In many cases the elderly do not wish to fall back on their family. If that cannot be avoided then the elderly expect to receive help from their children (especially from the daughters) (Qureshi and Walker, 1989; Finch and Mason, 2000). The classic remark by Peter Townsend (1957) states that "intimacy at a distance" is the ideal form of the relationship between the elderly parent and the adult children. The intimacy of a caring relationship could be experienced as a burden. The elderly parent wishes usually to maintain some independence. The carer may experience the intimacy as binding because being a carer for a family member means that the carer must be constantly available for the person in need of care (Gothóni, 1991).

A few studies have considered the decisive factors in selecting which one of the children should become the carer for the elderly parent. Three factors rise clearly above others: sex, distance and work. Caring is considered to be suitable and natural for women (Qureshi and Walker, 1989; Graham, 1983). The elderly parents themselves place more expectations about help and care on their daughters than their sons (Gothóni, 1991; Qureshi and Walker, 1989). Lorenz-Meyer and Grotheer (2000) state that the existence of a sister reduced the pressure of their young male interviewees to become a carer for their elderly parents. Women feel more often than men that they do not have a choice when it comes to caring for an elderly parent (Gothóni, 1991).

In a British study (Qureshi, 1996) daughters were found to become carers for a family member less frequently if they were also employed. Still, if a woman has a job her employment is not as easily acknowledged as a legitimate excuse for not caring as it would be for a man (Finch and Mason, 2000). The British interviewees also thought that it was easier for a woman to leave her job to become a carer than for a man (Qureshi and Walker, 1989). It seems that work and employment should be considered while thinking about who is the most suitable carer for an elderly parent. However for a woman her employment does not get the same significance in these considerations as for a man.

Also the geographical distance between the possible carer and the person in need of care has been seen to affect the choice of a carer (e.g. Gothóni 1991). Qureshi and Walker (1989) draw the line between those family members who live within the distance of a two hours drive and those who live further. The latter do not participate in the caring. But among the first group the distance does not explain the differences in the participation of the caring. In some cases the caring can affect the distance and not the other way around. A daughter may want to move nearer her elderly parent to be able to take care of him or her.

By representing the different factors affecting the choice of becoming a carer you get the picture of caring as some kind of a rational decision. It seems that family members contemplate together the different normative and material factors and decide then who should be the carer. However a typical experience of becoming a carer could not be seen as a conscious decision. Becoming a carer does not necessarily involve any reflections on the matter beforehand. With the help of the normative and material factors (such as sex and distance) it is possible to describe who the carers are as a large group. But knowing these factors does not facilitate answering the question *how* someone becomes a carer.

The family responsibility theory of Janet Finch and Jennifer Mason (1993) offers a useful way of examining the *process* of becoming a carer for an elderly parent. They approach the subject of family responsibilities from an interaction perspective, which makes it possible to put the experiences of caring into context and to make explicit the processes involved in becoming a carer. These two important factors – context and process – are often missing in the study of caring for an elderly family member. As I wished to examine realistically and accurately the process of becoming a carer and the experience of the room for manoeuvre of a daughter in the care arrangement, the theory of Finch and Mason suited my goals better than other approaches.

The theory of Finch and Mason will be represented here in broad outline as it was used as a background theory for analysing the data. The results of their study were compared with the results of the study represented here (Pyysiäinen, 2003). After reviewing the theory I will continue to discuss how the study was constructed and how the interviews were classified based on the theory of Finch and Mason. The rest of this chapter will be dedicated to the representation of the analysis of the data and the most important results of the study.

NEGOTIATING CARING COMMITMENTS: A THEORETICAL APPROACH

According to Finch and Mason, commitments within the family, such as caring for an elderly parent, are negotiated within its members over time. Family obligations cannot be explained merely as following normative rules (e.g. "a daughter is best suitable for taking care of her elderly mother"). The approach claims that purely material matters or norms do not explain the commitments between family members. Their effect is indirect and happens only through negotiations. Through analyzing extensive qualitative data, Finch and Mason found that there was no consensus among the interviewees on substantive matters concerning family responsibilities, but there was a consensus about procedural matters. In other words, the interviewees did not agree on *what* certain members of the family (daughter, son, daughter-in-law etc.) should do when a family member is in need of help; however, they did agree on *how* to settle what should be done. There were certain rules that the family members should obey while negotiating about the family responsibilities.

With the concept of negotiations Finch and Mason mean the processes of how the individual works out with others and which form his or her action will take. The concept of negotiation accepts that the individual has a certain freedom to define his or her action. But the freedom in question is limited by other factors. For Finch and Mason, the concept of negotiation contains both explicit and implicit negotiations. They claim that when it comes to family responsibilities, it is not enough to consider the explicit negotiations. Only a small amount of family responsibilities gets negotiated in the open; therefore, implicit and unspoken negotiations should also be considered while examining how the commitments to other family members form and develop.

Explicit negotiations are open discussions which may take place when a need for help arises in the family or is likely to develop in the near future. On the other hand, implicit negotiations take place when the family members involved work out who will be held responsible for a certain duty without actual formal negotiations taking place. Implicit negotiations happen in the course of time, gradually, and partly unnoticed. Open discussions are not always necessary, because as a consequence of implicit negotiations it might be clear to everyone which family member should help when a certain need arises. Accumulation is an essential trait for family commitments.

There is a specific kind of reciprocity which defines the commitments between the family members. The aim is to achieve a *proper balance* between giving and receiving. The services given have not only a material but also a symbolic meaning. It is important to acknowledge the fact that the receiver may come to feel herself dependent on the giver. Thus the help and the services should be arranged in a way that the receiver will not feel that he or she "becomes beholden to" the giver.

A moral dimension can always be seen in the background while people are negotiating – explicitly or implicitly – about the actual services provided for their family members. People are constructed as moral beings through the processes of give and take. Members of the family have created certain reputations during their common past. From the point of view of the individual, this reputation is a moral identity. The moral identities offer guidance in deciding which commitments one should accept. Different family members have accepted a different amount of family commitments during their common history. For example, an eldest daughter has taken care or her younger siblings already as a child: in this way, her family members have become accustomed to regarding her as a caring person.

From the point of view of the individual, at the core of the commitment there lies a consideration that withdrawal from the developing commitment might be too expensive in terms of the damage to the moral identity and in relation to the loss to his or her reputation within the family. Thus, a person may be willing to accept even a time-consuming commitment, such as caring for an elderly parent, because refusing would pose a threat to his or her moral identity. Not only is the moral identity of the giver at stake in the negotiations on family commitments, also the recipient of the favours has to protect his or her moral identity.

The theory of Finch and Mason does not claim that one has to act in accordance with his or her moral identity at all times. There remains a possibility for the individual to question the commitment that has been appointed to her on account of her reputation. But essentially, it is not necessary to have an open discussion every time a need arises within a family. Reputations in a family are absolutely important as a structure on which the negotiations are based. So, a reputation within a family is a result of the negotiations (explicit or implicit) of the past and a foundation for the negotiations of the future.

Using the theory of Finch and Mason as a model, I concentrated my study on the interactions between the parties involved in the care arrangement of the elderly parent. I examined the explicit and implicit negotiations of the care arrangement within the family. On the basis of these negotiations, I have tried to discover how much room for manoeuvre a daughter taking care of her elderly parent actually has. In the next section I present the method of data collection and data analysis.

How The Study Was Constructed

This study was a sub-project of a large quantitative study carried out by the Finnish National Research and Development Centre for Welfare and Health (STAKES), which examined the discharge of elderly people from the hospital into a home care arrangement (for details see Perälä, Rissanen, Grönroos, Hammar, Pöyry and Teperi, 2003). The study contained questionnaire data from the relatives of the elderly persons, with questions on care of the elderly person while in hospital and at home, and on their own participation in the homecare arrangement.

For the purposes of my study, the part consisting of the responses of daughters and sons was separated from the other data. With this data, a brief quantitative analysis was constructed before carrying out the qualitative part, that is the main part of the study. For the purposes of this chapter it will be sufficient to mention, from the results of the quantitative analysis, that carers of an elderly person were shown to be typically daughters who live near their parents. The interviewees were chosen from among the respondents on the basis that the interviewees were all daughters who lived near their elderly parent, and helped him or her frequently (at least once a week). In the data there were many daughters who filled these criteria. Finally the interviewees were chosen based on practical matters: the interviewees should not live further away than a three-hour drive from the interviewer. Two or three interviewees were always chosen from the same locality so that it would be possible to conduct two interviews on the same day.

Letters were sent to 12 chosen daughters telling them that they had the opportunity to participate in an interview-based study exploring their experiences of caring for an elderly parent. Seven of the chosen people agreed to be interviewed. A semi-structured interview seemed to best suit the purposes of the study. The aim was to let the interviewees guide the progress of the interview as much as possible, and to talk about the different aspects of caring and the care arrangement in the order they themselves wished. Nevertheless, it was important that certain themes were addressed with every interviewee. These themes arose out of Finch and Mason's theory of family responsibilities and the quantitative analysis constructed before the qualitative part of the study.

The interviewees differed in various aspects. Their ages varied from 35 to 59 years. Some lived in the city and others in the countryside. The geographical distance between the daughter and the elderly parent varied from 0.1 km to 18 km. The interviewees were also busy with several other activities other than caring for their elderly parent. Among the interviewees there was a working single-mother, a housewife, a self-employed person and a single career woman. One of them took care of an elderly father and the others of an elderly mother. The elderly parents all had some physical problems, but all of them were still mentally in good condition. All of them had problems in moving outside their own home. The main characteristics of the interviewees and the length of the interviews are summarized in Table 1.

Table 1. General information about the interviewees.

	Age	Work status	Age of the elderly parent	Length of the interview
1.	43	Full-time employed	68	1 h
2.	35	Full-time employed	73	1 h 10 min
3.	51	Self-employed	75	1 h
4.	58	Retired	82	40 min
5.	52	Full-time employed	76	50 min
6.	59	Housewife	85	1 h 30 min
7.	39	Self-employed	71	1 h

The seven interviews were tape-recorded and later transcribed on the whole, word for word. Laughter, sighs, long pauses and possible interruptions were also noted while transcribing[1]. After transcribing the interviews they were read many times and notes were taken about their content. The purpose was to read the interviews at first as free from preconceptions as possible and let the themes rise out of the material. Then I proceeded to group the themes into larger entities that focused on the same subjects. In this phase I realized that this preliminary classification consisted of two different kinds of concepts.

Some of the themes were describing the *substantive* issues of the caring or the content of the care arrangement such as the living arrangements or the medical treatment of the elderly. Other themes dealt with the *procedural* aspects of the care arrangement or the processes and interaction involved in caring. It was interesting to see that the interviewees considered the caring and care arrangement from many viewpoints, not only from their own but also from their family members and other participants.

CLASSIFYING THE INTERACTION

It was important that the classification dealt with the procedural aspects of the care arrangement as the aim of the study was to examine the process of caring and the room for manoeuvre in the care arrangement. By examining the interaction of the people involved in the care arrangement it was possible to treat the commitments of caring as a process.

In the classification, all the *open discussions* between at least two parties of the care arrangement on some aspect of the care were considered as explicit negotiations. Implicit negotiations were examined with the help of two different concepts. First, I searched for mentions of *non-negotiations*: specific statements that the interviewee had not talked with others about some aspect of the caring. Secondly, I picked out the *explanations* the interviewees had given for the care commitments they and their family members had made. These explanations implied that there had been interaction between the parties on the subject so that a certain reputation had been formed for a family member.

After classifying the data under the headings of open discussions, non-negotiations and explanations, the content of the different classes were carefully analysed. A record was made of every single text fragment, listing the traits of negotiations and explanations and examining

[1] The transcript notation is inserted in the appendix.

what was common in the negotiations and explanations. Again at this point of the study the aim was to let the important traits of the interaction rise from the data as free from preconceptions as possible – although the classification was constructed with the help of the background theory. On the basis of these findings it was possible to present an integrated interpretation of the interaction concerning the care arrangement of the elderly parent. It was possible to show that none of the daughters had made a conscious decision to become a carer. Instead they felt that they had in a way "drifted" into becoming carers. On the background of this drifting there could be seen the reputations and moral identities of different family members. A common finding was also the importance of the way of negotiating about the care arrangement. The analysis was developed further by examining the openness of the interaction between the elderly parent and the carer.

In the next section I will shortly describe in what kind of situations the interviewees were living. After that I present the analysis starting with the matter of becoming a carer. Then I examine whether it is possible to change the care arrangement once it has formed. The rest of the analysis concentrates on the *way* of negotiating about the care arrangement of an elderly parent. In this part the following subjects are tackled: exclusion from negotiations, the appropriateness of asking for help, the finding of the balance between dependence and independence, discretion as a main principle of the negotiations and the open negotiations as an exception.

THE CONTEXT OF CARING

Before presenting the findings on the negotiations in the care arrangement a general description of the situation of the interviewees and the elderly parents they cared for will be given. All but one of the interviewed daughters had siblings living in the same locality, but this did not necessarily mean that these siblings participated in caring for the elderly parent. All the interviewees had the main responsibility in their family for taking care of the elderly parent. The elderly parents in this study were also lucky to get some help from the municipality, such as regular visits by a district nurse. The professional helpers took care of some specific tasks, usually medical help, and the family members handled the rest. The interviewees made a large contribution to helping their parents in their daily activities, as the following quotation describes:

> My mother always says that she could not live at home if I did not help her. (I1)[2]

A common experience for the interviewees was that they were, in a way, bound by the caring. This experience was mostly mental, but it also meant that the daughters were required to make plans in advance in order to make room for the caregiving in their daily programs.

> (The interviewee sighs), well it [the caring] affects more like that, that I think about it all the time. And then I have to plan what I do, although I do not have so many things to do myself, but I always think that today at the latest I have to visit. (I2)

[2] The serial number of the interviewee is noted at the end of each quotation.

The daughters providing care were always concerned in some way for the parent in need of care. The concern the daughters experienced seemed to mean that they were always on a state of alert: ready to go when the least sign of alarm was raised. An illustrative example of the state of alertness is a story about what happens when the parent does not answer the phone. This type of story was told by more than one interviewee.

> Sometimes it happens that she does not answer the phone. Then someone just has to go and see what has happened. There have been some cases when the telephone plug has come off while cleaning. And we have rushed like little animals to see what is wrong with her... (I3)

BECOMING A CARER FOR THE ELDERLY PARENT

According to the data, the turning point, when the need for help arose, was usually the death of the other parent. A typical progression in the care arrangement was that the tasks that were previously taken care of by the other parent were *automatically* passed to the daughter. The daughters did not explain what they meant with this automatic transition. For them it seemed quite natural. The following quotations describe the turning points when these two daughters began to take care of their elderly parents.

> In our family it was our mother who took care of all the money matters. And when she died, they were automatically passed to me. So after that, I have taken care of, you know, the most important money matters. (I2)
>
> Well, her [interviewee's mothers] condition was not very good then, but she had a male friend, who was in good shape. And they did lots of things together; they had a car, so they went together to many places. And I am sure this man helped my mother a lot. But then he died, so it became more apparent that my mother needed help. Before it went okay because the man helped a lot, so before there was no need for home help [official help from the municipality]. And she did not accept our help either, or need it or whatever until then. (I5)

In the second quotation there is also a hint of an important theme: How hard it is for an elderly parent to receive help and thus admit that he or she is dependent on the children. This theme has been found in various studies concerning anticipations about future care by Finnish middle-aged or elderly people (e.g. Ervasti, 1996; Koskela, Kunnas, Salanko-Vuorela, Vaarama, Vanamo, 1991). In the Finnish culture the independence of the family members has been emphasized. Also Finch and Mason (1993) have noticed in Great Britain that the elderly value their independence and autonomy so much that it can be really difficult for them to ask their family for help. This theme will be considered more closely later on in the section entitled "The principle of not having to ask for help".

All the interviewees revealed that they had not discussed how to arrange the care of the elderly parent before the actual need arose. They did not question the absence of negotiations. They thought that there was no use discussing the care arrangement before there was a real need for help. One of the interviewees began to contemplate that a plan for care arrangement would not have actually been such a bad idea. In the following fragment, "J" marks the interviewer and "I" stands for the interviewee.

J: Did you talk beforehand with your family members about what will happen when your parents get old, who will take care of them?

I: I do not remember that there has been any talk like that. I don´t think so.

J: So, it has been more like let us see what happens?

I: Yes.

J: You do not make plans, because you do not know what will happen...

I: Yes. That´s how it is. Of course, it would be nice to have something settled beforehand. But... It is like, these situations change, everyone's family circumstances and everything... It would be good to have some kind of plan, but not too precise, if the plans change after all. So... you should think about the different options, I would say.

J: Do you have a feeling that you have been able to discuss these things with your siblings? There have been no problems?

I: Well, I guess not.

J: Or some have been more interested in these issues than others?

I: Well, yes... But actually we have not discussed that much about it. (I7)

Lorenz-Meyer and Grotheer (2000) have also pointed out this same situation from their study among young Germans: Although the children are aware that their parents' health will deteriorate and that the situation should be discussed and negotiated within the family, for some reason they avoid discussing the care prematurely (and in some cases even when the need for care has arisen). This absence of negotiations has its consequences: When the need for care arises, the caring is arranged automatically and the most self-evident carer among the family members takes the responsibility upon herself. The interviewees described the process of becoming a carer as natural and automatic, as a kind of 'drifting' into the responsibility.

J: Do you remember, have you talked with your family beforehand, who will take care of your mother when she needs help? Or how has the care arrangement formed?

I: Oh, I think it was just of itself. I guess I have some kind of a caring instinct (laughs)...

J: So, you have not exactly discussed it...

I: No, we have not. My father took care of my mother previously [before he died]. (I1)

The logic behind the process of becoming a carer without negotiations can be explained on the basis of Finch and Mason's theory (1993). Family members have accepted different amounts and kinds of commitments during their common history and have thus created different reputations. Based on these reputations they know what to expect from each other when a need arises. The reputation can be seen as a structure which guides who can be trusted for help in the future. Usually the individual does not want to risk her moral identity and will accept the commitments appointed to her. It is possible to act against others' expectations and one's own moral identity. But when a need—such as the need of care of an elderly parent—arises suddenly, someone has to act. This person will very likely be the one who regards him or herself—and whom the family members also see—as the carer in the family.

This interpretation of the process of becoming a carer fitted the data quite well. The interviewees explained their and other family member's positions in the care arrangement with quite stable characteristics (e.g. personality traits), not situational factors (such as who has most spare time at the moment). The explanations centred around the personalities of the family members or with their common past. In the explanations there could be seen an accumulation of similar tasks to a certain family member. There were almost no explanations dealing with situational factors, and where these kinds of explanations did appear, they were linked with some stable explanation. In the following quotations, an interviewee first describes her own position, and secondly the position of her siblings.

> I think it is because I am the eldest of the children and I have taken care of my siblings at home when we were little... it has just always been like that. And partly it must be because my work has to do with nursing. I have also had children in daycare at my home so I have been working at home and have been able to help my mother at the same time. I think that is also one reason. And when my sister was injured, I have been involved a lot with her care, so I believe it has also affected... Affected like that. So, this role has stayed. (I1)
>
> It is not like I am expecting their appreciation for what I do [care for the mother]. Because I know my sisters... They are not interested in it, so they do not appreciate it either. And they do not, sometimes I think that the real picture of our mother, the state she is in, they do not even understand it. They have their own businesses which are more important, their goings and their work. (I1)

People have differing abilities for getting their explanations of being unable to take care of a parent acknowledged as legitimate (Finch and Mason, 1993). These explanations are linked with the reputations and moral identities of the family members. The process of acknowledging has two phases: Others have to accept as legitimate the reason why someone will not participate in the caring, and be assured that the person is not avoiding the responsibilities on purpose. In the next quotation, the explanation given by the brother has been accepted as legitimate (at least the mother has accepted it). In the quotation it can also be seen that the daughters and the son have differing reputations.

> J: Can you say why it is so that your brother does not help as much?
>
> I: He is a self-employed man and his career has always meant a lot to him. And my mother has always supported it, in a way a lot more than ours... Mom has accepted that he works very late and does not have time. He does not have time to call me once a week or something like that. He calls once a month and that is enough for my mother. Or if there is something special she needs, like the TV is broken, and if it is like ten o'clock in the evening, she knows that now she can phone my brother because he will probably be home by then. So, it happens through quite natural choices.
>
> J: Is it like, she knows that you and your sister will be more available?
>
> I: That too. Besides, to tell you the truth, me and my sister are better in taking care of my mother than he [the brother] is. Really! Because he has not dealt with these kind of things before, so he couldn't, it would be a lot harder for him to do it. (I3)

Apart from explanations dealing with the personalities and abilities of different family members, the expectations and wishes of the elderly parent were also often used to explain why some participated in the caring and others did not. It seemed that the interviewees hardly questioned the wishes of the parent. On the contrary, they aspired to act according to them. More than one interviewee wanted to make it clear that the carer did not need any other reasons for helping the elderly parent than the fact that the parent needed help. They emphasized that they did not have to think about whether to give help or not; help was given automatically.

> I do not know [why I ended up as a carer]. One reason must be that I was at home with children a long time, so I was available during the daytime. It has been somehow quite

> natural, I have not thought about it so much. When she was still able to walk, I took her shopping and stuff like that. With her it has all been quite natural. It has somehow... Somehow it has, washing the clothes and all, it is clear that me and my sister take care of it. (16)

In light of the data, there remains the question whether the interviewees are always considering their moral identities before making a decision about becoming a carer and acting upon these identities. It seems that the concept of moral identity (and reputation) works best while comparing the participation of different family members in the caring, and when asking why one of the children helps the elderly parent more than the other children do. Like Finch and Mason (1993) have stated, the reputations offer a structure that guides the family members to ask for help from a certain family member.

Another question is why the daughters in this study so seldom refused to help. It may be, as Finch and Mason (1993) explain it, that they hope to maintain their moral identity as a helpful daughter. According to the data, it seems that the help is given *automatically*. So it seems that in many cases the daughters do not consciously pause to think how their behaviour (helping or not helping) will affect their moral identities and reputations. The concept of a moral identity is more useful in a situation where the daughter does not see her help as absolutely necessary. Then she might still choose to give her help because it is important for her to maintain her moral identity and reputation as the carer in the family.

In the next section it will be considered whether the interviewees were able to change their position in the care arrangement once it was formed or whether they feel themselves to be stuck in the position of a carer.

A Stabilized Care Arrangement or Continuous Negotiations?

When there were more than one family member participating in the care of an elderly parent, it did not seem to be problematic that there were no negotiations preceding the need for help, or that the care arrangement thus formed through a process of natural and automatic drifting. It was still possible for the siblings to negotiate among themselves and share the tasks. Three of the interviewees were, however, solely responsible for the caring even though they were not the only children in the family. For them, the non-existing division of labour was a problem, and they had thought more about the reasons why it was them who helped the elderly parent and not their siblings.

The care arrangements had stabilized in every family. The interviewees did not mention that some family member had in some phase or situation participated more in the care. It seems that the position in the care arrangement once formed will be reinforced by the accumulation of "natural" choices.

> And he [the father] calls me like, hey now I need some help, I need this and that. And it suits me, it does not suit anyone else but me. It´s because there are no siblings besides me and my brother, and dad's siblings have only two children. His own siblings are already dead. And that´s about everyone there is. And he does not have any friends, he has friends, but not the kind of friends who could help in these kind of things. So he will turn to me with his troubles.

I doubt that he tells everything, I think that he broods over most of them in his mind, but then sometimes there are some things... (I2)

The same interviewee also said that it was easier for her to take care of her father's wishes herself than to ask someone else for help.

> J: Do you feel that it is difficult to ask others for help, or...
>
> I: Well, I guess it is, apart from my brother. But I know I could if I wanted, if the situation needed that. Actually there are people if I come to think about it. But it´s so automatic, that it is easier in a way, for me it is easier if I do it myself than if I begin to call people and ask "can you come and help". (I2)

When asked directly could the interviewees see the situation changing in the future, they believed that the only possible change would be that the same persons who take care of the parent now would be taking more and more responsibility for the care in the future. None of the interviewees thought that they could reduce the amount of help given to their parent. Although some of the interviewees experienced their position as the only or the main carer as unfair, there were almost no examples of negotiations where they would have tried to change their position in the care arrangement. It seemed that the only times they had asked for help from their siblings were when they themselves were going away for a few days. It seems that the interviewees were so well aware of their roles in the family as a caretaker that they did not even consider it possible to change their position. There are also some fragments in the data suggesting that the elderly parent might not approve of any other care arrangements than the present one. The wish of the elderly parent is in some cases an important factor why the care arrangement gets stabilized.

In the data, there was only one example where an interviewee said that she had tried to talk to her sisters, suggesting that they should participate in the care of their mother a little more.

> J: Have you ever tried to tell your sisters that they could help you a little...
>
> I: I have tried sometimes but it won´t work. Promises are all that there is. They seem to sympathize when I tell them but it will not result in anything.
>
> J: So you cannot make them help...
>
> I: No I cannot and then if my mother lies sick in the hospital then they remember but it ends right there when she leaves the hospital. [Pause.] And luckily mother does not need more help, because I can still manage and make it on my own. (I1)

This interviewee had found it impossible to make her siblings help her more in the care of their elderly mother. Elsewhere in the interview she said that she was a bit worried about the future and how would she be able to manage the care on her own if her mother´s condition deteriorated. Because of the non-existent help on the part of her siblings she had already considered professional help. She had not yet dared to inquire for such help because she knew that her mother would not approve of others helping her than the daughter herself. In the next section I will move on to consider situations where someone is left out of the negotiations in order to maintain control over the result of the negotiation or to protect someone from inconvenient facts.

LEAVING SOMEONE OUT OF THE NEGOTIATIONS

While examining negotiations about family responsibilities, it is important to note who is negotiating and who is left out of the negotiations. The act of leaving someone out of the negotiations can have different functions that are not necessarily negative. One obvious function is gaining control over the result of the negotiation. In most of the data examples dealing with control, it was the elderly parent who had wanted to leave the children out of the negotiations concerning his or her own care. They wanted to decide for themselves who should take care of them and how, as in the following example where a daughter is left out of a negotiation arranged in the hospital.

> I would have wanted to participate in the planning in the hospital [about the care at home] but... It is possible that my mother has announced that she does not want me to come to the negotiation. It is very likely that it was like that... (I5)

In this case there was a discrepancy between the wishes of the mother and the daughter. The daughter was concerned about her mother and therefore wanted to have a say in the care of her mother. The mother interpreted her daughters concern as interfering in her life and her autonomy.

> And it's like she does not understand that we are concerned, that we do not want to impose or interfere with her life. But she does not understand that we are actually concerned. (I5)

It seems that a loss of independence or autonomy is such a difficult experience for an elderly person that some elderly people need to protect their right to decide about their own life sometimes even quite fiercely. This feature is apparent at least in Finnish and British cultures (e.g. Ervasti 1996, Finch and Mason, 1993). In a case where the opinions about the proper care arrangement might clash, the elderly person could opt for deciding by her or himself without any negotiations and thus maintain a sense of autonomy.

The same logic – a wish to control the result of the negotiation – appears in an example where, after many open but unsuccessful negotiations, the daughter refuses to negotiate anymore on the topic.

> My mum has finally accepted the visits of the district nurse, although we had a terrible fight about that in the beginning. She felt that I should take her every time to the health centre for these blood tests. But I do have my job, and I said that I cannot be absent from work so often. And then I just said that the district nurse is coming and I did not give up on that. (I1)

According to Finch and Mason it is also possible to use the exclusion from the negotiations as a means of protecting the receiver of the care. In the data there were a few examples where the desire to protect the elderly parent by leaving him or her out of the negotiations was apparent. One interviewee did not want to discuss in advance any future plans about the care with her mother so that her mother would not be disappointed if they did not come true.

Once I did consider, but I did not even talk to her [the mother], I only talked to my husband when our neighbour rented his apartment. I thought that what if we rented the flat and it would be on the same floor and everything... My husband was against the idea, he thought that it would have been too tight, and my friend said so too. And so I believed these two people and I did not even talk to my mother about it. But I had the idea that I bring her to live near us. But I didn´t talk to her about it. (I6)

Another interviewee said that she did not dare to talk about future arrangements for her mother's care or a possible move to an old people's home. Her motivation was to protect her mother from feelings of depression.

J: Have you talked with your sister or with your mother about the future, about what your mother wants?

I: Well [sounds surprised]. Yes, it is a very tricky thing, and I am a bit cautious about the subject, because she would not want by any means to leave her own home. But I do think about how long she will last at her own home...

J: Well, do you know what does your mother think about an old people's home?

I: Well. Yes... I have to say that I have not dared to ask her, to tell you the truth. There was a time when mother was... Actually now I could talk with her about the subject, she has been so lively for a long time. But at some time she was so depressed and like that that I would not have dreamed of asking her about it, you could almost have guessed the answer. (I7)

It seems that in a caring relationship between an elderly parent and the children there are topics that should be avoided. I will return to the subject of discretion more thoroughly after I have considered the theme of autonomy and independence of the elderly parent more deeply in the next two sections.

The Principle of not Having to Ask for Help

There seemed to be a silent agreement that the giver should always have ultimate control over the decision whether to give help to a family member or not. The interviewees shared the view that the initiative for helping should optimally be taken by the helper.

It is interesting that asking for help becomes an issue even in situations where the care arrangement has already stabilised. It was still difficult for an elderly parent to ask for favours from the daughter although the daughter had already committed to the care arrangement. The daughters explained this via their parents' way of thinking: You have to manage on your own and asking for help or depending on someone can even be experienced as a shame. In the next extract, the daughter describes how it used to be impossible for her mother to ask for help from her daughters when she was still living at home. After moving to an old people's home she had learned to ask for help from the nurses there.

I: And she would never ever call us. We always had to contact her ourselves. We still call her every day, my sister and I. I think it is a fine thing that there is someone she can call now and ask for things. She used to tell me that she would not have called my sister either. She thought that she should always make it on her own.

J: So now she prefers to contact the nurses?

I: Well, yes now it has been so for a couple of times. She has noticed that it is possible to ask for help. (I4)

The daughters in the data had realized how hard it is for their parents to ask for help. In some cases they had encouraged their parents to contact them and announce their needs directly. Still, asking for help seemed to be an unbearable thought for some parents.

And we have told her that if you need you can ask for help. But she is actually a kind of a proud person, so no... It is not easy for her to ask for any special help. (I5)

This kind of pride and hesitation to ask for help was not visible with all the elderly parents in the data. In any case the carers should take into account that it is not always easy for an elderly person to ask for help from family members. In the next section the function of the principle of not having to ask for help will be explained.

Aiming for a Balance between Dependence and Independence

According to the data, the most typical means for the elderly parent to avoid the loss of independence was to avoid directly asking for help. The typical approach for maintaining the balance between independence and dependence is by reciprocity. For the elderly people this may be impossible unless you think about reciprocity from the point of view of the entire lifespan. This means that the daughter has to interpret the elderly parent's communication and actions quite carefully.

But my mum never calls, she will never call me either, to ask if we could go shopping. She assumes that I will call and ask how she is doing and... Then I know if she calls, if she has called two to three times while I have been away, then I know that there is something wrong. But otherwise she will not, very rarely she calls and asks how is it going. It is not like mum at all that she would call. Least of all to ask for any help. (I1)

Thus, the acceptability of asking for help depends most of all on *how* you ask for it. In the quotation above, the mother may feel that a direct request would be too demanding for her daughter. The communication between the mother and daughter had taken such a form that the daughter had the ultimate control in deciding whether to give help. If considered from the point of view of the moral identity of the daughter, it could be questioned if there is any real choice. Hinting about the need for help is one means by which the elderly parent keeps to the principle of not asking for help and not expecting it automatically.

Well, there can be clean curtains just waiting to be ironed and hung up on the windows when I go there. And she might do some preparations there beforehand so that I will clean the windows or... Might be that some things are waiting for me when I go there, when she knows that I am on my vacation or have a day-off. Because I have always said to her that she should just tell me so I will do it. But she won´t necessarily say anything if I do not notice that there are some curtains lying on the living room chair. She feels that it is terribly hard to ask. (I1)

In the previous quotation it can be seen that the daughter has internalised her mother's wishes. The example raises the question does it matter to the helper whether help is asked for directly or given as a result of implicit negotiations and internalised expectations? In both cases the daughter seems to know what to do. In a way, direct and open requests are preferable from the point of view of the daughter: to a direct request the daughter is also able to react directly. An indirect request could actually be more compelling to the daughter than a direct one because it is more difficult to negotiate. An open request could be discussed from both the point of the view of the giver and the receiver of the help and thus an optimal solution could be negotiated. With an unspoken wish there are more possibilities for misunderstandings from both sides, as it will be illustrated below.

Discretion as a Principle of the Interaction

Asking for help was only one theme that usually remained unspoken. Several expressions were found in the data that described indirect negotiations such as "he did not say it out loud", "you could read between the lines", "there have been some hints" and "I interpret it from her tone". It was obvious that there were issues that should be left unspoken or which the daughter should handle extremely carefully. The condition of the elderly parent can in itself be a theme which does not occur in the discussions.

> I did think, because she always said so, that everything was OK, but then it was not always that OK... I think she could stay in an elevator for three days before she would call for help. (I6)

Another forbidden or avoidable theme was moving from home to an old people's home.

> I checked up what kind of possibilities there were for living arrangements when she was returning from the hospital. I somehow thought that she would not make it at home alone anymore. I wanted to find out what kind of different housing services there were. But she got really angry and hurt about that. (I5)

Discretion in the care relationship serves to maintain the balance between dependency and independence. On the basis of the data, discretion also seems to have other functions. According to Peter Townsend's (1957; Finch and Mason, 2000) classic remark, the ideal form of relationship between an elderly parent and his or her adult children could be described as "intimacy at a distance". When the relationship turns into a care relationship, the regulation of intimacy and distance becomes an even more critical task. There's a risk that the daughter (or son) who takes the care responsibility will land too close to the elderly parent. On the basis of the data another function of discretion seems to be the maintenance of the balance between intimacy and distance. For the elderly parent it is vital to maintain some degree of privacy, an area where others are not allowed to enter. The elderly parent may try to protect this area, sometimes quite fiercely. However, in a care relationship it is not always easy for the carer to follow the limits of privacy.

The balancing act between intimacy and distance and between dependence and independence seemed to be particularly important for the daughters who took care of their elderly parents by themselves. When there is only one person giving help, the dependency is more apparent. The following example describes how difficult it can be to achieve a balance between dependency and independence.

> I visit her and when she is in a better mood she says that you don´t have to come here so often. But then if I don´t go there the phone rings and she is like "good gracious, what is it with you, are you sick, are you sleeping..." Well, it is like that, she is an old person and she would not want to be a burden. But I have the feeling all the time that soon the phone will ring again. (I6)

It seems that in this case it could be easier for both of them if there were more carers. In this way the elderly parent could divide her wishes and expectations between more than one carer. Where there is only one carer she needs to develop ways in which to manage the situation so that the commitment of caring does not become unbearable. One such way—breaking the silence—is discussed in the next section.

BREAKING THE SILENCE

It is not always easy for the carer to follow the principle of discretion because the wishes and requests of the elderly parent have an impact on the carer´s own personal life. Some wishes are experienced as unreasonable. In these situations the daughter could not obey the principle of discretion but it was necessary for her to say aloud her opinion. In the following example it is interesting that the parent has not actually expressed his wish aloud and the daughter actually reacts to her own interpretation. Thus the quotation is at the same time another example of the meaning of the implicit, indirect negotiations.

> [...] and when there have been things like, he must for example go and see the doctor in the daytime, so he says, or I interpret it from his tone of voice, that I should go and take him there. But I say that no I will not, I am working and I just cannot leave there all of a sudden. In theory I actually could leave, my job is like that, but to tell you the truth I do not want to. For example I had my summer vacation, it was four weeks, so all my vacation went by more or less as I had to take him here and there. (I2)

From the example it can also be seen that discretion is employed when the daughter refuses to tell the real reason why she will not help. The reason is more discrete for both of them: The daughter will not seem to be indifferent and the father will not feel himself to be a burden.

The interviewees used the expression 'saying their opinion aloud' only as they recounted exceptional situations. This fact strengthens the idea that many aspects of the caring are carried out without any explicit negotiations. According to the daughters, help and care is given in the usual way - typically following the wishes of the parent - as long as it is possible, and any expression of the daughter´s own opinion is avoided.

> I have not experienced the caring so far as terribly heavy or anything. In my vacation, if I am completely honest, I did think about, it does not sound so nice, but I thought that I am

> running around doing this and that, and he had to get to the barber and things like that. But when I think about it, I have not felt it that way yet. (I2)

The act of saying an opinion aloud creates limits to one's own position in the care arrangement. If the parent asks for one particular favour, it is easier for the daughter to give a situational and more discrete reason for not helping. She does not have to say that the request is unreasonable and that she feels the caring relationship limits her own freedom. With such discretion it is possible to maintain sufficient distance between the daughter and the elderly parent.

More than one interviewee told about a situation where the parent had wished that the daughter could generally participate more in the caring. This request would affect their lives strongly and so the reaction of the daughters was also stronger. This meant breaking the silence and speaking their opinion aloud. Here speaks an interviewee whose mother rejected the idea of professional care services.

> J: Do you know did your mother wish that...
>
> I: I had taken care of her... Yes she did. I told her that I have only this one life and I am a selfish child and I will not agree to it that I would cook for you and rush here all the time washing your clothes if it is possible that the home help [municipal service for old people living at home] can do it. (I5)

The daughters in the data were lucky to get professional help from the municipality in the care of their parents. Although they were not themselves able or willing to take responsibility for all of the care, they could maintain their reputation and their moral identity as a responsible and caring daughter by providing their parent with professional help. The existence of municipal elderly care services therefore reduces the pressure on the daughters to participate more in the caring of an elderly parent.

There were also situations when even breaking the silence did not have an impact on the care arrangements. One interviewee said that her only option then was to act in a way where she was able to get some distance from the situation at least for a moment.

> And sometimes when it is not absolutely necessary for me to visit her every day and when I feel that I have been listening to her complaints on and on that she is so sick and when I try to tell her to go and visit the doctor for a change or get some medicine or get some kind of treatment... But when she does not take any of my advice and everything seems so difficult then I might take a break and it will help me in a way that... (I1)

For this interviewee the balancing between dependence and independence was not an easy task. However there were also interviewees who claimed that their communication with their elderly parent was almost totally open. In the next section the implications of this kind of open communication will be considered.

EXCEPTIONALLY OPEN COMMUNICATION

Two interviewees claimed throughout the interviews that their interaction with the elderly parent (although not with other family members) was totally open and unproblematic. This kind of open negotiation could not be described as the finding of a proper balance between dependency and independence. In these negotiations the only task seemed to be to handle the actual topic and get a satisfactory result. There seemed to be no need to avoid the showing of the dependence between family members. In the next fragment, the daughter emphasises also the importance of her mother's mental capacity as a crucial element for successful open negotiations.

> J: Can you make your own plans like before or do you have to take your mother's situation into account?
>
> I: We always pay attention to it, there's no problem in that. In fact I... The positive thing with my mother is that if she calls and asks and says that she has some need, and if I tell her that now I have this situation with my job and I have to go here and there, and ask her is it OK if I come after five o'clock. And normally it is OK with her. We can agree like that because she is still mentally so sharp. (I2)

The other interviewee who emphasised the meaning of directness in the negotiations said that she thought it would be impossible to try to make out her mother's wishes. She identified the directness of the negotiations with the altogether easy and unproblematic mother-daughter relationship.

> Well, I have always tried to make her tell directly what she needs... If you go figuring out what she means it usually goes wrong. Because you just cannot tell what another person wants. Even after we have discussed it, it can still go all wrong. But no... It has always been easy to handle things with her. When I have listened to some of my friend's stories about their relationships with their mothers, I have always wondered like, good heavens what kind of quarrels, like terrible... Like I have always had an easy relationship with my mom. (I7)

These exceptional interviewees regarded caring for their mothers as a natural and automatic course of action. They did not consider dependency between family members as something that should be avoided. The dependence could thus be shown openly. Therefore there was no need to negotiate in an indirect way that would hide the dependence of the elderly parent. One of these open negotiators also emphasised her feelings of duty towards her mother.

> I am aware of the problems involved in caring and all. But it happens to be so that she is my mother who has done a huge job with us kids. So that I do not... or I assume that it is my responsibility to do so. My sister has the same attitude. And well... my brother then he does what he does because... But I am sure it will fall on us, my sister and I, the caring in the future, that is for sure. (I2)

Finch and Mason (1993) however deny the fact that commitment to a family member could be explained as the direct result of a sense of duty. As has been discussed earlier they suggest that the family responsibilities are rather negotiated over time and these negotiations are based on the structure of different family members' moral identities.

It was interesting to see that everyone in the families of these two exceptional interviewees (who emphasized the directness of the communication) did not think the same way about caring and responsibility. The differences between the family members could be interpreted through the concepts of moral identity and reputation. The daughters have evolved a moral identity as a carer while the son has avoided the commitments because of his moral identity as a career-person. When these identities have been strengthened in real-life situations, the carrying out of family responsibilities has become more and more automatic for the daughter.

So the question is not that these families would be exceptionally close or that the daughters are following a general norm of caring for the elderly parent. What seems to be of significance is the relationship between the mother and the daughter. The commitments of caring have evolved in relationships and the history of these relationships has affected the content and the intensity of these commitments and the means of interaction. The moral identity should thus not be seen exclusively as an internal experience of the individual. It has developed by way of the interactions between family members. The moral identity could therefore be seen as a property of the relationship, not of the individual (Burr, 1995). Caring as an automatic course of action in this way becomes more understandable than if the moral identity was seen as a property of the individual. To behave according to the moral identity is not the same as a choice or a decision that the individual needs to make every time something such as help is expected from her (or him). The proper behaviour is evoked often automatically and unconsciously in the context of the relationship because of the common history and earlier commitments of the two people.

DISCUSSION

The aim of the study was to examine how much room for manoeuvre a daughter has in caring for her elderly parent. The concept of room for manoeuvre was comparable to the idea of limited freedom; the structure defines partially the position of an individual in a care arrangement, but the individual can to some extent influence her own position.

In previous Finnish studies about family caregiving (e.g. Gothóni, 1991), the experience of caring was described as binding. In this study, it can be seen that the moral identity—which has evolved during the common history of the family members—has a profound impact on defining the room for manoeuvre of the daughter who is involved in the care arrangement. This finding was compatible with the theory of Finch and Mason (1993). None of the interviewees had negotiated who should take care of the elderly parent before the need for care actually arose, and the care arrangement was said to have formed automatically and naturally. Seen from this perspective, the room for manoeuvre was limited for a daughter who had committed herself to being helpful around other family members, thus creating a reputation for herself as a carer. The expectations of the family were placed on her and this made it difficult for her to find legitimate excuses for not taking care of the parent.

However, it should be noted that having limited room for manoeuvre does not necessarily equate with a negatively binding relationship. It was not the experience of the daughters interviewed in the study that they had become carers against their will. None of them expressed a desire to stop participating in the caring, although some of them wished for additional help. The moral identity has evolved from the relationship with another significant person and it is a property of this relationship. Behaviour that is consistent with one's moral identity is a condition for the smooth functioning of the relationship. Thus the moral identity is not seen as a straitjacket that determines what an individual does. In a relationship with significant and close persons, one wants to act in a way which guarantees that the relationship will also continue as close and significant. In some cases, having limited room for manoeuvre can be experienced negatively from the point of view of the moral identity. This happened when the other family members totally withdrew from the caring because they saw one family member as the sole carer of the family.

For the daughter taking care on an elderly parent, having an opportunity to negotiate increased her room for manoeuvre. It was vital that the daughter was able to discuss the care of the elderly parent with other family members for her to gain any room for manoeuvre. If it was possible to negotiate directly at all times and on all subjects, then there was also greater room for manoeuvre for the daughter. Nevertheless, this was in fact rarely possible because the negotiations also had a moral dimension. The data clearly supported the idea that the way in which negotiations were carried out was as important to the process as the actual result of the negotiations. Through discretion and leaving things unsaid, it was possible to regulate the balance between dependency and independence, and intimacy and distance.

Conclusion

In this chapter I have presented the main findings of a qualitative study considering the caring for an elderly parent from the point of view of interaction. The concept of room for manoeuvre was used in describing the limited freedom that the daughter has in choosing her position in the care arrangement. The analysis was constructed with the help of Janet Finch's and Jennifer Mason's (1993) theory of family responsibilities. In the analysis I focused on the explicit and implicit negotiations about the care arrangement that take place within family. The main findings tackle the process of becoming a carer and the way in which family members negotiate the care arrangement. The daughters were shown to take the position of the carer automatically, without a conscious decision to do so. This process was analysed using the construct of moral identity. It was claimed that the moral identity is a property of the relationship, not the person. The way of the negotiations between the elderly parent and the daughter were shown to be extremely important; the openness versus the discretion in the negotiations and their functions for the carer and the elderly parent in need of care were specifically examined.

Practical Considerations and Recommendations

- The perspective of interaction is fruitful in studying the experiences of caring for an elderly family member.

- In the studies concerning family caregiving the context of caring and the nature of caring as a process should be recognized.
- The commitments of helping and caring tend to accumulate to the same persons within the family.
- The binding nature of the caring can be understood by considering the common history of the family members and the moral identities that they have constructed in these relationships.
- Not discussing the care arrangement before a serious need for care arises puts the pressure of caring on a sole family member.
- It is difficult to change the care arrangement (e.g. to get other family members participate more on the caring) once it has formed.
- Respect for the autonomy of the elderly parent affects the interaction in the caring relationship profoundly. The carer must be able to interpret the sometimes indirect or unsaid wishes of the elderly parent.
- The openness of the negotiations widens the room for manoeuvre of the carer by giving her (or him) the opportunity to react directly to the requests and wishes of the elderly parent.
- A certain amount of discretion is needed in maintaining the proper distance and independence between the carer and the elderly parent.
- A careful analysis is needed in studying the reasons and motivations why someone becomes a carer. It is not enough to point out factors such as gender and employment affecting the choice of becoming a carer.
- The care relationship is not exclusively a relationship of the carer and the person cared for, and the question of family caregiving should not be left exclusively as a problem of the family.
- The family caregivers need support from the society. Attention should be paid to the processes of becoming a carer in order to maintain (or even raise) the potential of the families to care for their elderly members.

REFERENCES

Attias-Donfut, C. and Wolff, C. (2000). The Redistributive Effects of Generational Transfers. In: S. Arber and C. Attias-Donfut (Eds.): *The Myth of Generational Conflict –The Family and the State in Ageing Societies*. (pp. 22-46) London: Routledge.

Burr, V. (1995). *An Introduction to Social Constructionism*. London: Routledge.

Ervasti, H. (1996). Kenen vastuu? Tutkimuksia hyvinvointipluralismin legitimiteetin näkökulmasta. Stakes, Tutkimuksia 62. Helsinki: Stakes. *(In English: Whose responsibility? Studies from the point of view of the legitimacy of welfare-pluralism.).*

Finch, J. and Mason, J. (1993). *Negotiating Family Responsibilities*. London: Routledge.

Finch, J. and Mason, J. (2000). Filial Obligations and Kin Support for Elderly People. In: J. F. Gubrium and J. A. Holstein (Eds.): *Aging and Everyday Life*. (pp. 194-213) Oxford: Blackwell.

Gothóni, R. (1991). Omaiset – loppuunpalaneita ihmisiä vai käyttämätön voimavara. Sosiaali- ja terveysministeriön kehittämisosaston julkaisuja 1991:4. Helsinki: Sosiaali- ja terveysministeriö. *(In english: Family members - suffering from burn-out or an unused resource.)*.

Graham, H. (1983). Caring: A Labour of Love. In: J. Finch and D. Groves (Eds.): *A Labour of Love: Women, Work and Caring.* (pp. 13-31) London: Routledge and Kegan Paul.

Koskela, K., Kunnas, M.-L., Salanko-Vuorela, M., Vaarama, M. and Vanamo, J. (1991). Ikäihmisten palveluiden vahvat ja heikot lenkit. Helsinki: Vanhus- ja lähimmäispalveluiden liitto. *(In english: The strengths and weaknesses in the services of elderly people.)*.

Lorenz-Meyer, D. and Grotheer, A. (2000). Reinventing the Generational Contract – Anticipated Care-Giving Responsibilities of Younger Germans and Turkish Migrants. In: S. Arber and C. Attias-Donfut (Eds.): *The Myth of Generational Conflict –The Family and the State in Ageing Societies.* , (pp. 190-208). London: Routledge.

Perälä, M.-L., Rissanen, P., Grönroos, E., Hammar, T., Pöyry, P., Teperi, J.: (2003) PALKO - Palveluja yhteensovittava kotiutuminen ja kotihoito: Koeasetelma ja lähtötilanteen arviointi *(In english: PALKO - Integrated services in hospital discharge and home-care: experimental design and results of base line evaluation)*. Research Report, *Aiheita*, 27. Helsinki: Stakes.

Pyysiäinen, J. (2003). Neuvottelut ja liikkumavara iäkkään vanhemman hoitamisessa. *(Negotiations and room for manoeuvre in caring for an elderly parent.)* Research Report. *Aiheita* 14/2003. Helsinki: Stakes.

Qureshi, H. and Walker, A. (1989). *The Caring Relationship. Elderly People and their Families.* London: Macmillan.

Qureshi, H. (1996) Obligations and Support within Families. In: Alan Walker (Ed.): *The New Generational Contract. Intergenerational Relations, Old Age and Welfare.* (pp. 100-119). London: UCL Press.

Townsend, P. (1957). *The Family Life of Old People*. London: Routledge and Kegan Paul.

Vaarama, M., Hakkarainen, A., Voutilainen, P. and Päivärinta, E. (2000). Vanhusten palvelut. In H. Uusitalo, A. Parpo and A. Hakkarainen (Eds.), Sosiaali- ja terveydenhuollon palvelukatsaus 2000. *(A report on the social and health services in 2000.)*. Stakes, Raportteja 250. Helsinki: Stakes.

Vaarama, M. and Kautto, M. (1998). *Social Protection for the Elderly in Finland.* Helsinki: Stakes.

APPENDIX

The transcript notation:

Sighs, laughter etc. are noted inside normal brackets. ( )

Author's comments that help the understanding of the fragment are noted inside square brackets. [ ]

Longer pauses where the interviewee stopped to think are noted with …

Unimportant sentences in the middle of a fragment that are removed are noted with […]

In: Family Caregiving for Older Disabled People
Editor: Isabella Paoletti, pp. 127-149
ISBN 1-59454-808-0

Chapter 7

FAMILY CAREGIVING WHEN RELATIONSHIPS ARE POOR

Lesley Baillie
Clinical Skills Development,
London South Bank University, London

INTRODUCTION

This chapter examines the topic of caring for older relatives where the relationship between the caregiver and care receiver is poor. This dimension of caregiving appears to be little explored or recognised, despite the wide range of literature addressing different aspects of informal caring for older people.

Paid professional carers are rightly expected to put aside any feelings of like or dislike for individuals they are caring for because they are paid to do a job and are working to a professional code of practice. There is much in the nursing literature about 'emotional labour' (e.g. Smith, 1992) – that nurses are required to care for people and appear caring despite personal feelings and emotions. Clearly nurses are not the only professionals who this applies to and indeed much of the literature draws on Hochscild's (1983) work on emotional labour and flight attendants. Family caregiving is unpaid (though there may be a will and property to consider) but, aside from this, there are a number of other differences between paid professional caring and family caregiving. Most paid caring is conducted over a limited time frame and can be concluded at any point. However in many instances family caregiving continues for an unpredictable but possibly very lengthy period of time. Indeed the Department of Health (DH) (1999) states that in the UK, nearly a quarter of carers have been looking after the person they care for, for at least ten years, and a further quarter have looked after them for 5-9 years. In addition while paid professional caring occurs in fixed weekly hours of work, informal care can be almost constant. For example, in O'Neill and Evans's (2001) study based in Ireland, most carers were involved in caregiving seven days a week, with one in ten providing constant care (168 hours per week). Thirty one per cent had provided care for more than ten years and 56 per cent for more than five years.

My interest in caregiving where relationships are poor, developed from many years of health care experience in an acute hospital setting. I noticed that staff consistently made assumptions about caregiving relationships; the notion that the relationship could be poor remained unacknowledged in most instances. I observed that there is an assumption that people care *about* their older relatives and will thus – willingly – care *for* them. On occasions I encountered patients being brought to Accident and Emergency, having been cared for by relatives, who would then refuse to have the patient home after treatment. I observed that staff responded negatively in such cases (though not directly to the patient and relative). Staff never appeared to consider the relationship between the caregiver and person cared for, but my view was: how could we, as staff, know what their relationship was like, or what had gone before? Yet the possibility never surfaced that the relationship might be poor and that, therefore, expectations of informal caring might be unrealistic. I also recalled no empirical research where this topic had been explicitly examined.

In my examination of this topic I first reviewed the literature, examining two main sources: current UK health policy, for facts and assumptions about caregiving relationships, and empirical research about caregiving, for any evidence that some relationships between caregiver and the person cared for, are poor. From this I identified aims for my study and I explain my methodology. The results, a selection of personal experience stories, are then presented. A discussion of these follows, in particular motives for caregiving when relationships are poor are examined in some depth, with reference to the stories. Finally conclusions and recommendations are presented.

Caregiving for Older People in the UK

Britain has an estimated 5.7 million carers, and half of all carers care for someone over the age of seventy five years (DH, 1999). Much of the literature about informal caring stresses that women are more likely to be carers than men and Walker (1983) argues that in political speak terms like 'community' and 'family' are 'euphemisms for female kin' (p114). However, the Department of Health (1999) identifies that 58 per cent of carers are women, while 42 per cent are men – clearly not such a marked difference between the genders as has sometimes been claimed. Most carers are aged 45-64 years, and 9 out of 10 are caring for a relative: 2 out of 10 for a partner and 4 out of 10 for parents (DH, 1999).

Wright (1983) describes an exploratory study with carers, which highlighted the varying and unpredictable nature of caring for older parents. In this study of single adult children caring for older parents, twenty two were sons and thirty six were daughters, challenging the supposition, even at that time, that only women care. However analysis of the care they undertook found women carers carried out more personal tasks than men, and that men were much less likely to give up work to care, perhaps because they were not expected to by society, while women were put under pressure to give up work to care full-time. Men carers were much more likely to get help, for example, a home help. Wright (1983) found that women had given up work thinking it would be temporary as the parent would only last a year, but many years later they were still alive. One woman who had had to change jobs for one which fitted better with caring for her mother, thus affecting her pension, said 'Society will penalise me in the future because at present I am doing what society is telling me I should do,' (p94) clearly highlighting feelings of an obligation to care. This is discussed later in this chapter.

As regards who older people wish to care for them, Qureshi and Walker (1989) report that, in general, close relatives are preferred to more distant ones, any relative is preferred to a non relative, and female relatives are preferred to male relatives. In 68 per cent of cases there was a hierarchy of preference: spouse, relative in lifelong household, daughter, daughter-in-law, son, other relatives, non relatives. Bond *et al.*'s (1999) study, based in four varying locations in England, supported these findings. They found that of 1127 people aged 65 years and over, 78 per cent had a key informal supporter who helped with activities of daily living, indicating that the majority of frail older people are supported at home by the family. Key supporters were: spouses (38 per cent), daughters (30 per cent), sons (9 per cent), daughters-in-law (4 per cent), other relatives (11 per cent) and neighbours (8 per cent). Thus the main informal carers of older people, in this study, were found to be spouses and daughters. Bond *et al.* (1999) note that although both men and women provide informal care, women below the age of retirement are much more likely to provide informal care than men of the same age. However the spouses who were carers, were just as likely to be husbands.

Finch (1989) makes the point that the issue of there being larger numbers of older people who need care is a new one due to people living longer, and that paradoxically it has arisen at a time when women who, she states, were traditionally expected to provide care, are in a less easy position to do so as they are much more likely to be working, than in earlier decades. Clearly in the last fifteen years since she wrote this, the numbers of women working, and working full-time, has increased substantially. However Finch also points out that working women are as likely as non-working women to take on caregiving, and that the relationship between paid work and care is not straightforward and is affected by many other factors, such as available care alternatives.

In 'Caring for Carers: a national strategy for carers', the Department of Health (1999) reiterates a number of times that its role is to support carers to continue to care. Clearly there are sound financial reasons for the government desiring to do this, for example, in 1995, the British Medical Association estimated that family care saves the state £40 billion a year. Bywaters and Harris (1998) identify that 'the major providers of care to older people in need of help are informal carers, working mainly without pay and very substantially reducing the burden of costs to the state while providing care, which on the whole, is preferred to purchased services by those who receive it' (p458). Smith *et al.* (2003) highlight that: 'Both government and the health care system in the UK have a major stake in the ability of families to support the independence of older people and maintain them in their own homes' (p13). They go on to identify that the developments and policies relating to community care have made the reliance of formal services on unpaid care increasingly explicit, with a shift in rhetoric from care *in* the community to care *by* the community. Smith *et al.* (2003) point out that with numbers of older people increasing, and cuts in taxation demanded, it is no wonder that the government wants to promote the role of carers. Emotive terms about carers and attempts to romanticise their roles are apparent, for example in 'Caring about carers: a national strategy for carers', Tony Blair, the current British prime minister, refers to carers as 'the unsung heroes of British life' (DH, 1999, p3). The Deputy Minister for Community Care, Iain Gray, in the Scottish Executive (SE)'s document 'Strategy for carers in Scotland' states that the SE 'acknowledges the vital contribution made to society by the many unpaid carers in Scotland' (SE, 1999).

Assumptions about the Caring Relationship

In the foreward to 'Caring about carers: a national strategy for carers' Tony Blair states 'Carers devote large parts of their own lives to the lives of others – not as part of a job, but voluntarily' (DH, 1999, p3). He goes on to refer to carers transforming 'the lives of the people they are caring for' by their compassion (p3). While such phrases could be considered merely apt and well deserved recognition of the valuable role caregivers play, Blair makes the assumption that all carers are compassionate and that their care is given voluntarily and through choice. Nolan and Dellasega (2000) comment on how 'notions of choice' have become common within the rhetoric in health care planning, with an underpinning assumption that carers have chosen to care and that the overriding concern is to ensure that they are able to continue to do so.

'Caring about carers' moves on later to list what carers want, with the list headed by 'wellbeing of the person being cared for' (DH, 1999, p5), which is another assumption, one which will apply in many, but not necessarily every instance. Later 'Caring about Carers' states 'We recognise that caring is founded on close relationships. The caring role grows out of the relationship and is one which most carers undertake by choice'(DH, 1999, p13), and then 'Most caring is based on close personal relationships' (DH, 1999, p17). Thus once again, it is presented that caring based on a close relationship is the 'norm' with caregiving chosen and desired by the carer. However, on this occasion the Department of Health does state that *most* carers take on the role by choice thus acknowledging, albeit weakly, that some carers do not care through choice. The possibility that some people may not want to care is thus barely acknowledged; the underlying assumption is that carers want to care, and support must be given so they will continue to do so. Furthermore, Long *et al.* (1998) asserts that caregivers are expected to undertake their role 'without regard for the positive or negative consequences of caregiving' (p1107).

It is not only in health policy that assumptions about the caregiving relationship are made. For example, it is common for nursing literature, when talking about carers to refer to those they are caring for as 'their loved ones'. In Benner and Wrubel (1989)'s discussion comparing professional caring with caregiving by relatives, they acknowledge that nurses' caring is temporary but for relatives it is ongoing, by stating: 'The patient's family must remain in a world altered or threatened by the illness of their loved one' (p393). There is no acknowledgement here that, in some instances, they may not in fact be 'loved' at all.

The Evidence of Poor Relationships Between Caregivers and those they Care for

Qureshi and Walker (1989) acknowledge that relationships between older people and their relatives are complex and difficult to measure, stating 'it is clearly not sufficient to take the existence of helping behaviour as an indicator of a good relationship' (p149).

However, they argue that asking families about the nature of their relationships is likely to evoke merely a socially acceptable response. This comment highlights the difficulty of obtaining reliable data on this issue. I examined the literature on caregiving for any examples of where relationships between caregiver and care receiver are poor, and found they tended to be embedded in general material about caregiving and given little attention or prominence. Nevertheless I did find some examples, outlined next.

Qureshi and Walker (1989) report that only 72.5 per cent of carers said they felt emotionally close to the person they were caring for. Especially where care was of a parent, 'liking' had little influence on whether or not care was given. They give a detailed example of a woman, caring for her ninety year old father, who said that she did not like him and that he had always treated her very badly, and was verbally and physically abusive – a really striking example of caring where the relationship is poor. Elsewhere, Finch (1989) starts by claiming that the quality of the relationship between the two people is central to support being given, stating that 'The idea that anyone would give significant social or practical support to someone for whom they had hostile – or even neutral – feelings seems inherently implausible' (p159). Nevertheless, she proceeds to review some studies which suggest that, particularly in relation to care of older parents, levels of emotional closeness can impact little on the care actually given, supporting the findings of Qureshi and Walker (1989). Finch (1989) discusses the reasons for this, for example is it that the obligation to care for one's parents is so strong that it overrides the quality of the relationship? She states that there is a lack of evidence as to how poor a relationship has to be before the usual obligation to care is overrided.

Lewis and Meredith (1988) studied women who were caring for their mothers on a co-resident basis. They identified that eight of the forty-one women interviewed expressed very little affection towards their mothers. Seventeen of the women described their relationships with their mothers as 'Bad'. The majority of these were women who were trying to achieve a balance between other activities and responsibilities and their caregiving, and were experiencing great tension. A significant minority had no support from either other family members or health professionals. In some instances a relationship which had been positive deteriorated during caregiving, as the women found their mothers increasingly demanding, manipulative and domineering.

Jansson *et al.* (1998) explored motivation for caring, her study sample of caregivers comprising fifteen daughters and two nieces, who were caring for ageing relatives (mothers and aunts) with dementia. While the majority expressed positive feelings about caring, two daughters had a poor relationship with their mothers and had no feelings of closeness, nor positive feelings about the caring role. They felt there was no alternative but to care due to the absence of other family members, thus implying they felt an obligation to be carers. They had had a poor and problematic relationship with their mothers throughout their lives and stated that caring was a duty. Interestingly, at the time of the study, both of their mothers were now living in care homes and thus their physical care was being carried out professionally. Yet they clearly still felt they should visit and support their mothers, despite their poor relationship. Jansson *et al.* (1998) propose that when interventions are planned the nature of past interaction between the caregiver and the care receiver should be taken into account as caregivers often experience more stress when their relationship with those they care for is poor. However professionals may find such conversations difficult; it is altogether easier to assume that carers want to care, unless the reverse is overtly discussed.

In Noonan *et al.*'s (1999) study, comprising of interviews with sixty five caregivers, there is just one example of a caregiver whose mother was absent for much of her childhood, thus preventing a relationship from forming, and she was brought up by her father, now diseased. This respondent described the burden of being a carer saying 'She wants me more and more and I have two homes....And sometimes ...you get tired'. However she also reports that caring for her mother has restored her to her: '[I] get overwhelmed when I think about the relationship now that I have with her...It's close. It's something you really should have when you're growing up and not when you're ...an adult'. Thus caregiving appeared to allow her to establish a relationship with her once-estranged mother. This caregiver was strongly opposed to nursing homes and determined that she would keep her mother in her own home, which seems a remarkable commitment given the history of their relationship.

A study by Opie (1994), based in New Zealand, examined twenty eight caregivers of people with confusion, of which eighteen were female (7 wives, 9 daughters, 2 daughters-in-law), six were husbands and four were sons. The study reported one example of a poor caregiving relationship. This was a daughter-in-law who had had a long and very bitter relationship with her mother-in-law and had refused, until just prior to the interview, to be involved in her care. There is no further information given about this example, in particular it would have been interesting to know what had made her ultimately decide to be involved despite the poor relationship. Opie states that each individual caregiver's situation is different, that stereotyping on the basis of gender should be avoided, and that caring is partially determined by individual life history. She suggests that how people care is also affected by personal disposition, gender and their caring career, and she identifies different affective positions caregivers may be placed in within the field of caring. One of these relates specifically to where there is a poor relationship. The four positions are:

Commitment to Care

Opie considers that the crux of this is the caregiver's relationship with the dependent person – its significance, historically and currently. She proposes that it is also affected by competing demands and where the carer feels they can make a positive contribution.

Obligation to Care

This is where caring is carried out as a 'social, moral and gendered duty' (p42) rather than a desire. Obligation lacks the absoluteness of commitment. Caregivers in the 'obligation' category often have more competing demands e.g. family commitments and work. Opie suggests that because of obligation in relation to filial obligation and duty, or in relation to marital duty, it is difficult to attempt to terminate or refuse to accept the obligation to care.

Dissociation

Here caring is carried out with psychological or physical restrictions on the level of involvement. Opie observed that carers sometimes went through this stage before withdrawing their care. She suggests dissociation does not reflect lack of concern but is a more limited commitment, with other responsibilities given priority and the demands contained. Relationships between caregiver and dependent are distantly friendly rather than close. She argues that establishing these limits in caregiving may reduce stress but may require some degree of rationalisation of the moral implications of adopting this position. She states that a dissociated position has tended to be defined as masculine, that it carries a negative undertone, and implies moral failure: that the caregiver does not care enough. However, this dissociated stance allows caregivers to evaluate their resources and responsibilities in a more rational way.

Repudiation and Caring

Here the caregiver has to actively care while repudiating any desire to do so. Relationships between caregiver and cared for are characterised by anger, fear and resentment, often due to their historical relationship (which may include childhood abuse or marital violence). This situation can, Opie advises, lead to depression in caregivers as they turn their anger inwards. Opie presents examples of carers who moved into this position because caring had become destructive due to its burden. She offers no examples of carers who started off in this position (as in the example cited earlier, from Qureshi and Walker, 1989). Opie notes that, despite this far from ideal situation, caregivers in this position were still unable to abandon caring due to their socially defined responsibilities and feelings of guilt. In fact, Opie claims that 'the greater the guilt, the greater the impossibility of withdrawing from the caring relationship' (p. 46). She argues that the interaction between relationship, gender, and social knowledge combine within a repudiatory position to make it almost impossible for the caregiver to stop caring.

Opie presents these categories as a matrix and states that people may move positions within it, or straddle across categories. Opie highlights the importance of health and social care professionals raising the quality of the relationship, acknowledging the positions from which caring is conducted and that caring relationships may fail. However, gaining the perspective of both parties, while desirable, may be challenging. In addition, if the professional becomes aware of a poor relationship between the caregiver and the person they are caring for, they are then faced with the dilemma of how to address the situation. If the poor relationship has led to abuse, and of course professionals should be alert to this possibility, then their action will be more clear cut but in many instances the care given may be quite adequate and the person cared for content with the situation.

Opie's (1994) paper was the only one in the literature examined which studied in detail the premise that people do care for others within a poor relationship, where there is a lack of closeness or affection. However, she does not explore why people feel they must be caregivers despite seemingly every justification not to do so in some instances.

In summary, the literature highlighted the extensiveness of caregiving for older people in society today, and that making assumptions that caregiving relationships are voluntary and loving is beneficial both politically and socially. Only one paper examined in the literature review (Opie, 1994) gave significant attention to the nature of caregiving relationships, and explicitly analysed the different forms of relationship acknowledging in some cases the relationship might be poor. Other examples of caregiving within poor relationships were identified, but not explored in any depth in the papers reporting them. There is clearly a dearth of research in this area, yet the literature review confirmed that such relationships do exist, despite being largely ignored and unacknowledged, it would appear, by politicians and professionals. In the next section I am going to describe my research method, it is certainly not an easy topic that can be studied through interviewing, for example; a more indirect approach seemed necessary.

THE STUDY

Due to the lack of research in this area, I believed an exploratory approach would be most appropriate, and I based my approach on the interpretative biographical method. This approach includes the collection and study of personal life-stories, accounts and narratives (Denzin, 1989). Denzin (1989) explains the biographical method as being an approach to studying human experience with the aim of grasping the meaning of people's experiences. He highlights that there are many forms of the interpretative biographical method and a variety of terms are used. He defines a 'personal experience story' as where people talk about their own personal experience, which are often anecdotal everyday experiences. My intention was to collect a small number of personal life experiences, which I could examine in depth, to offer insights which could be drawn on for future work in this area. The aims were:

1. To identify situations where people care for older relatives despite having a poor relationship with them.
2. To investigate the motives of people who care for older relatives when the relationship is poor.

The topic is a delicate one, and as discussed earlier, appears unacknowledged in health policy documents. Accessing people who could offer personal life experiences of the issue I was interested in would, I felt, be sensitive and potentially problematic. Therefore, at this exploratory stage, I informally asked the following questions of friends, with healthcare backgrounds:

- 'Have you ever encountered a situation professionally where a relative who is a caregiver for an older person, admitted to you that they have a poor relationship?'
- 'Do you personally know, or have known, anyone caring for an older relative within a poor relationship?'
- 'Do you have any personal experience of caring for an older relative, within a poor relationship'?

People who replied affirmatively to any of the above were then asked if they would be willing to provide a written description of the situation.

I was aiming to collect stories from people with direct or indirect experience of the situation I was interested in. Coffey and Atkinson (1996) claim that asking for stories is an obvious way for people to retell key experiences or events, as people commonly use stories in everyday interactions. I believed this could be an insightful way of exploring the complexity of caregiving where the history of the relationship may be of central importance. Interpretation of material gathered from the biographical method can take many forms. I attempted to make sense of the personal life experiences by examining them in relation to the literature, firstly by using Opie's (1994) categories to identify, from this theoretical framework, what type of relationship existed between caregiver and their relative. This analysis is presented within the 'Results'. Then in the discussion I examine motives for caregiving, in relation to the stories collected. Here I was examining the relationship between social processes and personal lives, which has been termed 'interpretative interactionism' (Denzin, 1989).

RESULTS

I found that most people I informally talked to had encountered situations in their professional practice where they and other staff had suspected that the caregiving relationship was poor. However, they confirmed my own experience, which was that it was a difficult, personal topic to raise, and that they felt that family relationships are private matters, and to ask direct questions would be intrusive. Some expressed that it is unusual for relatives to openly admit to not liking the person they are caring for as they tend to behave as they feel they are expected to. Outside their professional experience several knew of situations where people were caring for older relatives with whom they had a poor relationship. One person was herself in such a situation. From my informal questions I obtained one story drawn from professional experience, two stories drawn from people's personal contacts, and one story drawn from personal experience. All names and identifying details have been changed to maintain anonymity. Here they are analysed in relation to Opie's (1994) categories of caregiving relationships.

Story A. Doris and John

The person offering this story knew the couple personally, not as a health professional.

> I met the couple, Doris and John, when they were in their late sixties. John had advanced Parkinson's disease and Doris was his carer. I observed that she kept the house and garden immaculate and fed and clothed John. She did her duty as a carer. However I noticed that she rarely addressed a direct remark to him and never had a conversation with him. It seemed obvious that Doris resented John, and as I got to know the couple she admitted to me that she loathed him. She also told me about their lives together.
>
> The couple had met and married in their early twenties when John was in the RAF in the second world war. After the war, John had a job on the fringes of show business working for a company that sold scripts. The job involved lots of socializing in the West end of London, on which John thrived, while Doris looked after the home and children in the suburbs. The marriage became increasingly fragile as the couple lived separate lives. John was a catholic and Doris, though not a catholic, took her obligations to the catholic church seriously, making divorce out of the question. However at the age of forty five, John developed Parkinson's disease and by the time the couple were in their late fifties, John was very disabled and dependent on Doris. He had retired and although he managed one more trip abroad to visit a sister alone he was mainly housebound.
>
> John was over 70 years old when he died and until the last six months, when he moved into a nursing home, he was cared for by Doris. I always felt he lived so long to spite her. Somehow the relationship however negative seemed necessary for both of them. Interestingly Doris, an apparently fit woman, died eighteen months after John from breast cancer.

Clearly Doris and John would have been in contact with various professionals as John's illness progressed. However, it would no doubt have been difficult if not impossible for Doris to admit her true feelings towards John to any visiting health care professionals, nor to staff she might have encountered, had he been admitted to hospital. To most people Doris probably appeared to be devotedly and voluntarily caring for her much loved husband.

In relations to Opie's work (1994) discussed earlier, the caregiving relationship here appears to be one of 'obligation' – the expectation that, as John's wife, she would care for her increasingly disabled husband despite their hitherto poor relationship. Caregiving carried out as a marital duty makes it hard to refuse to care (Opie, 1994). Doris's caregiving also clearly fell into the category of 'repudiation'. From the story offered, it is difficult to identify whether her caregiving fell into this category from the start, or whether feelings of repudiation had increased during the period of time spent caregiving. It appeared her resentment derived and enlarged at feeling obliged to care for her husband with whom her relationship had been poor for much of their marriage.

Story B. Sandra and Alice

This story was offered by a close friend of 'Sandra'. She knew the difficulty of the relationship before Sandra became Alice's caregiver. Sandra explained her caregiving as being about duty, and not feeling she had any choice.

> Sandra (who qualified as a nurse, but is not currently working as one) and Phillip (both in their late 40s) married in their early twenties, and have two sons, both at university. Phillip's parents (his mother in particular) never liked Sandra from the start and were always unpleasant to her, because she did not match their expectations of who their son should marry. Sandra initially tried hard to form a relationship with them but found it impossible, and formed a strong dislike for them in return, particularly her mother-in-law, Alice. There were long periods when they had no contact at all, and Sandra was particularly hurt at the lack of interest they showed in their grandsons. However, when her father-in-law died, as Alice was now in her late 80s, and increasingly frail with developing dementia, Sandra and Phillip moved her in to live with them and care for her. Phillip works and lives away during the week so Sandra takes the brunt of the care for a woman with whom she has always had a poor relationship. Alice does have a daughter, with whom she always had an amicable relationship, but she plays no part in her care. Sandra feels she's expected to care for Alice because of her nursing background.

In relation to Opie's (1994) theory, this is clearly another example of 'Repudiation', with the poor relationship established at the start of caregiving, rather than developing because of it. However, the category of 'obligation' also seems strong here with filial duty playing a central role. It is interesting in this story that it was Alice's son and daughter-in-law who appears to feel obliged to care rather than Alice's daughter. How Alice treated Sandra in the past appears to have had no impact on feelings of obligation to care. Sandra, being a nurse by background, appears to feel that as she has knowledge and skills of caring, she is morally obliged to use them.

Story C. Carol

This story was the professional experience of 'Carol'.

> At work, as an Accident and Emergency nurse, I looked after an older woman who was accompanied by her middle aged daughter who was her main carer. The patient was querulous and demanding, both of me and her daughter. The daughter became angry and started to shout at her mother. I intervened, I can't remember exactly how, and the daughter and I left the cubicle. I empathised with the daughter. I told her that my mother had lived with me for five years before she died and I understood how difficult it could be, living with a parent. The daughter then said that she didn't like her mother, with whom she now lived and cared for. She was, she said, difficult and manipulative – and always had been - and the daughter felt trapped, resentful and embarrassed by her mother's behaviour. The incident passed. However, sometime later I met her daughter in Accident and Emergency again. I didn't recognise her although she remembered me, and said she remembered I had been kind to her.

The daughter (and others in a similar situation) might have felt afraid that staff would judge her for her actions and words towards her mother. The empathetic response from Carol probably felt supportive, which was why the daughter remembered her as being kind, and also why she openly admitted to her that she disliked her mother for whom she was caring. This story was different from the others so far discussed in that it resembles more of a 'critical incident' – a brief snapshot of experience. This is the sort of story staff particularly in acute care experience repeatedly. They rarely know the full background and history leading up to an event like this, and may not wish to draw firm conclusions from an event lasting just a few minutes. However, as suggested earlier, to openly admit dislike for the person a relative is caring for is uncommon. In relation to Opie's categories, obligation (filial duty) could be assumed to be relevant here, but the patient's daughter is also in a position of 'repudiation', from what she said to Carol.

Story D. Gina and George

This story was the personal experience of one person asked, who is a nurse.

> My father died when I, and my siblings, were very young. Two years later my mother married George, who was some years older than her, out of financial necessity. She often said that she knew within two weeks of being married to him that she had made the worst mistake of her life but she remained married to him until she died, as she did not believe in divorce.
>
> My stepfather was a difficult man. He was very jealous of my father and would allow no photos or mention of him in the house, hard for my mother who continued to grieve for him until the day she died. He disliked noise and we had to keep very quiet when he was around. He was an unsociable man who disliked visitors or visiting, and my mother was frequently embarrassed by his rudeness to her friends. He expected my mother to devote her life to him and spend no time with anyone else. He disliked holidays so she wasn't allowed them either. He had a fierce temper and frequently shouted very loudly which frightened me as a child and this fear has never left me as an adult; I still do anything to avoid causing voices to be raised. He also hit us although, for the 1960s in England, this was probably no more than many

biological parents did. As I went through my childhood my mother used me, her only daughter, as her confidante. I was brought up to despise my stepfather as she did and from an early age had no dialogue with him at all. As I entered my teens I looked for employment which would enable me to leave home as soon as possible, which I did, and I married at eighteen years old.

After I left home I did of course visit my mother regularly but never again stayed under her roof. She continued to express her misery to me. As my stepfather got older we expected that eventually she would have a few years of freedom and we planned what she would be able to do. He was considerably older than her so it never occurred to us that she might die first. But she did, dying after a short vicious illness leaving my stepfather, now in his eighties, living alone. He was at this point reasonably physically fit but had failing eyesight and had never looked after himself even when he was younger. I only lived a few miles away, I had no excuse and I simply fell into a caregiving role for him.

I can honestly say I never envisaged having to care for him but I have done so for several years now. To start with he would accept little paid help – in the house or garden – and although this has improved, it is still minimal. I carry out gardening, housework and laundry – filling in for what the small amount of paid help can do. I handle his finances as he can see very little now, I deal with his post and oversee health care. As he has become frailer, I have taken on more personal care. I have to be present when he has a bath as he has fallen several times, I help him change his clothes, I shave him and I wash his hair. I often cannot believe that I am doing these things for him. This is the man with whom I had no relationship and who I was brought up to hate. This is the man who I am convinced drove my mother to an early grave through the stress of living with him. This is the man who shortly after my mother died embarked on a series of infatuations with young women causing me embarrassment and fury. He even manipulated to spend the first anniversary of my mother's death with one of these women, causing me great distress.

The year after my mother died I went to visit an old friend of my mother's. She had been talking to George on the phone and he had told her about the care I was giving. She said to me: 'Why are you doing this? You have more than enough to do. You have your own family to care for. He wasn't a good stepfather to you and he made your mother's life a misery'. I didn't know what to say because I didn't know the answer. Why was I looking after him? It certainly wasn't because I cared about him. I wasn't doing it for my mother either. In fact sometimes I feel guilty – like I'm betraying her.

One health care professional I involved early on was the health care advisor for older people. I have had a number of conversations with her and she visits regularly to monitor his coping alone at home. I honestly think she assumes I am a loving daughter and refers to George in an affectionate way as 'Your Dad'. Last year he was very ill and was admitted to hospital. As always, I carried out my duties impeccably. I visited at least daily, liaised between the hospital staff and his other relatives. I took his washing and brought him in food he liked. At one point when he was extremely ill the doctor hinted that they would need to decide how far they took his active treatment. I feared that the doctor would involve me in the decision – after all it is considered good practice to involve relatives in such decisions. Luckily the situation did not arrive.

These days I carry out the care in, I believe, an objective, resigned and efficient way, and to some extent, I feel proud that I have managed to do it. I have learnt how to talk with him and basically how to survive the situation, and in some ways I feel we have, despite everything, developed a sort of relationship. He does always thank me and I know he speaks well of me to other people.

This account resembles more a 'life story', defined as a person's story of their life, or a part thereof, often in a narrative, storytelling form (Denzin, 1989). It might also be considered a chronicle, defined by Coffey and Atkinson (1996) as an account of events and decisions, such as those which led up to Gina becoming a caregiver for George. A chronicle type of narrative can give insights into how the past relates to the present (Richardson, 1990), and this is evident within the story above.

This story highlights many issues relating to caregiving. For example, Smith *et al.* (2003) state that: 'Older people often prefer to be assisted informally'. George needed care but was reluctant to have formal, paid care, preferring to be given unpaid informal care from his stepdaughter, despite their poor relationship. But the central question arising from Gina's story is: why is she caring for George? Gina herself has no explanation; she simply does it. In relation to Opie's (1994) categories of caregiving, it appears that Gina started from a position of repudiation but has moved to one of dissociation. But straddled across both of these is possibly 'obligation' as she appears to suggest it was just something she had to do.

Opie's (1994) categories, used to examine the caregiving relationships in the stories above, highlighted the complexity of the caregiving relationship as it was clear that no one category represented any of the relationships. The framework gave little insight, however into motives behind caregiving other than that obligation seems a powerful factor. The discussion centres on examining why people are caregivers to older people with whom they have a poor relationship.

DISCUSSION

The Department of Health's (1999) view is that carers care 'for reasons of love, loyalty, friendship or support for others' (p11), which presents a very positive perspective of the motives for caring. However the stories presented above provide a different perspective, and an examination of the literature reveals a more complex situation too.

Ungerson (1983) analyses why women care, arguing that caring *about* someone, and caring *for* someone, are two different things. Caring about someone relates to an emotion, but caring for someone may have little to do with caring about. She identifies that caring for someone might be based on affection, but could be based on any of the following:

- payment
- feelings of compassion for all people
- societal expectation.

She also points out other differences between caring for and caring about. Caring for someone takes time while caring about someone may not. Caring for someone entails addressing their needs and may arise through a socially (rather than affectionately) based obligation, through payment, or through social norms. Gina, in story D, is a nurse, and therefore a professional carer as well as an informal one, and Sandra also qualified as a nurse. As nurses, it could be even more difficult to resist the social norm of caring for a needy ageing relative.

Ungerson's (1983) point out that caregivers may choose to care because of a general (rather than specific) feeling of compassion is an interesting one and several writers have presented the view of caring as being part of being a human. For example, Graham (1983), in exploring the nature of caring (in the context of informal family caring) states that an analysis suggests that caring requires both love and labour and is seen as a basic human emotion, part of everyday life and which all humans wish to experience. Thus the caregivers featured in the stories might have been afraid of not appearing human, had they declined to take on their caring roles. Roach (2002), a nurse who writes about nursing, and caring within nursing, from a Christian perspective, proposes that caring is the human mode of being, stating that: 'An individual cares not because of his or her particular role but because he or she is a human being' (p38). Roach believes that to care is integral to being human and that it is essential to human development. From this viewpoint, then, some people might become caregivers because of a general feeling that is the right thing to do, as one human to another. This introduces a moral dimension to family caregiving. These issues are discussed in other chapters in this volume, in particular Katila in chapter 2 and Paoletti in chapter 1; the moral dimension appears quite central to the caregiving experience.

Finch (1989) argues that where members of a family are caring for another it should not be assumed that the motive is obligation or duty but that the reasons may be more complex than that. However, she asserts that the quality of the relationship does not appear to determine the strength of obligation to provide support, and this certainly seems to be so in the stories examined earlier. She argues that simply asking people their motives for caring does not necessarily give the full answer as people often wish to present themselves and their family in the best light. Thus even if health professionals raised the issue of Gina's relationship with George, she may not wish to divulge her personal feelings. Lewis and Meredith (1988), in their study of co-resident women caring for their mothers, found a variety of reasons but expectations of other family members were a major motivator. However many women saw caring for their mothers as 'natural' and simply drifted into it. Affection and obligation were identified in a varying balance, and reciprocity featured strongly. A common response was 'Well, it's your mum'.

In an Ireland-based study, carers interviewed stated that they took on caregiving out of loyalty and love for the family member, and they expressed satisfaction with their role and said it gave them a purpose (Lane *et al.* 2003). However the interviewees were a self selected sample. In a study by Pickard and Glendinning (2001), of older people caring for older people with dementia, some carers expressed that they saw their caring as the continuation of the close relationship they had enjoyed during their marriage, highlighting again the significance of a relationship in caregiving. For example one respondent had been married to his wife who had Parkinson's disease for over sixty years and only once had they been apart when he had to work away for six weeks. Kane *et al.* (1999) studied caregiving by families following hospitalization for a stroke or a hip fracture by carrying out telephone interviews, using open-ended questions, with 307 caregivers. The study found that few experienced no or little satisfaction in their caring role, with fifty per cent of all the respondents mentioning a sense of achievement and they frequently mentioned the sense of affection experienced while giving care as a source of satisfaction. They also referred to reciprocity and closer family bonds. Clearly, for some people motives for caregiving are positive in nature, and if these are common emotions it makes it even more difficult for people experiencing more negative feelings to admit to their very different emotions. Kane *et al.* (1999) also found that approximately 20 per cent of respondents mentioned a sense of duty as being their motivator. This is looked at in more detail later.

In Jansson *et al.*'s study (1998), which applied attachment theory to understanding motivation for caring, eleven of the daughters expressed positive feelings about caring. Many of the caregivers felt they had experienced personal growth, for example, they had become more mature, a feeling hinted at by Gina, when she talks of feeling proud that, despite everything, she has managed to care for George. However, this is clearly not her motivation for caring, merely a positive if unexpected effect of the situation. The motives for caregiving of the women in Jansson *et al.*'s study, were commonly cited as affection, reciprocity, and duty. Most of the daughters had warm and affectionate feelings towards their parent, had had a good relationship with them throughout their lives and found caring for them to be natural. Jansson *et al.* suggest that these feelings derive from childhood experiences. In many other instances of caregiving, however, the relationship – good or poor – is formed as adults so this theory is not applicable to these situations. In Gina's story, her childhood experiences with the man she is now caring for were predominantly negative ones and attachment theory appears to have no relevance to motives for her caregiving.

Two particularly dominant motives arising from the literature about reasons for caregiving are reciprocity, and duty/obligation, and these are discussed in more detail next.

Reciprocity

Finch (1989) writes extensively about the notion of reciprocity, noting that historians view reciprocal exchange as the essence of support between kin. However, she observes that this has varied during different historical periods, and therefore support across the ages cannot be compared. She suggests that support must be seen in the context of interpersonal relationships between those concerned, as each relationship has a past, a present and a future. In a later publication Finch (1995) highlights that reciprocity in relation to parents can vary widely between siblings, depending on the amount of care and help given from parents to individual children in the past. Thus adults who had the greatest levels of support from their parents felt the strongest commitment to caring for them in return. But as health care professionals, this knowledge is something we are rarely party to: we do not know (unless, exceptionally, as in story C 'Carol', relatives choose to tell us), what the relationship between caregiver and care receiver has been, and we should not make assumptions about this, for example, judge it in the light of our own family relationships. It seems that none of the health care professionals involved in George's care are aware of the background to his relationship with Gina (story D). Thus when health professionals are supporting informal carers they should be open-minded about relationship histories, their impact on caregiving and reciprocity.

In a study by Bornat *et al.* (1999a) interviewees were asked about willingness to care for their parents when they became older and unwell. Reciprocity featured highly in their responses. For example, one woman is quoted as saying she would look after her mother if the need arose commenting 'she's always been there for me'. However she did not feel the same desire to care for her father who had left home when she was a teenager, commenting he 'can rot'. But another woman, whose mother had left home leaving her young children behind, and with whom she continued to have a poor relationship, still thought she would care for her if needed because 'At the end of the day she's still my mum'. It should be noted that none of these people were currently caring for their parents, and might behave differently should they encounter the situation. In story B, Sandra may have thought she would not be prepared to care for Alice, as their relationship had been so poor, but when the situation arose she ended up doing so. Similarly, Gina herself states she had never contemplated she would end up caring for George.

Finch and Mason (1993) propose that responsibilities to care are built up over time, resulting from reciprocity in giving and receiving help. In studies examining motivation for caregiving, reciprocity often emerges strongly, and was mentioned in several of those reviewed earlier. For example, in Heenan's (2000) study of thirteen older people who were cared for by daughters or daughter-in-laws in a farming community, a typical comment was: 'She spent the best years of her life looking after my husband and family so it is not much to expect us to look after her'. Walker (1994)'s work on caregiving focused on the care daughters give to their aging mothers and her findings suggested that caregiving occurs against the backdrop of intergenerational assistance. She highlights the impact of the quality of the relationship, and states that although this might seem obvious, the literature has not taken this approach, focusing more on the burden of caregiving without considering its context. She identified most mother-daughter relationships are not stormy or conflicted though she describes a few whose relationship was conflicted and which were unrewarding. She argues that there is an overemphasis on caregiving burdens and that the impression given is that caregiving is fraught with anguish, misery and suffering but that the situation is much more complex with caregiver daughters who are caring for women who loved them, and who cared for them as dependent children and to whom they are very attached.

In examining the stories, reciprocity does not appear central to motivation for caregiving, but it may still have relevance. In story A, Doris may feel as John provided for the family financially she should care for him in return. In story B, while Sandra has not experienced care and support from Alice, she may feel that she is caring on her husband's behalf, as Alice brought him up as a child. In story 'C', the daughter may feel that as her mother cared for her as a child, she owes her care in return, despite their poor adult relationship. In story D, while Gina gives no impression of reciprocity in relation to care being relevant, it is implied that George did provide for her mother and family financially. In none of these stories does reciprocity in the form of love and affection appear to be motivation for caregiving.

Obligation/Duty

Finch (1995) identifies that there is a specific obligation to care entered into as part of the marriage contract, which is a step taken voluntarily in adult life. In story A, Doris clearly took these marriage vows seriously, and carried out her obligation to John, despite their poor relationship. However caring for older relatives in most other situations carries no such obligations.

Finch (1989) notes that formerly, the issue of caring for older relatives rarely arose as few people lived into long infirm old age so whether people today have less or more obligation to care for older relatives is not a valid question. Finch argues therefore that the 'golden age' which is often referred to, when family responsibilities were stronger than they are today, is clearly a myth, without any historical foundation. Obligation, or duty, as a motive for caregiving is prominent within the literature, and will next be examined in relation to story D: is Gina obliged to care for George, despite the poor relationship? Smith *et al.* (2003) state there has been little attention paid to the perceived obligations of adult children towards their parents.

Up until 1948, there was a legal requirement in Britain for adult children to provide for their parents financially thus the concept of family obligations was embodied within the law (Finch, 1989). The origins of these family obligations lie in the Poor Law, established in 1601, and remained little changed until 1948. Since 1948, only legal obligations between spouses, and between parents and immature children, remain. However Finch notes that obligations for giving practical (rather than economic) care to adults have developed from social and economic policy rather than the law. Finch proposes that there was a widely held belief (though not explicitly stated) developed in the 1950s, and sustained afterwards, that it is the responsibility of women to stay at home and look after dependent people. She argues that policy documents in the 1980s gave a clear message that care by family and friends should be considered the normal situation with care by the state supplementary or provided if no care by family was available. There is pressure, she states, for unpaid care to be provided by people sharing a household with older people, or adult children; both these categories held obligations under Poor Law until 1948. She considers that although this obligation is not now enforced by law, direct pressure can be applied by professional workers. Other countries also have a history of there being a legal obligation for adult children to care for their parents, for example Sweden (Jansson *et al.*,1998), and Germany (Dallinger, 2002). As in the UK, this obligation no longer exists but there remains a strong social expectation for such responsibilities to be upheld.

Finch (1989) discusses the obligations between different members of families identifying linear links (parent – child) as stronger than lateral links (siblings) and that obligations to one's own kin take precedence over a spouse's. In Finch's exploration step-families are never referred to, and in fact are rarely mentioned in any of the literature in caregiving. Finch (1989) discusses the 'special' nature of kin relationships and identifies the 'blood tie' as one aspect of this. Thus, should Gina feel a reduced sense of duty or obligation towards George because he is her stepfather, with no blood tie, rather than being her biological father? It is impossible to identify whether obligations to step-parents, in relation to caregiving, are seen as identical to those of biological parents. Clarke (1995) discusses the impact of changing family structures on informal care for older people, identifying that familial obligations in such circumstances are complex, and implications for care unclear. Bornat *et al.* (1999b) debate the nature of stepfamilies and propose that they vary extensively, from being a step-parent who has, as in Gina's case, been present through most of her life, to those who may be present for a few months only. The people they interviewed in their study of families who had undergone change, did not like using the prefix 'step', as it appeared to carry a stigma. They give few examples specifically relating to step-parent-child relationships but cite one older man who said he sees more of his step-daughter than of his own daughter. However he still intended to leave all the inheritance to his daughter, highlighting the strength of blood ties.

Jones *et al.* (1995) identify that step-relationships are usually more distant, involve more conflict and are less satisfying than relationships with biological parents, with bonds between children and stepparents weaker. The blood tie, they state, is still hugely symbolic but younger children more easily develop a bond with stepparents. However this clearly varies according to each family's dynamics and was not the case in Gina's experience. Jones *et al.* cite studies demonstrating the negative impact that having stepparents has on children but these studies were done with children of divorced parents and it is not possible to discern whether it is the divorce or the remarriage that causes the problems. Similarly Miles (1994) lists a number of detrimental effects of step-parents on children but again the analysis is linked to families affected by divorce, rather than death. Allen and Perkins (1995) note that caregiving in stepfamilies may be affected by resentments from the past, as well as lacking the important factor of reciprocity. The number of reconstituted families is increasing and though the literature about stepfamilies has grown, much remains unknown (Coleman *et al.*, 2000).

Qureshi and Walker (1989) identified that people felt society would judge them if they did not care for their parents, giving examples of media articles which have cast criticism in such situations. Several researchers have attempted to explore whether there is a general view in society that people have a duty to be caregivers. Wenger *et al.*'s (2002) study, based in a rural area of North Wales, found that support from children to older parents was still seen as normative behaviour. Smith *et al.* (2003) also carried out a survey in Wales to ascertain the public's views of obligations to care. The questions asked included whether respondents would regard the provision of care a duty, an obligation and a personal responsibility. Only seventeen respondents (all females) of the 174 respondents were currently involved in giving informal care. Of these, eight were happy to do so, four were resigned to doing so and five were very unhappy about it. The results indicated that females were consistently more willing to provide informal care than males even if the older person was ill or disabled. The reasons cited for providing care were pleasure of the older person's company, and to enable contact with the respondents' children. Only 16 per cent of respondents had made plans to care for older relatives implying that the possibility of becoming a caregiver, as in Gina's case, may not really be thought about. When asked who should provide care for older people, 70 per cent believed the state should do so while 30 per cent thought it was the family's responsibility. However, in relation to themselves, only 43 per cent of males and 33 per cent of females expected the state to care for them, and 44 per cent of women expected their children to look after them – a sizeable minority. The majority of respondents (80%) believed that the burden of care falls mainly on daughters yet 92 per cent stated it should be shared by men and women. The survey found that two thirds of women would feel guilty about putting an older relative into a home. Smith *et al.* highlight that guilt is a powerful emotion and that informal care should not be exploited to meet political and fiscal objectives.

The social acceptability of caregiving has also been identified in Ireland, with O'Neill and Evans (2001) finding that members of the public who were not carers had a favourable attitude to informal care: 71 per cent stated that they would be prepared to provide care. Heenan (2000) highlighted that the women in her study were very aware of cultural norms about giving care for one's own family and felt proud about being able to do so. When asked about reasons for becoming a carer, the strongest theme to emerge was that it was natural and not questioned, and part of being married to a farmer. Comments were made like: 'Families care for each other don't they?' Lane *et al.*'s (2003) study, also based in Ireland, found that although, as referred to earlier, carers identified loyalty and love as reasons for caregiving, in some instances they had felt they had no choice to care, for example, 'I was the oldest in my family, the only girl, I was the one who was left'. Some carers' sense of obligation was so great that they made amazing sacrifices, living away from their families. Despite this, some of the study's participants stated that in Ireland the strong culture that people should care for their families has gone.

A survey by Finch and Mason (1993) found that 57 per cent of respondents felt that there were circumstances under which it would be reasonable to refuse to provide personal help for a sick or elderly relative, while 37 per cent disagreed (implying that whatever the circumstances, help should be given). Another question they asked related to an older person living alone with no relatives except for a niece and nephew living nearby. The question asked whether they should help with shopping and providing a little help in the home. Sixty eight per cent of respondents believed they should and only 21 per cent disagreed. Respondents were also asked to respond to this statement: 'Children have no obligation to look after their parents when they are old'. Only 39 per cent agreed, with 58 per cent disagreeing with the statement. All these results give strong support to the view that a sizeable number of people do believe there is an obligation to care for older relatives. Thus even if there is a poor relationship, people may prefer to take on the caregiving role as expected by society rather than face possible criticism. There is, however, as discussed by Finch (1995), no consensus on the exact nature of the obligation between an adult child to their parents.

In story D, Gina stated that when she took on the caregiving role she had 'no excuse' and in particular she 'lived only a few miles away'. Finch (1989) states that it is common sense that the geographical distance between relatives will affect whether support can be given, but that there is no simple equation between geographical distance and level of support. What would a legitimate excuse be not to care? Finch and Mason (1993) examine this issue in relationship to family responsibilities, identifying employment, other family commitments, competence, geographical distance, and lack of resources as possible legitimate excuses. However, the quality of relationship between the parties (past or present) was not identified as a factor. Both gender and genealogical relationship were found to affect the acceptability of excuses. For example, women and people belonging to a parent-child relationship were less likely to have excuses for not caring being accepted. Finch and Mason believe legitimacy is important because people want others to see their excuses as legitimate (thus preventing judgement). In stories B and D, the caregivers, being nurses, might have felt excuses not to care would be less likely to be accepted as people may consider they have the attributes and skills to care due to their professional backgrounds. One question Finch and Mason posed to respondents concerned a woman who had a poor relationship with her mother, who had cut her out of her will. The question asked whether if the woman was too frail to live alone anymore whether her daughter, who has room, should take her in. A sizeable minority, 37 per cent, believed she should. This result confirms that many people would not see a poor relationship as an excuse not to care.

The Decision to Care

Finch (1989) argues that decisions about supporting relatives require negotiations about all aspects, for example who by and for how long. What is negotiated is about the need of one person for support and the capacity of the other to provide it. However Opie (1994) states that 'most caregivers have little active choice in whether or not they accept caring obligations' (p39). The reality of decision-making about care-giving is that, as examined earlier, obligation to care is such a strong force, it is hard for many people to resist the caregiving role unless they have an exceptionally legitimate excuse. Thus the decision to care is made passively rather than actively.

Brereton and Nolan (2000) comment on the 'growing consensus that the transition into a care-giving role is a crucial phase' and that when it occurs suddenly, carers need to be able to make an informed choice about whether to become a carer. They state that the notion of choice is emerging as a key concept but they acknowledge that the reality is different. They go on to note that for each individual, the circumstances in which they become a carer are unique, with no simple route into the role, and that it can occur very suddenly (with little time to prepare), or more gradually. In story D, Gina became a carer suddenly because George's carer, her mother, had unexpectedly died, and she certainly does not imply that she felt she had a choice – it was just something that happened. Brereton and Nolan (2000) note that most potential carers are relatives and many feel bound by love and obligation, with emotional attachment driving the wish to care. They carried out interviews with seven carers, all spouses of people who had had a stroke. All felt morally obliged to become carers in the absence of any suitable alternatives. There was no indication in the results as to whether any choice about caring had been offered or even discussed.

Finch (1989) identifies five normative guidelines relating to the decision to care:

- The genealogical relationship with the person.
- The quality of the relationship with them.
- The pattern of exchanges with them in the past.
- The affect of giving assistance on the balance between dependence and independence in their family relationships.
- Whether it is the right time in both lives to offer this type of assistance to this particular person.

When looking at Gina's decision to care, in story D, it appears that none of these guidelines are particularly applicable but she still took on caregiving. Finch goes on to discuss how support is negotiated (often subtly and unspoken) within families. She proposes that matters concerning duties and obligations in families are the type of situations where people feel able to make strong moral judgements about others' lives, and knowing what people are likely to say, can be a powerful influence on the decision to care. These judgements may arise from people both inside and outside of the family, and people often do take public opinion into account when making moral decisions. This is because, Finch argues, people need to maintain their reputation as moral beings to prevent the undermining of their social position, see Pyysiäinen in chapter 6 for a detailed discussion of the concept of "reputation". For some people, their self identity depends on being seen as the type of people who 'do the right thing'. For Gina, being a nurse, this might have been even more pressing, particularly as George became frailer.

Conclusion

This chapter aimed to examine a little discussed dimension of caregiving, that is caregiving for older people where there is a poor relationship. From an economic viewpoint it suits both the government, and society, very well to present the view that caregiving is an actively made choice and a freely chosen activity, performed on the basis of love and affection. Thus, caregivers simply need additional support to enable them to continue. Whilst there is plenty of evidence that many caregivers do take on their role at least in part through love, and based on a long-standing close relationship, this chapter has demonstrated that this is not always the case. There are many other reasons for taking on a caregiving role, but undoubtedly some people do so through lack of an alternative pathway, because they fear the judgement of others, or through the mere fact of being the closest available human being who has some connection with the person concerned. While there may be little that health care professionals can do in such situations they should at least try to avoid making assumptions about caregivers and be prepared to listen when caregivers feel safe enough to talk to them. We also need to see through the government's rhetoric about carers and caregiving, and while many of the initiatives to support carers are to be applauded, we should not forget the government's self interest here.

Recommendations

- Assumptions and expectations relating to caregiving relationships should not go unquestioned.
- Health and social care professionals should be alert to caregivers who may care for, but not about, the person they are caring for.
- Professionals should acknowledge that they do not know the history of the relationship pre-caregiving, and should restrain from making judgements about those who make the difficult decision not to care.
- The debate about the expectations of society and government about caregiving for older people should continue.
- More research into this dimension of caregiving is needed; ways of accessing caregivers in these situations need to be found.

References

Allen, I. and Perkins, E. (1995) Discussion. In Allen, I. and Perkins, E (Eds.) *The future of family care for older people* (pp. 221-234) London: HMSO.

Benner, P. and Wrubel, J. (1989) *The primacy of caring: stress and coping in health and illness*. Menlo Park: Addison-Wesley Publishing company.

Brereton, L. and Nolan, M. (2000) 'You do know he's had a stroke, don't you?' Preparation for family care-giving – the neglected dimension. *Journal of Clinical Nursing* 9, 498-506.

Bond, J., Farrow, G., Gregson, B.A., Bamford, C., Buck, D., McNamee, P. and Wright, K. (1999) Informal caregiving for frail older people at home and in long-term care institutions: who are the key supporters? *Health and Social Care in the Community* 7(6), 434-44.

Bornat, J., Dimmock, B., Jones, D. and Peace, S. (1999a) Generational ties in the family: changing contexts for traditional obligations. In Silva, E.B. and Smart, C. (Eds.) *The new family?* (pp. 115-128). London: Sage publications.

Bornat, J., Dimmock, B., Jones, D. and Peace, S. (1999b) The impact of family change on older people: the case of stepfamilies. In McRae, S. (Ed.) *Changing Britain: families and households in the 1990s* (pp. 248-262). Oxford: Oxford University Press.

British Medical Association (1995) *Taking care of carers*. London: BMA.

Bywaters, P. and Harris, A. (1998) Supporting carers: is practice still sexist? *Health and Social Care in the Community* 6, (6), 458-63.

Clarke, L. (1995) Family care and changing family structure: bad news for the elderly? In Allen, I. and Perkins, E (Eds.) *The future of family care for older people* (pp. 19-49) London: HMSO.

Coffey, A. and Atkinson, P. (1996) *Making sense of qualitative data*. Thousand Oaks: Sage Publications.

Coleman, M., Ganong, L. and Fine, M. (2000) Reinvestigating marriage: another decade of progress. *Journal of Marriage and Family*. 62, (4), 1288-1307.

Dallinger, U. (2002) *Elderly care in the family in Germany*. Paper presented at COST 13A Meeting in Copenhagen.

Department of Health (1999) *Caring about carers: a national strategy for carers*. London: DH.

Denzin, N.K. (1989) *Interpretive biography*. Newbury Park: Sage Publications.

Finch, J. (1989) *Family obligations and social change*. Cambridge: Polity Press.

Finch, J. (1995) Responsibilities, obligations and commitments. In Allen, I. and Perkins, E (Eds.) *The future of family care for older people* (pp.51-64) London: HMSO.

Finch, J. and Mason, J. (1993) *Negotiating family responsibilities*. London: Tavistocl/Routledge

Graham, H. (1983) Caring: a labour of love. In Finch, J. and Groves, D. (Eds) *A labour of love: women, work and caring* (pp.13-30) London: Routledge and Kean Paul.

Heenan, D. (2000) Informal care in farming families in Northern Ireland: some considerations for social work. *British Journal of Social Work*. 30, 855-66.

Hochscild, A.R. (1983) *The managed heart: commercialisation of human feeling*. Berkley: University of California Press.

Jansson, W., Almberg, B., Grafstrom, M. and Winblad, B. (1998) A daughter is a daughter for the whole of her life: a study of daughters' responsibility for parents with dementia. *Health Care in Later Life*. 3, (4), 272-84.

Jones, C.L., Tepperman, L. and Wilson, S.J. (1995) *The Futures of the Family* Englewood cliffs: Prentice Hall.

Kane, R.A., Reinardy, J., Penrod, J.D. and Huck, S. (1999) After the hospitalization is over: a different perspective on family care of older people *Journal of Gerontological Social Work* 31, (1/2), 119-141.

Lane, P., McKenna, H., Ryan, A. and Fleming, P. (2003) The experience of the family caregivers' role: a qualitative study. *Research and Theory for Nursing Practice: an International Journal* 17, (2) 137-151

Lewis, J. and Meredith, B. (1988) *Daughters who care: daughters caring for mothers at home*. London: Routledge.

Long, K., Sudha, S. and Mutran, E.J. (1998) Elder-proxy agreement concerning the functional status and medical history of the older person: the impact of caregiver burden and depressive symptomatology. *Journal of American Geriatrics Society* 46, (9), 1103-11.

Miles, R. (1994) *The children we deserve*. London: Harper Collins publishers.

Nolan, M. and Dellasega, C. (2000) 'I really feel I've let him down': supporting family carers during long-term placement for elders. *Journal of Advanced Nursing* 31, 759-67.

Noonan, A.E., Tennstedt, S.L. and Rebelsky, F.G. (1999) Getting to the point: offspring caregivers and the nursing home decision *Journal of Gerontological Social Work* 31, (3/4), 5-27

O'Neill, S. and Evans, D.S. (2001) Carers in the community: the nature, extent and needs of informal care provision within the Western Health Board. *All Ireland Journal of Nursing and Midwifery* 1, (6), 201-205.

Opie, A. (1994) The instability of the caring body: gender and caregivers of confused older people. *Qualitative Health Research* 4, (1), 31-50.

Pickard, S. and Glendinning, C. (2001) Caring for a relative with dementia: the perceptions of carers and CPNs. *Quality in Ageing – policy, practice and research* 2, (4), 3-11.

Qureshi, H. and Walker, A. (1989) *The caring relationship: elderly people and their families*. Basingstoke: MacMillan.

Richardson, L. (1990) *Writing strategies: reaching diverse audiences*. Newbury Park, CA: Sage Publications.

Roach, M.S. (2002) *Caring, the human mode of being: a blueprint for the health professions*. 2nd revised edition. Ottawa: CHA Press.

Scottish Executive (1999) *Strategy for carers in Scotland*. Edinburgh: Scottish Executive.

Smith, P. (1992) *The emotional labour of caring: how nurses care*. Basingstoke: MacMillan.

Smith, S., Snelgrove, S., Armstrong-Esther, C.A. and Clark, J. (2003) Is there a future for the informal homecare of older people in a changing society? *Quality in Ageing – policy, practice and research* 4, (1) 2-21.

Ungerson, C. (1983) Why do women care? In Finch, J. and Groves, D. (eds) *A labour of love: women, work and caring*. London: Routledge and Kagan Paul, 31-49.

Walker, A. (1983) Care for elderly people: a conflict between women and the state. In Finch, J. and Groves, D. (Eds) *A labour of love: women, work and caring* (pp. 106-128). London: Routledge and Kagan Paul.

Walker, A.J. (1994) You can't be a woman in your mother's house: adult daughters and their mothers. In Sollie, D.L. and Leslie, L.A. (Eds) *Gender, families and close relationships* (pp. 74-94) Thousand Oaks: Sage Publications.

Wenger, G.C., Scott, A. and Seddon, D. (2002) The experience of caring for older people with dementia in a rural area: using services. *Aging and Mental Health* 6, (1), 30-38.

Wright, F. (1983) Single carers: employment, housework and caring. In Finch, J. and Groves, D. (Eds) *A labour of love: women, work and caring*. London: Routledge and Kagan Paul, 89-105.

In: Family Caregiving for Older Disabled People
Editor: Isabella Paoletti, pp. 151-176
ISBN 1-59454-808-0

Chapter 8

MEN, MARRIAGE AND CARE: CARING FOR A PARTNER WITH MS

Elizabeth A. Watson
College of Education and External Studies,
University of Nairobi, Kenya

INTRODUCTION

This chapter explores some of the ways in which the lives of both carer and care recipient have been shaped by a chronic illness, multiple sclerosis. It focuses on that particular caring relationship as it finds expression in later life, often in a context of a longstanding marriage in which the provision and acceptance of care, in some form, has become an accepted part. The data on which it is based form part of a study of men's caring and the original sample included men of various ages and in an array of caring situations. Here I have restricted my discussion to a subset of this group - those now in their fifties or older. The number of male carers is small (17) but the examination of the caring experience is a detailed one and suggestive of issues which need to be incorporated within the larger picture of care. Such studies continue to have value in helping us question and reassess the body of theory we have constructed around care and caring. They also have value in helping develop more adequate policy responses.

Participants were selected because they were caring for a wife with multiple sclerosis, and while the research is about care and focuses on the experience of caring, it is not possible to understand that caring circumstance without some insight into the nature of MS. Multiple sclerosis[1] is a highly variable, baffling and unpredictable disease that affects adults,

---

1 Multiple Sclerosis is a highly variable and unpredictable disease. The symptoms usually occur in early adult life although it has been found among younger and older individuals. Women are more likely than men to develop the condition. Diagnosis has been difficult. This was especially so in earlier years. before the availability of the Magnetic Resonance Imaging (MRI) scan.
MS causes damage and deterioration of the myelin covering which surrounds nerve fibres in the central nervous system. Myelin acts as an insulator and helps conduct nerve pulses or messages from nerve endings to the brain and visa versa.

predominately women, and typically 'strikes' between the ages of twenty and forty. The symptoms and the deterioration may include loss of balance and co-ordination, diminished vision, weakness of limbs, extreme fatigue (especially during hot weather), impaired speech and loss of bladder (and, sometimes, bowel) control. A person with MS might experience one, several or all of these symptoms, depending on the location and extent of damage to nerve tissue which is the mark of MS (www.msaustralia.org.au). It is important to stress that no two cases of MS are identical. At one extreme, it is a chronic, progressive and debilitating disease. At the other, it is a sudden, short-lived annoyance such as temporary blurred vision. Among those included here, there were no cases which might be described as mild. This has meant that, from the time of diagnosis and, indeed, in a number of cases from before that moment, the couples in this study were engaged in a process of reassessment of their lives and their futures which had to take account of the likelihood of increasing disability on the part of one partner and of increasing caring responsibilities on the part of the other. By the time they had reached their fifties or sixties, these impacts were clearly evident and, in a number of cases, severe.

There are a number of important elements in this study. These carers are men doing work which is essentially gendered in nature; they are involved in care that has continued over an extended period; the care is for someone with a chronic and disabling condition; that 'someone' is their partner. While all these elements are significant in the account provided here, this chapter focuses most particularly on care giving as an activity that has shaped the life of both carer and care recipient. Because we are here concerned with a sub sample of older male carers, the aim has been to understand what this extended and often demanding care has meant in everyday 'domestic' terms, what impact it has had on their paid work, what support they have received, how they have managed to care in this way for so long, what has been the impact on their marriage and how they explain what is perceived by some as a sacrifice of their own life to care for their partner.

All the elements listed above represent aspects of care that have featured less prominently in the literature on care and caring. In the first place, there are not many studies that have been devoted to the study of male carers. (The exceptions include Cahill 2000, Brown 1996.) There

---

The scarring of the myelin causes a slowing down, distortion or, in severe cases, complete blockage of the flow of messages from the nerves to the brain and back again (www.msaustralia.org.au).

The results of this deterioration or blockage and their severity are completely unpredictable and differ enormously. As noted above in the text, the physical affects include loss of balance and co-ordination, diminished vision, weakness of limbs, extreme fatigue (especially during hot weather), impaired speech and loss of bladder (and, sometimes, bowel) control. Someone with MS may experience one, several or all of these symptoms, depending on the location and extent of damage to nerve tissue (ibid.). For some who develop the disease there are also mental impairments.

The cause of MS has not yet been established, although there have been numerous theories proposed. Neither is it known what causes an exacerbation, although it is clear that certain conditions or factors may increase the likelihood of one occurring (e.g., hot weather, stress or pregnancy). Nor do we know why some people experience very few exacerbations and these are slight, while others may experience exacerbation upon exacerbation with little reprieve. The effectiveness of treatments has improved in very recent times but there is still considerable debate about appropriate treatment programmes. And because it is a highly variable disease, some treatments that work well with some patients are less useful in other cases. Uncertainty, unpredictability and a high degree of variation characterise MS.

There are two additional issues – environmental and genetic factors - that are important to note here. In general, it can be argued that the rate of occurrence of MS within populations increases as one moves further from the equator (McDonnell & Hawkins 2000). There is almost no MS among populations in tropical regions. On the other hand, among peoples living in cold climates the rate is relatively high (Kurtzke 2000; Forbes et al. 1999; Hernan et al. 1999). Thus the rate in Tasmania is considerably higher than in the far north of Queensland (van de Mei et al. 2001; Hammond et al. 2000). There is also a debate about genetic links and the propensity to pass MS on to one's children or for them to be at greater risk because a parent has developed the condition (Ebers et al. 2000; Rasmussen & Clausen 2000; Kahana 2000).

are certainly references in the research literature to male carers and there are quite a number of cases included in larger studies (Ungerson 1987; Parker 1993). However, there are few pieces of research which set out to explore the experience of being a carer from (for want of a better expression) a male perspective, i.e., few studies which attempt to explore what caring involves when you are a man and, more particularly, what sense of that experience you make, how you might explain it to others, how you perceive that others understand what you are doing and how they treat you, especially family and service providers. Informal caring is, of course, a gendered activity: (in many significant respects formal caring professions and areas of work have had to contend with that gendered association). Yet the reality is that many men do take on major caring responsibilities. In Chapter 2 Katila described the case of a male caregiver in a Finnish farming community, indicating that, given the difficulties of farmers in finding a spouse, this is relatively common occurrence. Male carers actually dominate in some sectors of the caring community, i.e., among aged couples, in the case of HIV/AIDS and, at least potentially, within the MS community. In this last case, it is because more women get MS than men (almost three times as many) and typically MS strikes in early adult years when most people are in a relationship of some kind, at least for the greater portion of the time. It would seem that people with MS tend to be in long-term partnerships and marriage relationships, or have been[2].

Detailed, phenomenological studies of this kind which have explored the caring work of men have tended to concentrate on older men caring for a spouse who is also relatively elderly and where the period of care has, typically, been confined to those later years of life and of a marriage (Bytheway 1985). There has been less attention paid to caring which has been a feature of an ongoing partnership, something which has become a 'given' in that relationship over many years, in some cases over almost the entire period of the marriage.

It is also important to note here that even though there has been a greater emphasis in the literature on care in later life, there has been a surprising lack of attention paid to spousal caring as a specific and important caring relationship. This neglect has been especially apparent in the theoretical literature. Some have argued that the very fact that male carers feature in large numbers among spousal cares may explain the apparent lack of interest on the part of feminist researchers in caring between partners. For example, Diane Gibson, writing about aged care, notes:

> 'The role of spouse carers has been less commonly articulated in connection with feminist analyses. While spouse carers figure in some of the empirical analyses, they have received less attention at a theoretical level. Yet spouses are the single largest category among carers of frail and disabled older people, and their apparent neglect in feminist work may be indicative of the 'geronto-phobic' explanation for the neglect of certain aspects of research on the aged… The fact that both sexes have been shown to care for extremely dependent spouses may also have made spouse carers a less obvious subject for feminist analysis' (1998: 73).

There are a number of other gaps and 'thin patches' in the literature on care which have been the particular concern of this study. In the empirical research on caring, the emphasis on burdens or difficulties has meant that the possibility of satisfactions or rewards or 'good

2 It is difficult to check whether this is in fact the case as the MS Society database does not include marital status and, in any event, membership includes both people with MS (PwMS) and others. A recent interview survey of PwMS may provide a clearer picture but again the survey does not directly address this issue and the information that has been collected is thus incomplete (Tribe & Tribe 2002).

times' in a caring relationship has been less likely to be explored (Nolan *et al* 1996: 3). Just how carers cope with or manage their care work and fit it into their life as a whole, is poorly understood (ibid.) There has been little research attention paid to care involving a chronic condition, one where continuing deterioration is assumed and becomes part of the adjustments required of both carer and care recipient. Studies of caring where the chronic condition is MS are especially rare and have tended to be concerned with quantitative measures of burden or of coping strategies (Gulick 1995) rather than with the 'everyday/everynight' lived experience of carers and care recipients.

Furthermore, the ways in which care has been conceptualised have tended to be limited to task based conceptualisations and the physical dimensions of caring and this has led to rather static models of care (Nolan et al, *op cit.*). Studies over time, or looking back over extended periods of care, do allow for the possibility that the more dynamic and fluid aspects of care, the ways in which caring relationships (and marriages) change over time and are renegotiated and reinterpreted, can be acknowledged and better understood.

In this chapter I introduce the study, its methods, sampling strategy and mode of analysis. I then turn to the actual findings of the research and take the reader through the diagnosis and the period following diagnosis, looking particularly at the problems of continuing in paid work and of organising suitable accommodation. The kinds of support sought and used, both formal and informal, are then considered and the question of how accessible and useful this help has been. Finally I turn to the impact of the MS and the caring role on the marriage itself. This section of the chapter deals with the men's assessment of the effects of the MS on their life and marriage, how they consider the relationship to have changed with time and increasing dependency, what have been the gains and the losses, and how they would explain the reason for sustaining a caring role over so many years.

I begin with questions of method and methodology looking particularly closely at the way in which the auspice of the study by two local MS societies has determined the method of recruitment and influenced the content of the interview guide.

The Study

This is an interview based study which, in keeping with the tradition of qualitative approaches to research, has sought to explore a particular experience with those placed in that set of circumstances and to do so in some depth. Each of the seventeen participants included in this sub sample was interviewed only once but the interviews were lengthy and detailed, most taking several hours. The interviews took the form of a focus question interview which employed an interview guide. This ensured specific questions and issues were covered but allowed for a degree of flexibility in the way interviews were conducted and, in large measure, permitted each man to tell his story as he wished. The questions were set out under nine main headings - the background or history, the nature and extent of support received (informal and formal), the impact on both lives (and, indeed, the entire family) of the MS diagnosis, the stress and emotional strain in caring, the notion of altruism or of an ethic of care, the choice to care, limits to caring, men and caring, the things that would make the greatest difference to the carer's immediate circumstances. Interviews were taped and then transcribed. The analysis made use of a coding framework which attempted to reflect both the questions and theoretical concerns which had framed the research from the outset and those themes and issues which had emerged as the research progressed. This chapter draws on only a small number of the coding categories, specifically those relating to diagnosis, and decisions taken following diagnosis, formal and informal support, the impact of the MS on the marriage, and the reasons for caring.

The study was conducted in the state of New South Wales and the Australian Capital Territory. While the research was enthusiastically supported by the MS society[3] in each region, it was not commissioned by either body. Nevertheless, their support made it possible to recruit participants through the two organisations - using newsletters, direct approaches by staff and through a presentation (by the researcher) at one of the NSW Society's regional seminars. The sample reflects this particular recruitment strategy.

This group of MS carers and their wives had chosen to join and identify with a self help and advocacy organisation. Although not all were particularly active or involved, all had sought information from the Society and continued to receive monthly newsletters and, over the years, most had made use of some of the services and supports offered by the two state-based Societies. Whatever the other implications of this selectivity it does seem apparent that this recruitment strategy has resulted in a sample with a higher proportion of those whose condition might be described as more severe than might otherwise be expected. As noted above, MS is a highly variable condition and its manifestations, their frequency and severity, and the very course of the disease vary considerably. The sample reflects some of this variation but, perhaps inevitably, there are fewer cases where the MS might be viewed as 'mild' and none where the symptoms could be described as a short-lived annoyance occurring only very rarely. One might speculate that it is less likely that such individuals will choose to identify with an MS Society for a whole range of reasons not the least being a desire to keep to a minimum their contact with those with more virulent forms of the disease or to avoid as much as possible being labelled as someone with MS.

In addition, in selecting carers through this means, I have interviewed men who have 'stayed' in a marriage to someone with MS[4]. Thus they have chosen to stay in a marriage (although many rejected the idea that they had any choice in the matter) as well as to care for someone with a chronic and disabling condition. All the men who self-selected for this research

3 The MS societies in Australia reflect the federal political structure of the nation. There is a national body and a number of state societies: all are not-for-profit, charitable associations. The national body, MS Australia, coordinates and assists the functioning of the state societies. Its primary focus is on research, both the funding and auspice of research in Australia and keeping abreast of developments overseas, and national fundraising, shared services, strategic direction and branding. Direct client services are managed and delivered at a state level. Services are offered to those with MS and allied neurological conditions and to their families and carers. The MS Society of New South Wales is the oldest of the MS organisations in the country. It has operated for fifty years and now has a budget of more than $A11 million. The MS Society of the ACT is a smaller organisation. It has operated since 1978. Both societies are staffed by full time and part time employees, contractors and volunteers.

4 Almost all the men, both in this subset and in the larger sample, commented on how 'most men' behave in such circumstances. And a considerable proportion of those who made such comment used the quintessentially Australian phrase, 'to shoot through', to describe this behaviour: thus 'most men' were characterised as 'shooting though' or 'shooting through on their wives'. The men in this study, on the other hand, had not 'shot through'. The phrase 'to shoot through' was originally part of the expression 'to shoot through like a Bondi tram'. Bondi was the end of the line for those trams travelling from the central business district of Sydney to this Eastern Suburbs destination. It is essentially a Sydney colloquialism although its meaning was widely understood and appreciated by those living elsewhere in Australia. The expression was meant to suggest 'taking off' with great alacrity along with the notion of not looking back, of complete disengagement or desertion, of 'absenting oneself improperly' (The Macquarie Dictionary, 1981). Sydney did away with its trams in the mid 1950s. So, over time, the phrase 'like a Bondi tram' was dropped from this expressive description.

were in *de jure* (from all appearances), heterosexual marriages: there were no homosexual or *de facto* couples in the sample.

There is another interesting feature of the sample as a result of the process of recruitment of participants. The MS Society of New South Wales had a particular interest in the situation of their clientele who live in regional and country areas. Of especial interest was the northern region of the state, a region that was seen to be particularly poorly serviced both in relation to community-based and medical and related services. Because of their concern, they had requested that I seek as many participants as possible from country areas and from the northern region, in particular. For this reason, couples living in rural areas are prominently represented in the sample. This feature of the sample is of particular significance. Most phenomenologically based research on carers has employed convenience samples which typically are urban based as that is where most researchers live. As a result, our understanding of rural populations and of the impact of rural living, including of being distant from the specialist services rarely available outside larger towns and cities, has been very partial. As will become clear this inclusion of a large proportion of participants from outside urban areas was of considerable importance and has provided insights about family support as well as formal service provision which flow directly from this circumstance.

Fifteen participants continued to care for their wives at home. The remaining two had had finally to move their wives to a nursing home so difficult had the caring become.

The interviews were conducted in a variety of locations but quite a high proportion were conducted in the couple's home. As a consequence the wife with MS was present for a number of the interviews. While this might be judged far from ideal it was not something I could control and, indeed, having explained that the interview might raise issues which were difficult and stressful for the wife in the partnership I had to leave it to them to decide what they wanted to do. I could hardly have directed the wife to leave the room while I discussed the business of her care with her husband. Nevertheless, there are significant ethical issues here. Even allowing for the established ethical safeguards we put in place, it is important to recognise that participants cannot really know before the interview how they will respond to this kind of exploration or even what they may find themselves revealing. They cannot know whether they or their wife will find this intervention supportive or distressing. Nor can they know whether that impact will be fleeting or more enduring and what the implications of this might be. The ethical questions of concern here relate to a researcher's duty of care for those who participate in our research. While the chapter does not discuss these ethical concerns, I nevertheless note them here because they are important especially in research of this kind, because they remained a concern throughout this particular study, and because these are ethical issues we often fail to resolve very satisfactorily.

The analysis of the data collected in this study involved a careful and detailed coding of each interview transcript and then a further sorting and resorting of these coded pieces of transcript across all the accounts and under larger overarching headings. The final stage in analysis has taken the form of the 'writing up' of these results under those headings.

The reporting of the research findings has taken several different forms, addressed different audiences and featured different areas among the findings. One of the accounts has been the report to the MS Society of NSW. Another took the form of a doctoral thesis. Still others, such as the present account, have been shorter pieces focussing on particular aspects of the study. In each case, the structure of the report has been built up from the transcripts but in such a way as to allow for the empirical and policy issues which had prompted the research in the first place (and the questions that arose as the interviews progressed) to shape the final outcome. In this present account, I have taken selected coding categories and a sub sample of participants in order to explore a number of significant issues related to the experience of men caring for their partners in later life and where that care has extended over many years, as outlined above. In this account of the findings of the study, as in all the other cases, I have included quotes from the men themselves. Pseudonyms have been used and other identifying details changed.

In the next section, I present the results of the analysis.

The Analysis

I begin this account with the period before diagnosis and then move to the diagnosis itself. This is where the interviews began.

Diagnosis and Major Life Decisions

It would be difficult to exaggerate the importance of the definitive explanation that a diagnosis represents. All participants spoke of the need to find out what lay behind the worrying, on again and off again, recurring symptoms. For many in this group of older carers the diagnosis had been delivered many years before, still vivid but in terms of the caring experience but less to the fore than for those for whom it was more recent. Others in this group had had to live with numerous unsatisfactory diagnoses over decades until they had been given a final definitive diagnosis in more recent years with the benefit of MRI (magnetic resonance imaging) techniques. For this last group the adjustments the couple found themselves having to make were sometimes resented by a partner who was both disturbed and irritated by such symptoms as recurring tiredness. Because these symptoms would disappear for a time it could seem that this was more a question of some mental condition or personal characteristic of a partner than of some chronic physical condition. At least two of the men had questioned whether there was much point in remaining in a marriage which seemed to offer so little. However, once a clear diagnosis was delivered, their commitment to the marriage and their partner became unassailable: they saw their futures as inextricably bound together and the MS as something they would confront together.

All the men described how, once the condition had been identified, there followed a period of 'taking stock' including a thoroughgoing re-assessment of the future and what the wife's illness implied for both their lives. In this process of coming to terms, two areas featured prominently - the question of suitable accommodation and, in numerous cases, whether a move might be necessary or desirable, and the viability of continuing employment (both the wife's and the husband's) or of employment of a particular kind. Not surprisingly, there was also considerable concern about the financial implications of the choices that might need to be made in relation to these two critical areas, in particular in relation to employment.

The Question of Continuing in Paid Employment

Trying to ensure that their wife could continue to work for as long as possible had proved to be very difficult in most cases. None of the women were in paid employment at the time of interview. Some had been able to work for a little time following diagnosis but, for most, the time between diagnosis and withdrawal from paid work was very short. A few had not worked at all from that time onwards.

For the carers I interviewed there had also been issues around employment. Of the seventeen included in this sub-sample of older carers, six had continued in paid work, all but one, full time. For these six men the primary question was how to juggle the demands of a job with the task of caring for their wife. In earlier years that juggling had often included the demands of children as well. Continuing in paid work had also required adjustments in the work environment itself, in the kind of work that might be undertaken and in their own expectations about career paths. So these men had had to cut back on travel, especially overnight stays, or move to a job which did not require travel or where it was possible to work more flexible hours. One man had to give up work as a field geologist, a type of work he loved, and settle for a desk job. They had felt unable to contemplate promotions or further training where these might require a permanent move or too much time away from home. These adjustments were often difficult to make and involved regrets and costs, both professional and financial. Nevertheless, these men made clear that their view was simply that 'this is the way the cards had been played' and one adjusted and just 'got on with it'.

The remaining eleven men faced even greater adjustments in the area of employment. They had found themselves with little alternative but to 'retire' from paid employment to take up a full-time caring role. All but one had retired at an earlier time than might have been chosen had circumstances been different. For two men in this group, this represented a *very* early retirement. For another two, the choice to retire had been taken early but only slightly earlier than would otherwise have been the case. One man retired at a time that was much as it would have been in 'normal' circumstances. Nevertheless, he was retiring to care full-time.

The decision to leave work was described as necessary, as something that became inevitable: there was no choice.

> (I)t was starting to get to the stage where it was unsafe to leave her. I used to get all the kids to school and everything, and set her up for the day where she had a limited mobility and then get home and do all the domestics at home that evening and that's the way we survived for a while. But it was... quite obvious that it was getting to the stage where you couldn't safely leave her on her own, so there was no (choice).

When these decisions had been taken early, in their thirties or forties, they had had a profound effect upon both husband and wife. Needless to say, decisions about paid work and accommodation were closely linked. In a number of these accounts, participants related how once it had become clear that they would need to relinquish paid employment, this had prompted a further decision - to move to the country and to establish a different lifestyle for themselves. Some participants stated quite explicitly that, in making a decision of this kind, they were attempting to make the most of what they knew were likely to be difficult times ahead: others simply implied it. If they were both to be at home and living on a limited income, then let it be in pleasant surroundings. A number related how they had often dreamed of moving to the country and so they had decided to make that move at that time. They saw themselves as laying claim to some part of the shared future with which they had started their life together even though the diagnosis would almost certainly mean that many dreams would remain unfulfilled. Others spoke in terms of needing to live somewhere where house prices were more reasonable than in the large cities and so had chosen a country move on that basis.

> We left Sydney, built this house with wheelchair ramping, (and we) sit around receiving the pension... (We made the decision) almost straight away. About a year after the diagnosis Anna could not walk very well, so we decided that we would move.
>
> How difficult was it to make that decision?
>
> Pretty easy. We had been wanting to live in the country anyway.
>
> So in a way it prompted you to do something you'd always wanted to do.
>
> Yes, there was no reason for us to be in the city...

The primary reasons for the decision to leave paid employment was anxiety about their wife's increased level of disability and about her being left on her on her own during the working day. But in addition, many husbands had found it more and more difficult to carry the double load of paid and domestic work plus the demands of caring. The sheer quantity of work and its particular demands, physical and emotional, together with the long hours involved, had made it impossible to continue in the workforce.

> My day then was getting up at 5 o'clock in the morning and going to work, coming home at half past 5, 6 o'clock... cooking tea, cleaning up, 9 o'clock at night (falling into bed)... I was working six days a week. On the Sunday I'd have to wash and iron and vacuum and polish to keep the house clean... So, it was too big a week and I was getting too bloody tired and plus the fact that she was getting worse … It's not worth it. I've been offered a couple of jobs, good jobs, because in my game it's word of mouth... But it's not worth it. Peace of mind. Money is not worth anything if you haven't got the peace of mind. I'd be worrying (all the time) about what would be wrong with Mary… It was very good money and there were bonuses as well, but money is not everything.

With one possible exception, all those who were no longer in paid employment missed their work. Both those who left work in their thirties or forties and those who retired in their fifties, would have preferred to keep working rather than leave their jobs when they did. Many spoke of really enjoying their work, of the recognition and sense of achievement they had had, of the camaraderie of the work place. Being a full-time carer can be very isolating and that had been so for several of these couples. In circumstances where one simply cannot afford to run a car (as was the case in at least one instance), that sense of isolation was a marked feature of the caring experience. Most of all, they spoke of the straitened financial circumstances that they had had to contend with as a result of this early retreat from paid employment.

> We wouldn't have had the problems that we've got now had I worked for another ten years and that's all it would have taken to (set us up with a degree of security)... Yes, well it didn't happen... And, of course, on the pension you lose all your potential to earn extra money. Like I was just about doubling my wages on overtime. Once you go on the pension, you've got none of that potential at all. It has all meant a major upset in our financial circumstances.
>
> A trimming of expectations?

> *Yeah, very much so. Well, (actually) a wiping out of expectations...*

Self funded retirees who had had to retire earlier than expected were also struggling financially and were often worse off than those receiving the aged pension.

> We did our maths recently and found that, per fortnight, we are on something like about $14 or $15 less than a full pensioner couple.

There were other costs and losses. A number of the men were in senior positions and were expected to do very well in their careers. Being forced, through circumstances, to retire very early had meant a loss of a sense of achievement and of the recognition that had been there in their paid work. There was, also, for most, the loss of stimulation that was a part of their work environment. One man described how the knowledge that he would have progressed to the top of his profession had not helped his wife cope with their new life style and his full-time caring role. It has also been difficult for him to accept although he felt that he had been able to do this. Even for those who were now well past retirement age, the losses they had experienced as a result of such an early retreat from paid work were still keenly felt and they reflected on the way in which their lives had shaped by the need to make this critical 'choice'.

Life shaping and generally negative though these decisions had been, there had also been positive outcomes. In several cases the wife's health had improved when they had taken on her care full time and in one instance the condition had seemed to stabilise: at the time of interview, there had been no further exacerbations. Beyond these improvements, two men commented on benefits associated with being able to explore other areas of life or pursue a hobby and develop additional skills. One spoke of the enjoyment he had found in physical work, work with his hands, after a high-powered career in the private sector. The second man related how he had discovered a love of woodwork which had given far greater satisfaction than anything he had experienced in his paid work.

Decisions about Long Term Accommodation and their Consequences

Decisions about long term accommodation had also to be made. These had often followed fairly swiftly upon the diagnosis. While quite a number had remained in their homes (six in all), the rest had decided to move as a result of their wife's condition. In both cases they were attempting to ensure that the house was one in which she could move with ease and safety. Those who remained had had to expend considerable amounts of money in making major structural modifications to their homes such as widening doorways, redesigning bathrooms and kitchens for use by someone in a wheelchair or on sticks or crutches and providing for wheelchair access into the house and onto decks and verandas. Those who moved had sought a more suitable house and made further modifications or they had started from scratch and designed a house that they saw as meeting their needs into the future. All spoke of the need to ensure the greatest quality of life for their wife that it was in their power and their financial means to provide.

Two important consequences flowed from these decisions. The first affected all of these couples. The financial investment involved in making the necessary modifications to their homes had been considerable and in most cases was met my the couple themselves. Money that would in other circumstances have funded a retirement, paid for an overseas trip, helped children in setting up their own homes or provided an inheritance, had been used up and, quite literally, lost. While government assistance had been available it had not been adequate in most cases or the couple were not eligible for this support because of the husband's income at the time. The most important outcome of this major investment in house modification is not always acknowledged. There is no financial return on the investment that these couples had had to make in modifying their homes so that the wife could continue to live with some degree of independence: there will be no capital gain and no 'value adding'. If they sell at a later date (as most people do) the modifications, especially major alterations, are likely to be viewed as detracting from the value of the house.

The second consequence was one experienced particularly by those who had decided to move to rural areas and in so doing to place themselves at a distance from family and longstanding friends. As noted above, isolation is not an uncommon experience among carers but this kind of geographic isolation is rather unusual. There were others in the study who also experienced geographic isolation and those whose isolation had nothing to do with rural living. Isolation had resulted from factors such as frequent moves associated with particular careers, for example, service in the armed forces. Then there were couples who had spent the greater part of their adult lives in one country town. Isolation was not an issue for them: they had established significant networks of friendship and support. Even so, children had moved to larger cities to pursue further study and find suitable work and so important support for the caring effort was no longer to hand. The group of couples who had made a deliberate decision to move to more isolated settings must have made some calculation about its possible consequences further 'down the track'. Yet, there appeared to be few regrets and no complaints beyond those associated with obtaining good, reliable services in country areas.

Nevertheless, because of the wife's MS, overcoming isolation and distance posed greater problems than might otherwise be the case. Travelling to and fro and visiting other family members was more difficult because of mobility problems (and, in a number of cases, incontinence). A more permanent move was also problematic. The possibility of relocating nearer to one's family was likely to be constrained by two factors – by the need to live in the right climate, one where the summers were not too hot for the wife with MS, and, in some cases, by the investment already made in modifying a house. As already noted, this kind of capital investment could not be recouped and any new home would need to be modified as well. Undertaking two lots of home modification was an expense that few in this sample would have been able to meet.

> All of Alana's people are in (Large Town) in Queensland. We've often thought with me now out of the (armed services), there is no reason to stay in (Southern city). But where would we go? Having sunk a lot of our money into this house, we're not just going to sell it. We've over capitalised, in real estate terms. You're going to sell it at a loss and then have to spend it all over again. But, as I said, where do you go? You can't go to Queensland because the heat up there would kill her. She suffers badly from the heat even here in (Southern city)... All my brothers and sisters are up there as well. No, we don't have any family whatsoever south of the border. We're on our own. It is as simple as that, really.

Regardless of the reasons for the isolation and the history that lay behind it, being removed from your kith and kin had incurred particular costs for these carers and their wives. This issues is discussed in the next section.

Support From Family and Friends

The first and most obvious costs was the lack of support, especially immediate physical assistance, from those who might otherwise be willing and able to give it. Nine of the couples in this sub-sample lived too far from family to be able to count on any practical help from family members. Of course, family and friends who live at a distance may keep in regular contact and continue to provide moral support but in this study it was apparent that this was not always forthcoming either, even from close family members. In some cases this was the direct result of major rifts within the family but in other cases the family simply had little idea of how difficult things had become for their siblings or parents. Where there is frequent contact family members are better placed to develop an understanding of the condition and the prognosis: infrequent contact in more likely to result in a limited comprehension of these things.

There were other reasons why relatives might not understand the nature of MS nor see the difficulties that it posed for both the wife and husband. A number of participants made explicit comment about the importance of getting on with your life, about not imposing on others and about allowing your children, who had their own kinds of problems and pressures, to get on with their own lives and not feel burdened by their mother's illness. They also spoke about not allowing the MS to take over and determine everything else. It is important to recognise that these men gained a sense of worth and identity from managing the caring situation competently, of coping well. But of course there is a paradox here. This very strategy may increase the possibility that others outside the immediate situation, and most particularly those who have only intermittent contact with the couple, will remain unaware of the demands of MS and of MS caring. As participants themselves commented, the fact that a couple are coping well may help others in the family, especially children, to cope ('Mum and Dad are okay') but it may mean that relatives are less ready or able to acknowledge the nature of the demands involved. This is speculative, of course. It is possible that those who observe a couple dealing with the particular circumstances without drama or self-pity may respond with admiration and affirmation. But if you add distance and infrequent contact to this set of circumstances, then there are likely to be some relatives who have no understanding of what is going on. It may be the case that the better one copes, the less likely are others to take notice. As one participant put it:

> What they don't see, they don't have to worry about.

Not all of these men lacked support from family. Four spoke at some length about the support they received from their children, and of how willingly and warmly it had been given over the years. Others were in constant contact with children who lived at a considerable distance. They felt they had been able to talk about some of the difficulties they were having to contend with and to feel acknowledged and supported. As to parents of this group of older carers, not surprisingly they were either elderly themselves or had died. Nevertheless, a number of parents had provided substantial financial help at various critical times over the years of caring. Not only support from family and friends, but also access to formal services and specialist medical services had been affected by distance and isolation.

Use of Formal Services

In theory there is a considerable range of services available to those with MS and their carers: in practice these were not always readily accessible or were unsatisfactory in one way or another. Those services specifically for the MS community are provided almost exclusively by the state based MS societies. They include the provision of detailed, up-to-date information and advice, counselling services and assistance from field officers and social workers, some limited financial assistance especially in the form of loans, and visiting specialist teams that travel to country centres and provide information and practical help with problems such as incontinence or appropriate exercise. The Society also provides residential and respite support. A number of these services (such as the provision of respite care) are government funded. General or mainstream services and supports are almost entirely government funded although most are provided though the 'not-for–profit' and community sectors (including many church based organisations). The primary financial support available is a Commonwealth funded Carer Payment which is subject to an income and assets test and a Carer Allowance which is not means-tested. The Commonwealth Government also funds respite provision. The Home and Community Care Program (HACC), which is a joint Australian, State and Territory cost-shared program, provides a range of basic maintenance and support services to those with MS and their carers including personal and nursing care, home modification and maintenance, transport and counselling. The state based and national carers associations which comprise Carers Australia provide information, counselling and advice to carers.

It is important to note that actual levels of use of services and the degree of reliance on professionals were surprisingly low among this sample of MS carers. Given the demanding nature of much MS care and the more tenuous family connections in many instances, I had expected more intensive and extensive service use than was apparent. In other demanding caring situations, such as dementia care, there tends to be much higher use of services, especially respite services, than is evident here (Schofield et al, 1998: 71). However the findings of this research may be less at odds with the findings of other studies where the focus has been upon physical disability and care. Compared with other categories of carers, those caring for someone with a physical disability are less likely to register an explicit need for services. Schofield and her colleagues, in their survey of Victorian carers, note that fewer of these carers (compared with those caring for someone with dementia) 'reported *needing* one or more of these services', that is, the range of community services (ibid: 70). Among the group of older carers included in my study most described themselves as being able to 'get by' most of the time.

In these accounts of caring, the theme of self-reliance was a recurring one. Nevertheless, many of those in this group of carers did consider that having access to good, reliable services was important and saw themselves as managing well *in spite* of the lack of outside help. The reality for many in this sample was that needed support was inadequate in one respect or another. Coverage was patchy; agencies were poorly funded and unable to meet the level of demand; many had high rates of staff attrition or turnover; they were unable to provide adequate or appropriate respite or emergency back up; and staff had little or no understanding of MS. There were notable exceptions. One of the couples who had had very extensive support reported that all of it had been satisfactory. Others had made use of fewer services but had also had excellent service from those particular agencies. And among others, who had used a range of services over time, there were examples of good service provision even if others had been less satisfactory. Nevertheless, the generalisation reflects accurately what the majority of the couples in this sample encountered most of the time.

In the accounts of this group of carers, one particular area stands out as presenting difficulties for carers and care recipients alike – the provision of respite care, day care and emergency or crisis care. Taking a break from caring, having an opportunity to pursue your own interests and hobbies, being able to rest and relax away from the caring situation and freed of the caring responsibilities, is regarded as very important. For many carers, the need for nights of uninterrupted sleep can become a pressing need. The discussions of support for carers in the literature (Hubert 1993; Montgomery and Borgatta 1989; Schofield et al. 1998) and in policy statements about and analysis of carers' needs (Gibson et al. 1996), lay stress on this provision. Yet few in this group of MS carers had access to respite or day care or, if they had access, felt able to make use of those services.

While the need for respite was not something raised by everyone in this sample, among those who had sought to make use of respite services only one couple had found an arrangement that might be judged satisfactory. A number had simply 'given up on the idea' because what was available was seen to be so unsuitable. In most country areas, respite services are available only in nursing homes among elderly people most of whom suffer from some form of dementia. Travelling to Sydney to use the respite services run by the MS Society posed its own difficulties.

Contact with doctors, especially specialists, was for the most part, very irregular and brief. With general practitioners, the contact was more frequent but did not appear to be a regular feature of the lives of most of these couples. Participants related how actual consultation times tended to be short and focused on the immediate physical condition of their wife. In a surprising number of cases the wife was described as being in remarkably good physical health apart from the MS and this might, in part, account for infrequent medical visits. But the most likely explanation is that the most pressing needs were not medical or were not able to be addressed by medical professionals. As for doctors being responsive to the needs of carers, there was little comment on this area, yet a number of the men related how they had suffered from recurring depression, constant fatigue, high blood pressure and a range of medical conditions.

Putting to one side, the difficulties in locating suitable services and the experience of unsatisfactory provision, most of these carers did acknowledge that, even though they might not need particular forms of assistance at this moment, the knowledge that such services existed, were accessible and affordable and staffed by competent professionals was essential to one's peace of mind. If you are to cope in the present you need to know that needed supports will be there in the future, if and when you need them.

This picture of the caring experience makes clear just how thoroughgoing have been the changes wrought in the lives of this group of couples – carers and partner with MS alike. Such major changes have clearly had significant consequences for the marital relationship.

The Impact on the Marriage

Many of the adaptations had been made gradually but their cumulative effect had been considerable. For some couples, however, the progress of the disease had been relatively swift and its disabling impacts had required significant and rapid adjustment on the part of both husband and wife. But, whether gradual or rapid, the necessary changes in life style and expectations were difficult and sometimes very confronting.

The impact of these fundamental changes and reassessments on the marriage itself resonated throughout the interviews. These were very poignant stories and although there was no self pity, a deep sadness pervades these accounts. In no other interviews with carers have I been so conscious of the person who was being cared for: even when she was not present, her presence haunts the interviews.

For all the considerable adaptation and the difficulties that attended such adjustments, most men described their marriages in positive terms – 'good', 'sound', 'solid', 'strong', 'very, very close'. Two relationships were defined by the husband as difficult or strained. Nevertheless, they, too, were presented as based on a strong bond, and a high level of commitment. It was clear that the two husbands involved were not prepared to take themselves out of the marriage. Most participants also depicted the essential core of their relationship as unchanged.

For all that the 'base relationship', as one man expressed it, might remain the same, there were changes and losses in these marriages that were of a greater magnitude than one might expect to be part of the ordinary adjustments of any ongoing relationship or of simply getting older. The losses included loss of sexual relations and, in a few cases, physical closeness; the loss of intellectual companionship in several instances; losses associated with lifestyle adjustments, with shared elements of the relationship, or of certain kinds of reciprocity and of particular 'gifts' to one another in the exchanges that typify all relationships; and loss of the expectation of a particular and shared future, of the dreams with which the marriage had begun. These men described how they had had to rethink their priorities and re-order all the elements of their life together. The wife's needs had become the central focus of the marriage and everything else had been given a lesser priority. At least that would appear to be the case in most of these relationships, most of the time. In the picture that is constructed here, the husband's needs are certainly of much less importance. In many of these marriages, they hardly even rate as a secondary element in the marriage equation. They simply do not feature in these marriage narratives.

Listening to these accounts, it would seem that the presence of MS had contributed to greater stress in all the relationships although the ways in which this impact was registered were less to the fore in some accounts than in others. Those participants who reflected more directly on these issues commented that, as a result of this additional strain, the 'downs', the times when things were not going so well or when there were disagreements, were more likely to be exaggerated. While this chapter does not explore the issue of depression, it is a recurring theme in the interviews. Many of the men and their wives suffered from depression including serious clinical depression. As well as this response, a number of men described their wife's emotional withdrawal, moodiness, or general low spirits. Some men described their own difficulties in keeping 'buoyant spirits'. At least one wife was reported as suggesting that her husband should leave her, find himself someone else and start afresh. Other participants spoke of the pressures created, on the home front, by the substantial increase in workload, physical and emotional. They spoke of the constant demand entailed in caring, of the need always to be available and, consequently, the restrictions on what you could do in the way of pursuing your own hobbies or leisure interests or individual pleasures. This had meant that, in these relationships, it had become much more difficult and, in some instances, impossible for the two individuals to lead their individual lives, to pursue separate activities especially where these involved physical exertion or travelling about.

In her study, *With this Body*, Gillian Parker describes one of the tensions in the marriages included in her sample of couples in a caring relationship as 'the strain of being too much together' (1993: 97). John Bayley, speaking of his marriage to Iris Murdoch, refers to that 'happy apartness which marriage had once taken wholly for granted'. The 'new marriage', which emerges as Iris Murdoch gradually succumbs to the ravages of Alzheimer's disease, was one that, of necessity, demanded far greater physical and emotional closeness.

> 'Life is no longer bringing the pair of us "closer and closer apart", in the poet's tenderly ambiguous words. Every day we move closer and closer together. We could not do otherwise. There is a certain comic irony – happily not darkly comic – that after nearly forty years of taking marriage for granted, marriage has decided it is tired of this, and is taking a hand in the game. Purposefully, persistently, involuntarily, our marriage is now getting somewhere. It is giving us no choice: and I am glad of that' (1998: 183).

Several writers have argued that good care also entails an element of separation or distance. This is important for many reasons but not the least is the importance of recognising that the carer may not question his own perception of what the needs of his partner are and may believe he knows simply because of the closeness of the relationship between them.

> 'If I see myself as "indistinct" from you, or you as not having your own being that is not merged with mine, then I cannot preserve a real sense of your well-being as opposed to mine. Care and understanding require the sort of distance that is needed in order not to see the other as a projection of the self, or self as a continuation of the other' (Grimshaw, 1986: 183 as cited in Engster, 2004: 116).

In these marriages, where MS had assaulted the health and well being of one partner, the increased closeness between the couple was certainly remarked upon. But, the differences between their circumstances and those of Bayley and Murdoch are significant. Even where there had been a decline in mental acuity, there was nothing approaching the confusion, loss of functionality and childlike dependency of dementia. Mentally these wives remained alert and involved and contributing to the relationship albeit, at times, in ways that differed from those of the past. Apart from the physical deterioration, they remained the same person and, despite high levels of dependency in some of these cases, the wives continued to relate to their partner as an equal and to be committed to the relationship (even in the case of the wife who apparently was urging her husband to leave and start afresh). That, at least, is what is conveyed in all but one of these accounts.

There was one relationship where the commitment of the wife to the marriage would appear to be in question. In setting out his own account of the marriage, the husband's commitment was made very clear. The strains in this relationship were considerable. He sought greater closeness: she wanted 'her space'. He expressed his distress at seeing her in pain and losing her independence: she rejected his concern, declined his help (most of the time) and denied he was a 'carer' in any sense. She saw him as weak and herself as strong and self sufficient, a characterisation with which the husband, in some measure, agreed. She did not want others to know of the MS and was suspicious of his talking to anyone: he had a desperate need to talk to others. When he had spoken to a counsellor about his feelings and his marriage, the counsellor had passed on this information to his wife. This serious breach of professional ethics had further increased the tensions in the marriage. Both the man and his wife were socially isolated. They knew very few people in the town to which they had moved since diagnosis. They were also living at a considerable distance from any close family. The husband felt very alone and depressed: I can only imagine that the wife had similar feelings. The picture developed here is, of course, the husband's view of the plight of his marriage. I do not doubt that the wife would have constructed a different picture but, no doubt, one that was equally negative. I also do not doubt that the husband's anguish was utterly genuine and the hurt deeply felt. For all these tensions and difficulties, he described his marriage as being sustained by 'a different love'. Interestingly, the same term was used to describe the nature of his marriage bond by the other man in a relationship that was under considerable strain. It is worthwhile exploring what kept these men in such difficult relationships.

The Commitment to Care

In attempting to describe what they were doing and to provide an explanation for their commitment to care (and thus for remaining in the relationship), this group of men were almost universally uneasy with explanations or descriptions that relied on notions of moral worthiness, goodness or altruism. Yet, in describing themselves and their actions, they spoke in terms such as, 'I'm not the kind of person to walk out', or 'I'm just a loving husband', or of not being able 'to do that to my wife', or of how it would be worse or more difficult if they left than if they remained. They spoke of guilt and of not being able 'to live with themselves'. Many also made it clear that they knew that, if the situation were reversed, their wife would care for them. With that knowledge how could they not remain to care for her? They espoused notions of 'duty', 'responsibility', and 'doing the right thing'. A number did talk of personal values and morality and used this as grounding for their actions. However, this language was not something most were comfortable with. One man stated explicitly that he did not think his decision had anything to do with goodness, that he did not regard himself as a 'good person'. Most particularly the majority eschewed any suggestion that what they were doing was from altruistic motives or could be viewed as an example of altruism. The strength of feeling about this notion and the objection to using it to describe their actions was very strongly expressed by some participants. Altruism was seen to involve notions of 'choice', of choosing to do something selfless: most of these men saw themselves as having no choice. This is interesting in light of their repeated accounts of 'most men' as making the choice to leave wives who had been diagnosed with MS and thus of avoiding taking on, what could turn out to be, onerous caring responsibilities. In this construction of their situation, 'most men are seen to be exercising a 'choice' which these men simply did not see as being theirs to make.

What then were the kinds of explanations provided? What language was seen as acceptable when it came to describing motivations and actions? Participants seemed most comfortable with a way of speaking about their situation simply as a job that needed to be done and their own actions as a response to that need. They were just doing what needed doing. They took on the job because it was theirs to do; it had fallen to them. A number stated baldly that they were the only one who could or would undertake the care and that, if they didn't do it, their wife would need to go into institutional care immediately. As stated already, there was some (and for a few, considerable) irritation with any suggestion of heroics, self-sacrifice, altruistic motives or notions of worthiness. There was also a disinclination to pursue the idea that they might be possessed of a caring nature, that they were a caring person. Only one man used such language. He described how he had grown up in a family where there was a tradition of caring. He felt that those who had taken on caring responsibilities in his family had 'generally been of a kinder and more gentle nature', that they were more likely to be 'altruistic' and 'selfless'. He also saw himself as somewhat in this mould.

The language of 'care' was here a language of doing, of undertaking a necessary job. It might well be that these participants would have been unwilling to do this for anyone else or for anyone who was not a very close relative, a parent or child, several said as much, but they did not want to be seen to be doing anything extraordinary. They might want the acknowledgement that caring was demanding and sometimes unremitting and that what they were doing was sometimes hard. But their accounts are often very matter of fact and the tone clipped – 'I'm just doing it!' In Parker's study there were also carers who didn't provide or want to provide explanations of a moral kind and who, instead, simply stressed the fact that 'one just did it and got on with it' (op cit: 93).

As already noted, the care being offered, 'the getting on with it', was seen to be something which, had the situation been reversed, the wife would have done for the husband . As one participant commented…

> I know in every bone of my body that, were the circumstances reversed, she wouldn't hesitate to do the same for me. It wouldn't occur to her. She's that kind of person. So how could I not care for her.

In marriage relationships of this kind where there are high levels of dependency on the part of one party, such 'hypothetical reciprocation', as it might be named, was a critical element in the re-negotiation of notions of mutuality and exchange. While other factors were mentioned, this took centre stage. Negotiation and re-negotiation assume a degree of choice but there was not much room to move in these circumstances. Nevertheless it is important to recognise the ways in which these couples (or most of them) had worked out an ongoing relationship of equals. Where it has become impossible to restore a balance which is based on physical exchanges or equality, couples may devise other means for retaining a sense of equity. They may set about altering the views they hold about the kind of balance that is acceptable to them; they may re-evaluate the balance itself. Married carers 'might ascribe more value to the relationship, as a relationship, or see their partner in a more positive light than previously' (Parker, op cit: 90-1). A spousal carer might acknowledge, almost tally up, the past contributions of a partner, as wage earner, or homemaker, or parent and, perhaps, attribute greater import or value to these contributions than they might otherwise have done. The fact that his wife is placed in the situation she is and her manner of coping with pain and discomfort and loss of independence may also be part of the 'calculation' in the 'giving/receiving equation' (ibid.). In at least two instances, the past contributions of the partner had involved providing care for a partner who has now become carer and this was seen as a significant element in the balance. This reciprocity was real and palpable even if the caring had been of shorter duration.

We cannot conclude this account of men's caring without acknowledging the fundamental significance of gender in any consideration of care. Men caring for their wives do not neatly fit the various schema developed in research of caring (for example those of Gillian Dalley (1988) and, later, Joan Tronto (1994)), nor does their experience reflect the gendered nature of the different dimensions of care. The findings of this study are not exceptional. In more recent writing about care, numerous researchers have shown how obligations within families and marriages 'are not gendered in a straightforward way' (Elliot 1996: 128). In their work on family responsibilities, Finch and Mason (1993) found that, at least in their publicly expressed beliefs, men would appear to be saying essentially the same things as women about the kinds of assistance that should be offered to kin and the circumstances in which that help should be provided. Furthermore, in relation to the particular issue of disability within the context of marriage, it would seem that husbands, like wives, are defined as the primary source of care (Qureshi and Walker 1989). Spousal care is not gendered in quite the same way as other kinds of care may be. Faith Robertson Elliot sums up the current understanding of the different caring roles and relationships of men and women...

> 'The research literature... suggests that although women are more often carers than men, gender differences in caring commitments are not as significant as had once been supposed. At the same time, the circumstances in which women and men care – and are cared for – appear to differ markedly: the evidence shows that the majority of male carers are husbands caring for a spouse and unmarried men caring for a parent with whom they have lived for most of their lives. Male caring most often takes place in later life and in the context of a shared life whereas women more often care in the context of a filial or sibling relationship, more often provide extra-residential care, and more often engage in caring in middle age. Conversely, most older men are cared for by their wives whereas older women are more often cared for by daughters, daughters-in-law or sisters and are more likely to be in institutional care' (op. cit.: 137).

DISCUSSION

The sample of male carers discussed here is comprised of older men most of whom have been in their present relationship for some considerable time. We are viewing their lives after a good many years of care and when the impacts of a wife's disabilities and of his caring for her have re-shaped almost everything in their lives. If we consider Tronto's dimensions of care (1994), this group of carers have been involved in all of them save the final one of care-receiving (although two had experienced this in the past). Many had had to relinquish paid employment so as to be better able to care for their wife. By taking on the care of their wife they had become less 'powerful' than they might have otherwise been. If caring activities are devalued and occupied by the relatively powerless in society, as Tronto and other have argued, then this is borne out in the experience of a majority of these men. The one man whose income enabled him to continue to work and to 'buy in' care was not exempt from caring work. On the contrary, he undertook some caring and much domestic work. When the paid help was not there he took over the 'hands-on' care. It is also noteworthy that, in his case, the emotional labour was significant. Of the others with generally good incomes, it could be argued that their higher income had enabled them to purchase expensive aids such as motorized wheelchairs but this is only partially true. In several cases the income was no buffer and several had been left in straitened circumstances. In addition, higher incomes had meant that they were deemed ineligible for certain kinds of support. It would seem that caring work marginalises all but the very wealthy. Where the level of care required is great, money is not able to offer any real amelioration of the demands on the husband. The income would need to be exceptionally high or the support offered exceptionally ample and cheap, for the partner not to be involved in considerable amounts of hands-on care. As to the impact of income on the emotional load associated with caring, the evidence from this study would suggest that it is negligible. It might be argued that ample and reliable income can help allay anxiety about immediate financial concerns but the experience of this group would suggest that once you drop out of the labour force to care, former high income is no insurance against future financial worries. The marginalised may be more likely to become carers but, equally, those who take on demanding caring roles may well experience a degree of marginalisation. Sometimes the extent of that marginalisation is very great.

One final reflection on what this research might suggest about our understanding of care and caring work. The emphasis on care as work and as a practice rather than focusing on caring as a disposition takes on particular significance in this study. Joan Tronto takes up this argument in her landmark book, *Moral Boundaries. A political Argument for an Ethic of Care* (1994). What these accounts would seem to suggest is that, regardless of your disposition, caring is essentially about actions, about what you actually do rather than the kind of person you are. Their objection to talk of dispositions is that it tends to 'make you look special' or as though you were possessed of a particular temperament. This was not how they viewed their caring. Had they had a choice, they would much rather not be caring. They were doing it because it needed to be done and it was their job rather than anyone else's. Tronto argues that the focus on dispositions or personality types is a rather unproductive avenue to pursue in any attempt to enhance our understanding of care or to disentangle the complex and diverse nature of 'caring'. She argues against the preoccupation in the writing of theorists such as Blustein (1991) with the emotional investment that has to be made in order to care. For Tronto this is problematic.

> 'To think of care in dispositional terms allows us to think of care as the possession and province of an individual. It makes any individual's ideals of care fit into the worldview that the individual already possesses. This perspective allows care to be sentimentalized and romanticized, permitting the divisions in care…' (ibid: 118).

In re-conceptualising the nature of care, Tronto makes use of Sara Ruddick's argument concerning the importance of understanding care as a form of practice. The emphasis on dispositions, personality types and emotions also reinforces the traditional gendered expectations associated with caring whereby women are seen to be more caring by nature than men. Men are considered simply to be not as good at caring as women and much less likely to take it on with ease. In addition, men are seen to be more rational so that if they do take on caring roles, their caring is 'limited to the achievement of their rational plans (one of which is taking care of their families)' (Tronto, op. cit: 119). Tronto is not arguing that care has nothing to do with dispositions or emotions but rather that these dimensions are only a part of caring.

> 'Unless we also understand care in its richer sense of a practice, we run the risk of sentimentalizing and in other ways containing the scope of care in our thinking' (ibid.)

So what can we conclude about 'MS marriages', about the 'new marriage' (to use Bayley's term) which emerges as the impact of the MS is registered and the demands of caring take their toll. It would be accurate to say that the same rather matter-of-fact tone used in speaking of care and the so-called 'choice' to care, is evident in the comments on marriage in these interviews. Yet, it is clear that all these marriages were, in a sense, thrown out of kilter by the diagnosis of MS. As a result these men and their partners were prompted to engage in quite a deal of reflection on if not a re-appraisal of their marriage, of how they felt about the marriage relationship, about commitment to a partner, about the future.

Not surprisingly, reflection and reassessment becomes an ongoing part of such marriages. The future will require different and, perhaps, even more thoroughgoing reassessments. If we may assume that such constant and thoroughgoing re-evaluations are not part of most unions, then, perhaps, we can argue that this characterises MS marriages, it becomes an inbuilt part of how such marriages operate. Change and adaptation tend to follow: sometimes the change and adaptation precede and prompt the reassessment. Here there is considerable variation – variation in the kinds of change, in the pace at which change occurs and in the capacity to cope with such change and adjustment. In those few cases where the decline in the wife's health had been swift and the realignments in the marriage relationship had been considerable, it would seem that those adjustments were made almost in automatic mode. There was limited time to negotiate how best to rework their marriage relations and, as I stated before, there really was no room to move (surely a precondition of genuine negotiation).

Renegotiation, of course, assumes an ongoing commitment to the relationship by both parties. This group of men believed in marriage and was committed to sustaining their own relationship. But there was no elevated language about the nature of commitment as such. Instead there was an emphasis on 'not shooting through on your wife', on doing what needs to be done, on working with the 'hand' you've been dealt. There were other significant elements in their view of marriage. While participants did not emphasise the contractual element of marriage or dwell on its reciprocal nature, they did speak of their certain knowledge that their wife would care for them in similar circumstances (what I have called 'hypothetical reciprocation'). One or two spoke of doing what they would want others to do for them if they found themselves in a similar situation. The idea of marriage as involving mutual obligation was also expressed in notions of 'duty' and 'responsibility'. Several used the term 'love' and one spoke of being a 'loving husband'. How you behaved in a relationship, what decisions you took, were seen to be tied inextricably to the kind of person you are. These were men who would not 'walk out' of a marriage because 'things had got tough'. They could not abandon someone who was now, more than ever, in need of their continued commitment to the relationship. For all the resistance to the language of morality, there is a strong moral narrative running through all these accounts. That moral narrative is concerned with the practice of a responsibility, one that is expressive of our identities, our values and our ways of understanding our connections to others. Margaret Urban Walker, in writing about how we might best understand the nature of morality, says:

> 'Morality adheres in those ways we acknowledge and constrain each other that show that we are responsible for certain things to certain others. In learning morality, we learn who we are, to whom we are connected, and what matters enough to care about and care for' (1998: 201).

Conclusion

This chapter explores the experience of a group of men caring for a partner with a chronic condition, multiple sclerosis. All seventeen of these male carers were in their later years and most had been caring for a considerable time. This exploration of care is thus concerned with a particular caring circumstance and with what that might reveal about the nature of care. What is highlighted here are the ways in which the lives of husband as carer and wife as care-recipient are bound inextricably together. Most marriages might be described as intimate relationships in which the well being of one is tied to the well being of the other, where the decisions made and the actions taken by one rebound upon the other. But in the 'general case', the two in the partnership retain the capacity for independent action and decision making. In these marriages, on the other hand, it is as though there were a third party to the union – the MS – and it is this which has shaped (and continues to shape) the lives of both husband and wife. Clearly the wife's capacity for independent action, her ability to pursue a career and achieve her own goals, has been more greatly constrained than his. Nevertheless, the impact of the MS on her husband's life has also been very great and in some cases the 'shaping' and determining effect of the condition has become a highly constraining and confining one for him as well.

The chapter examines the nature and extent of that shaping and determining influence. It begins with the critical choices concerning accommodation and paid employment. While some of these men had been able to continue in paid work, most had had to retire earlier than would otherwise have been the case. Few wives had continued to work for long after the diagnosis. A number of couples had chosen to move to the country and set themselves up in such as way as to enable continued care at home for as long as possible. Many couples had experienced a degree of isolation from family and longstanding friends as a consequence or because of the moves associated with a career in the armed services. There were also a number of families where serious rifts had occurred and had resulted in separation from one or more family members. Whatever the reason for the isolation it had invariably meant that there was no immediate practical help from family members and often no moral support either. Some had not sought help from their children because they felt they had their own worries and pressures and did not want to add to them. There was constant worry about money for all but a few of the couples. Where family members had been able and willing to provide support it was primarily children who had given this help. On the other hand, in relation to financial help, it was principally parents who had provided this assistance: a number had done so on numerous occasions over the years.

In only a few cases had couples been reliant on formal services. Most of the couples included here made only marginal use of these services. They gave accounts of their experience with community and other services that were not always particularly positive. Much provision was seen to be unreliable or inappropriate with little capacity to provide emergency backup. There were high rates of attrition and staff turnover especially in rural areas. Knowledge of MS and its 'treatment' was often very limited. Inadequate provision was especially marked in relation to respite provision. To seek respite in country towns or regional centres almost invariably meant being accommodated in an aged care facility where the majority of residents were suffering from some level of dementia. Reliable or regular day care was not available to any of the carers included here.

These men spoke of their situation in matter of fact terms but they were acutely aware of the costs and losses involved. For all but one man there was a sense of loss associated with the need to retire early from paid employment. For some of the men this was especially marked: there was no substitute for the rewards associated with work. While they took pride in caring competently and well, quite a few men found domestic work difficult and stressful. Other costs featured in their accounts. Many of these were the direct result of the impact of MS on their wife's health, for example, the absence of a sexual relationship and the loss of certain shared elements of the marriage and of a future which had been jointly planned and anticipated. These were a loss equally for husband and wife.

The shaping impact of the MS and of the caring responsibilities is evident at every turn in these stories but the focus is upon the wife, her needs and the importance of finding ways to ensure these are met. It is this concern that lies at the centre of these accounts: this is the priority and it is this that has shaped all else. Of course, this is one perspective, that of the husband, and I cannot know whether there were other more negative elements to these marriages – for example, resentful and exploitative aspects. Nevertheless, this was not how it seemed and I do not believe that, beyond the ordinary 'ups' and 'downs' of all marriages, there was a darker side to these unions. As with so many other accounts of care, these stories underline how all encompassing care may become and how inextricably the lives of carer and care recipient may become bound together. But this is particularly graphic here. In most of the cases in this study, the care has extended over decades. This is care in a context where things will inevitably become more difficult and the care more and more demanding. These men might take exception to a language of altruism, goodness and sacrifice but they did not question the rightness and necessity of giving priority to the needs of someone they loved even when that might involve putting aside their own needs and desires and doing so over many years, indeed in some cases for the greater part of their married life. As for the reasons for this commitment, there were two that featured in these accounts, first, that it was a job that needed to be done and it had fallen to them to do it and, second, a conviction that, had the situation been reversed, their wife would, just as surely, have cared for them.

Practical Considerations and Recommendations

1. In undertaking research in the area of social care, there is particular value in joint research involving academe and an 'industry partner' – a community based agency, charitable organisation, advocacy body, etc. The mutual benefits include the contribution of workers in the field to the design and conduct of research

particularly in the analysis phase, and the ready communication of research findings to those who can put them to immediate and practical use.

2. The importance of developing more dynamic, fluid and open ended conceptualisations of care is underlined in this study.
3. Here is further evidence of the importance of workplace flexibility of a kind that enables working carers to continue in paid work for as long as possible. Workplaces also gain from having experienced workers able to go on working while they care.
4. There is a need to reassess 'means-tested' government provisions and benefits which exclude many working carers. The result is that working carers often struggle on without assistance or are forced to draw on superannuation savings or rely on relatives for financial help or decide they cannot continue to work. When working carers drop out of work, they become eligible for many of the supports that would have helped them to stay in paid employment.
5. It is important that the training of medical and paramedical professionals includes an emphasis on the crucial role of family carers in the health care of many disabled and elderly patients. In addition doctors need to be ready to listen carefully to carers and care recipients and to respect and draw on their knowledge.
6. Doctors also need to pay attention to the health of the carer as well as the care recipient. In particular, they need to be alert to mental health issues especially the possibility of depression.
7. Real estate institutes should be encouraged to establish special services for people in wheelchairs or with other mobility problems who are looking for suitable housing, including providing separate listings of homes that meet their requirements.
8. The importance of good, accessible and affordable respite is underlined again in this study – short-term, full-time alternative care, day care, and emergency or crisis care. There is an urgent need for ample and separate respite provision (of all three types) for younger disabled people.
9. There is a need to assess the extent to which country areas are being disadvantaged in terms of provision of community services and health services, the nature of the gaps or areas of inadequate provision, staff turnover, staff training, etc. These inadequacies should be widely publicised and pressure placed on governments, particularly on politicians in rural electorates, to address these shortcomings.
10. Consideration needs to be given to providing special training for counsellors to enable them to work effectively with couples where one individual (or both) in the partnership is in need of ongoing care. Training programmes of this kind should be developed in consultation with spousal carers and their partners (and those already working closely with them), for example through carers' organisations.

BIBLIOGRAPHY

Bayley, J. (1998). *Iris. A Memoir of Iris Murdoch.* London: Duckworth.

Blustein, J. (1991). *Care and Commitment: Taking the Personal Point of View.* New York: Oxford University Press.

Brown, P. (1996). Caregivers - the invisible workforce: Caregiver and gender issues. In Department of Human Services and Health, Aged and Community Care Division and Office of Disability, Towards a National Agenda for Carers: Workshop Papers (pp. 68-89). Canberra: AGPS.

Bytheway, B., Keil, T., Allatt, P., and Bryman, A. e. (1985). *Becoming and Being Old: Sociological Approaches to Later Life.* London: Sage.

Cahill, S. (2000). Elderly husbands caring at home for wives diagnosed with Alzheimer's Disease: are male and female caregivers really different? *Australian Journal of Social Issues*, 35 (1), 53-72.

Dalley, G. (1988). *Ideologies of Caring.* Basingstoke, Hampshire: Macmillan.

Ebers, G. C., Yee, I. M., Sadovnick, A. D., and Duquette, P. (2000). Conjugal multiple sclerosis: population-based prevalence and recurrence risks in offspring. *Annals of Neurology*, 48 (6), 927-931.

Elliot, F. R. (1996). *Gender, Family and Society.* Basingstoke, Hampshire and London: Macmillan.

Engster, D. (2004). Care ethics and natural law theory: toward an institutional political theory of caring. *The Journal of Politics*, 66 (1), 113-135.

Finch, J., and Mason, J. (1993). *Negotiating Family Responsibilities*. London: Routledge.

Forbes, R. B., Wilson, S. V., and Swingler, R. J. (1999). The prevalence of multiple sclerosis in Tayside, Scotland: do latitudinal gradients really exist? *Journal of Neurology*, 246(11), 1033-1040.

Gibson, D. (1998). *Aged Care: Old Policies, New Problems*. Cambridge: Cambridge University Press.

Gibson, D., Butkus, E., Jenkins, A., Mathur, S. and Liu, Z. (1996). The Respite Needs of Australians. Prepared for the Respite Review undertaken by the Aged Care and Community Care Division of the Commonwealth Department of Health and Family Services. Respite Review Supporting Paper 1, Aged Care Series No. 3. Canberra: Australian Institute of Health and Welfare.

Gulick, E. E. (1995). Coping among spouses or significant others of persons with Multiple Sclerosis. *Nursing Research*, 44(4), 220-225.

Hammond, S. R., English, D. R., and McLeod, J. G. (2000). The age-range of risk of developing multiple sclerosis: evidence from a migrant population in Australia. *Brain,* 123 (Pt. 5), 968-974.

Hernan, M. A., Olek, M. J., and Ascherio, A. (1999). Geographic variations of MS incidence in two prospective studies of US women. *Neurology*, 53 (8), 1711-1718.

Hubert, J. (1993). At home and alone: families and young adults with challenging behaviour. In J. Bornat, C. Pereira, G. Pilgrim and F. Williams (Eds.), *Community Care: A Reader* (pp. 107-113). Basingstoke, Hampshire: Macmillan in association with the Open University,.

Kahana, E. (2000). Epidemiologic studies in multiple sclerosis: a review. *Biomedicine and Pharmacotherapy*, 54 (2).

Kurtzke, J. F. (2000). Multiple sclerosis in time and space - geographic clues to cause. *Journal of Neurovirology,* 6 Suppl. 2, S34-40.

Mc Donnell, G. V., and Hawkins, S. A. (2000). Multiple sclerosis in Northern Ireland: a historical and global perspective. *Ulster Medical Journal*, 69 (2), 97-105.

Montgomery, R., and Borgatta, E. (1989). The effective of alternative support strategies on family care giving. *The Gerontologist*, 29 (4), 457-464.

Nolan, M., Grant, G., and Keady, J. (1996). *Understanding Family Care. A multidimensional model of caring and coping.* Buckingham and Philadelphia: Open University Press.

Parker, G. (1993). *With this Body. Caring and Disability in Marriage.* Buckingham and Philadelphia: Open University Press.

Qureshi, H., and Walker, A. (1989). *The Caring Relationship: Elderly People and Their Families*. London: Macmillan.

Rasmussen, H. B., and Clausen, J. (2000). Genetic risk factors in multiple sclerosis and approaches to their identification. *Journal of Neurovirology*, 6 Suppl. 2, S23-27.

Schofield, H., with Bloch, S., Herrman, H., Murphy, B., Nankervis, J., and Singh, B. (1998). *Family Caregivers. Disability, Illness and Ageing.* Sydney: Allen andUnwin, in association with Victorian Health Promotion Foundation.

Tribe, K., and Tribe, G. (2002). MS Society statistics and profile of membership. (Personal communication.)

Tronto, J. (1994). *Moral Boundaries. A Political Argument for an Ethic of Care*. New York and London: Routledge.

Ungerson, C. (1987). *Policy is Personal: Sex, Gender and Informal Care.* In. London and New York: Tavistock.

van der Mei, I. A., Ponsonby, A. L., Blizzard, L., and Dwyer, T. (2001). Regional variation in multiple sclerosis prevalence in Australia and its association with ambient ultraviolet radiation. *Neuroepidemiology,* 20 (3), 168-174.

Walker, M. U. (1998). *Moral Understandings. A Feminist Study in Ethics.* New York and London: Routledge.

In: Family Caregiving for Older Disabled People
Editor: Isabella Paoletti, pp. 177-200
ISBN 1-59454-808-0

Chapter 9

MOTHER-DAUGHTER RELATIONSHIPS WITHIN THE CARE PROCESS OF ALZHEIMER'S DISEASE: THE DAUGHTERS' PERSPECTIVE

Catherine Ward-Griffin
School of Nursing, The University of Western Ontario, London, Ontario, Canada.

INTRODUCTION

By the year 2031, 750,000 Canadians will be diagnosed with dementia (Canadian Mental Health Association, 2000). The prevalence rate of dementia nearly doubles with every 5-year increase in age from the age of 60 years, rising to 32% in those aged 90-94 (Hofman et al., 1991), and the probability of developing Alzheimer's Disease (AD) is higher for women than men. AD is an insidious pervasive debilitating disorder that destroys the affected person's capacity for self-care (Wuest, Ericson and Stern, 1994). It not only has a profound impact on individuals diagnosed with the disease, it also affects the lives of family members caring for them. At the same time, recent changes in patterns of care provision, including health care restructuring, the closure of long-term care facilities and under funding of home care (Chappell, 1999) have led to an increasing reliance on family care. Currently, it is estimated that between 75% and 85% of all types of care received by elderly people comes from the family. Among adult children, daughters and daughters-in-law provide over three quarters of parental care (Stone et al., 1987). Providing care to a parent with AD can involve a progressive increase in care responsibilities over a period of years while the caregiver continues to fulfil the demands of multiple roles (McCarty, 1996; Mui, 1995).

Planning for the care of increasing numbers of elderly persons with dementia has become an urgent health concern in Canada and elsewhere. Given the longer life span of women and the gendered role expectations of women as family caregivers, intergenerational caregiving between mothers and daughters will become increasingly common. It is essential that we understand the lives of women across the generations in order promote the health of both caregivers and care receivers. More importantly, understanding the care process within AD and other dementias is critical for the identification of appropriate types of programs and policies in order to strengthen the necessary supports that promote the health of both caregivers and care recipients within dementia.

LITERATURE REVIEW

AD and Caregiving

While family caregiving can be a deeply meaningful experience (Allen and Walker, 1992), it may also incur substantial physical, emotional and financial costs upon the caregiver, such as physical exhaustion (Aronson, 1994), depression and isolation (Wuest, 1997), and missed employment opportunities (Martin Matthews and Keefe, 1995). Most of the research in AD and caregiving have focussed on the negative consequences of caregiving. The literature is replete with studies of the problems of caregiving, many of which view the individual with AD as a significant source of caregiver burden (Beeson et al., 2000, McCarty, 1996, Pallett, 2000; Stevenson, 1990), with a few exceptions (Butcher, Holkup, and Buckwalter, 2001).

Other researchers have studied the process of caring for a family member with dementia. Chenoweth and Spencer (1986) found that most caregivers of family members with AD experience a great deal of stress throughout their relative's illness, but the stress varied and took on different forms depending upon the phase of illness. MacRae's (2002) qualitative study showed that family members found the loss of self in the member with AD particularly stressful, refusing to let go of what remained of the loved one's former self. Similarly, in a grounded theory study of 15 caregivers (1 son, 3 husbands, 1 sister, 5 daughters and 5 wives), Wuest, Ericson and Stern (1994) found that caregivers and care recipients with AD interact on a continuum from intimacy to alienation through dimensions of dawning, holding on and letting go. Spousal and adult child caregivers while awaiting placement of cognitively impaired members also reported a high degree of burden and fatigue in Strang and Koop's (2002) interpretative descriptive study. They also found that there was a deeply embedded bond between the family caregiver and the member with dementia. This bond nourished the caregiver's desire to look after the person with dementia at home and it continued to do so after long-term care placement.

Although these studies increase our knowledge about the process of caregiving within dementia, they fail to illuminate a range of caregiving outcomes, both negative and positive. Furthermore, most caregiving research has relied solely on the perspectives of the caregiver, but has rarely examined the perceptions of the care recipient because of the dementia of the care recipient (Cotrell and Schulz, 1993) and difficulty in recruiting care recipients (Long, Sudha, and Mutran, 1998). However, recent research demonstrates that individuals with mild to moderate cognitive impairment are able to answer questions about their own care with a high degree of accuracy and reliability (Whitlach and Feinberg, 1999). As well, most studies tend to obtain a diverse sample of family caregivers in one study even though there is strong evidence that male and female spouses and adult children have very different caregiving experiences (Matthews, 2002; Parsons, 1997). The literature also suggests that stress is mediated by both the type and quality of relationship between the primary family caregiver and the elderly relative with dementia (Pallet, 1990). Gender and type of family relations is important to consider when the focus is on relationships rather than roles. Clearly, it is important to focus on and understand women's experiences in an intergenerational relationship, and how that bond may change within a caregiving situation over time.

Family Ties and Caregiving

Although the caregiving literature is extensive, research has tended to segment the life course, with women giving care receiving more visibility than women receiving care (Aronson, 1991). In addition, as described by Poirer and Ayres (2002), caregiving is relational, and cannot be separated from people's experiences of each other in the past, present, or even the anticipated future. As explained by Pallett (2000), family caregiving takes place within the historical context since bonds of affection and reciprocity that sustain caregiving are rooted in past relationships. Walter's (1991) study of 48 caregiving daughter /mother dyads (without dementia) suggested that the more peer-like the mother-daughter relationship at the time of the caregiving experiences, the less stress that adult daughter experiences as a caregiver. Although this study included both caregiver and care recipients within the sample, it tended to focus on the perspectives and outcomes of the daughter.

Another limitation of the published research is that the relationship between an aging mother and her caregiving adult daughter has tended to distort the reciprocity in their relationship (Allen and Walker, 1992). Neufeld and Harrison (1995) found that 20 women (wives, daughters, daughters-in-laws, and granddaughters) caring for older adults with cognitive impairment described reciprocity as "give and take". However, caregivers were unable to establish the same kind of reciprocal relationships with the person with dementia as they did with others. Keefe and Fancey (2002) also explored the importance of giving and receiving for caregiving daughters and their older mothers without dementia. They found that mothers and daughters have different perspectives about reciprocity with mothers minimizing their past contributions. In contrast, Talbot's (1990) study of 55 older widowed mothers without dementia suggested that mothers give much and receive little, which may contribute to the negative effects of these relationships on the mothers. Finally, Carruth (1996) explored reciprocity among adult children of parents with dementia and without dementia and found that the diagnosis of dementia did not contribute to the explained variance of caregiver reciprocity. These study findings suggest that it is the exchange received rather than given that is more predictive of the nature of the reciprocal relationship; however, further research in this area is warranted.

Pohl, Boyd and Given (1997) studied mother-daughter relationships through the first year of caregiving (without dementia) and found that for many daughters, caregiving was a somewhat fixed extension of their life long relationships, but for others, caregiving provided an opportunity to develop closer mother-daughter ties. In their sample of 29 mother-daughter pairs, Allen and Walker (1992) found considerable evidence for both positive caregiving outcomes and the active role of mothers in intergenerational dyads. Aronson (1991) concluded from her study of 14 middle-class older women that the relationships between women of different generations are heavily loaded with constraints and expectations that are sometimes manifest in the form of interpersonal strain. In addition, she found that the limited availability of publicly provided services and supports was a significant ingredient in producing such strain. Although these studies help us better understand the relationships between adult daughters and their mothers, we can not assume that these qualitative experiences would be found within dementia care.

Strain and Blandford (2003) in their cross sectional study of caregiving networks of older adults found that individuals with cognitive impairment were significantly more likely than those who were cognitively intact to receive assistance with care; however, the types of network were similar for both types of care receivers. Fast, Keating, Otfinowski and Derksen (2004) reported that network characteristics, such as small size, geographically distant members, and male, placed frail seniors at risk of receiving inadequate care. Using the National Survey of Families and Households Database, Uhlenberg and Cooney (1990) reported that adult children without siblings in the United States were found to report lower quality relationships with their mothers, and this association was statistically significant only for daughters with two or more siblings, suggesting a possible negative connection between high obligation to a mother and feeling positive about the relationship. Although the results of this study are not generalizable to situations in which mothers suffer from cognitive impairment, one wonders how caregiving within AD contributes to the development of the mother-daughter relationship, as well as how contextual factors, such as care network and access to appropriate publicly supports and services, influences caregiving and care receiving outcomes for mothers and daughters.

In a rare qualitative study of 17 daughters who cared for parents with AD, McCarty (1996) found that the availability of sibling support and/or spouse support was identified as meaningful assistance. While this grounded theory study expanded awareness of the interrelationship between caregiver stress and the contextual aspects of social support, such as sibling network and the nature of filial relationship, it is unclear if daughters caring for mothers compared with daughters caring for fathers had similar or different experiences.

In summary, what we know about mother-daughter relationships within the care process of AD is primarily based on quantitative, cross-sectional designs. As well, the lack of longitudinal research has been identified as a gap in the family caregiving research (Pohl et al., 1997). There is limited research about the specific relationships between adult daughters and their mothers with AD, how their relationship changes over time, or how the care process influences their health and well-being. Moreover, if we are to broaden our understanding of the care process of AD, future research needs to focus on caregiving as a dyadic process, one which considers both perspectives of the caregiver and care recipient (Lyons, Zarit, Sayer, and Whitlach, 2002).

METHOD

In order to address the resulting lack of knowledge on which to base practice and policy, the purpose of this longitudinal, qualitative study was to develop a better understanding of the experiences of adult daughters and community-dwelling older women with AD who receive this care. Evidence suggests that the caregiving experience differs by gender, by the relationship of the family member to the care recipient, and by the health status of the care recipient (Dupuis and Norris, 2001). Therefore, this study focused exclusively on adult daughters caring for mothers with mild to moderate cognitive impairment. Specifically, we were interested in the following research questions: 1) How do daughters describe their experience of providing care to their mothers with AD?; 2) How do mothers with AD describe their experience of receiving care from their daughters?; 3) How do mothers with AD and their adult daughters describe their relationship?; 4) What contextual factors (e.g. living arrangement, employment status of caregiver, use of professional services) influence the care provided/received? ; and 5) What is the impact of care provided/received on women's health and well-being over time?

Theoretical Framework

This qualitative study, guided by socialist-feminist theory and a life course perspective, was used to explore the perceptions of adult daughters and their mothers diagnosed with AD. This type of inquiry gives primacy to individual subjective perceptions of their care experiences, while at the same time, seeks to understand the fluctuating nature of the mother-daughter relationship over time. Feminist scholars have identified the importance of the tie between mother and daughter. Given their skills and expectations in maintaining social ties, it is not surprising that mothers and daughters share stronger relationships than fathers and sons in adulthood (Fingerman, 2001). Feminist theorists have also questioned the premise that autonomy is the final virtue to be equated with maturity. Instead the emphasis in feminist writing has been on the bond that mothers and daughters share (Fingerman, 2001). .

Social-feminist scholars, most notably the writings of Ungerson (1990) and Stoller (1993) have provided explanations for the ways in which caring is defined, and the way it is organized. Since a feminist perspective recognizes women's everyday caring experiences as inextricably connected to the larger political, social and economic environment (Hall and Stevens, 1991), elicitation of women's narratives about the intergenerational care process identify larger cultural values and ideologies. As discussed earlier, the caregiving literature tends to portray elderly mothers as burdensome to their overworked daughters. Feminist inquiry offers an alternative view-that caregiving is an intergenerational journey between two women. Finally, the goal of feminist research is to develop knowledge, which is capable of creating positive changes with the aim of improving the lives of women in this intergenerational relationship.

This study also took a life course perspective in order to understand the interactions and exchanges between mothers and adult daughters throughout their lives. This perspective is appropriate since it assumes that the meaning of care (giving and receiving) is based on a lifetime of experiences rather than on the current event or situation that is being addressed (i.e. mother with dementia) (Finch, 1987; Fingerman, 2002). In addition, since a life course perspective is particularly interested in the dialectic between employment and family life over time (Rossi and Rossi, 1990), as well its contributing socio-cultural factors, this approach may help to detect changes in patterns of employment among employed daughters. It also captures the impact of those changes at various stages of family life, and on the health and well-being of caregiving daughters and mothers receiving their care.

Recruiting and Sampling Methods

Building on the theoretical perspectives outlined above, the accounts of mothers and daughters were treated as both individual perceptions of caregiving and care receiving and "points of entry" into social processes far beyond participants' realities (Smith, 1987). After gaining approval from the university's Ethics Review Board, multiple recruitment strategies were used to obtain a purposive sample of 25 mother-daughter dyads. Key community agencies, such as the Alzheimer Society, Day Hospital Programs and Memory Clinics were approached to identify potential participants. In an attempt to reach participants who may not access these services, colourful flyers and notices about the study were sent and posted in family physician offices and community sites, such as libraries, YWCA, and senior centres. Health professionals who worked with seniors and/or their families, such as clinical nurse specialists, community nurses and social workers, were also contacted by telephone or in person to enlist their help in identifying potential participants. Follow-up letters and telephone calls to agencies were made two to three weeks later. Finally, using a snowball technique, some daughter participants introduced us to other interested women, usually their sisters. Consequently, three mothers had more than one daughter who participated. Regardless of the method of recruitment, all women interested in taking part in the study were asked to contact a member of the research team.

Daughters/mothers willing to participate in the study were asked to provide names of their mothers/daughters who were then contacted by one of the researchers. Inclusion criteria for mothers with AD included: 1) consents to participate; 2) English speaking; 3) receives at least 2 on average hours of care/week; 4) receive a score of 17 or higher on the standardized mini-mental status examination (SMMSE); and 5) has good verbal and comprehension skills (e.g. able to state birthdate). According to Molloy and Clarnette (1999), a score of 21-24 is indicative of early dementia and a score between 10 and 20 is indicative of moderate dementia. Based on previous clinical experience of one of the investigators, the "cut off" score was set at 17 to ensure accurate reliable interview data. Once consent was obtained, one of the investigators administered the SMMSE to the mothers with AD. Inclusion criteria for daughters included: 1) consents to participate; 2) English speaking; 3) regular contact with mother (i.e. provides at least on average 2 hours of care/week). All potential participants were given written information about the purpose and nature of the study, and were asked to take part in two interviews, six to nine months apart. Written consent was obtained immediately prior to the interview and confidentiality was promised to all participants (e.g. use of pseudonyms).

The mean age for the daughters in the study was 52 years, although there was a range of ages from 36 to 64. Majority were Canadian (75%), married (71%), had at least a post-secondary education (50%) and were employed, either full-time (42%) or part-time (25%) in various sectors, such as education, business, or retail. The average household income was evenly distributed amongst the participants who completed this demographic question: $0-$19,999 (4 daughters); $20,000-$39,999 (6 daughters); $40,000-$59,999 (6 daughters); $60,000-$79,000 (3 daughters); above $80,000 (3 daughters); undeclared (2 daughters). The sibling network of the daughters also varied, ranging from no siblings to nine children in the family: only children (5 daughters), one sibling (2 daughters), 2 siblings (9 daughters), and 3 or more siblings (8 daughters).

Daughters reported that they had been giving care to their mothers for an average of 45 months, with a range of less than one year to greater than six years. The mothers receiving care ranged in age from 75 to 98 years (mean age=87) and obtained SMMSE scores of 10-28 (mean 20.5/30). The majority of the mothers were widowed (76%). All daughters, with one exception, lived in the same city as their mothers. At the time of the first set of interviews, four of the mothers lived in their own homes, four mothers lived in their daughters' homes, and eleven of the mothers resided in retirement homes. On average, the daughters provided regular assistance to their mothers (three days per week), ranging from daily to weekly contact. The length of time that the daughters had been providing assistance to their mothers also varied: seven were in the early stages of caregiving (i.e. less than two years), seven were in the middle stages of caregiving (two to five years), and ten were in the later stages (more than five years). As will be discussed in the findings, all daughters provided help with transportation, housekeeping and meal preparation while many assisted with personal care.

Data Collection

If both mother and daughter in a dyad gave consent to participate in the study, separate in-depth interviews were arranged at a mutually convenient time and place. All interviews were audio-taped. At the time of writing this chapter, a total of 25 interviews were conducted with the daughters, averaging 75 minutes each. The majority of these were conducted in the participants' homes. The remainder of the interviews with the daughters occurred in a quiet room at their mothers' residences, or at the daughters' workplaces. On one occasion, a daughter from out-of-town requested that the interview be held at one of the researcher's offices. Given the sensitive nature of the interview, eight daughters openly expressed sadness (i.e. weeping) as they recounted their past and current experiences about their mothers. Eleven interviews, lasting approximately 45 minutes, were conducted with the mothers who scored a SMMSE of 17 or higher. One mother was interviewed twice because needed extra time to discuss her relationships with her four daughters fully. All of these interviews were held at the mothers' residence. At the end of the interview, all participants were also asked to complete a brief demographic questionnaire. Finally, full field notes were written after each interview.

The decision to not conduct conjoint mother/daughter interviews was largely based upon the belief that individual reports may be more forthcoming. Furthermore, since there is considerable less research documenting the perspectives of persons who receive care, it was important to capture voices previously unheard (Allen and Walker, 1992). However, on three occasions, mothers required or requested the presence of a relative, usually the daughter or grand-daughter. During these interviews, the mother or daughter occasionally drew one another into the conversation to confirm or verify some information. Therefore, it is possible that the mothers' responses in these situations were influenced by the presence of her relative. However, one advantage of the conjoint interviews was the opportunity to collect observational data with respect to mother-daughter interactions. Thus, interviewing the mother and daughter together did not necessarily yield a more complete picture of the relationship, just a different one.

Using an in-depth focussed interviewing approach (Merton, Fiske, and Kendall, 1990), the participants were asked non-directive questions designed to trigger dialogue about their experiences in providing/receiving care, the mother-daughter relationship, and the factors influencing process of care. This approach encouraged participants to discuss what they thought were the most important aspects of the care process and of their relationships. As well, our approach to interviewing was also informed by the work of feminist researchers and scholars (Oaklkey, 1982; Reinharz, 1992). All three interviewers strove towards building rapport, and giving support and information during the interview if requested. For instance, we provided information at times to daughters about accessing community resources or discuss possible alternatives when service deficiencies were identified. Thus, the study created the potential for consciousness-raising and personal empowerment consistent with feminist goals.

Also in keeping with a feminist inquiry, preliminary study findings were taken back to the daughter participants in a focus group forum for discussion, clarification and refinement. Following the procedures by Krueger (1994), two audio-taped focus groups with 17 of the 24 original daughter participants were conducted and led by one of the investigators. In addition, the focus group data served as a means to assist with the development of the second round of interviews. Finally, the focus group discussions provided an opportunity for daughter participants to offer mutual support and tangible strategies to other daughters who are providing care to mothers with AD.

Data Analysis

The major procedures for qualitative data analysis followed the guidelines of Lofland and Lofland (1995). The data analyzed for this chapter consisted of interview transcripts and corresponding field notes. After each interview, full fieldnotes recorded perceptions, insights and observations (Morse and Field, 1995). The fieldnotes, commonly used in qualitative research, added richness and depth to the data, and guided the planning for future interviews. As the data analysis proceeded, memos or notes kept track of insights and included justifications for making analytic decisions. For instance, it became apparent that the daughter's sibling network directly influenced the care that she provided to her mother. Consequently, additional questions about siblings and other relatives will be asked in subsequent interviews.

Gathering and analyzing data were simultaneous processes (Lofland and Lofland, 1995). Transcription and initial analysis of the interviews began immediately after the first interview and proceeded concurrently as data were collected. Shortly after each interview, individual researchers read the transcription of each interview and independently made a preliminary analysis of the transcribed data, focusing on the key phrases and concepts that emerged from the data. Team analysis further clarified concepts (e.g. independence, dependence), themes (e.g. being in control), and patterns (e.g. regulation). Shortly after the completion of the last interview, the principal investigator prepared an overarching conceptual interpretation of participants' experiences which was finalized through subsequent team analysis and focus group discussions.

Strategies to promote credibility, dependability, confirmability and transferability of the qualitative findings (Lincoln, 1995; Miles and Huberman, 1994) included: a) maintenance of an audit trail of the researchers' activities; b) collection of both observational and interview data; c) audiotaping and verbatim transcription of all interviews; c) member-checking with a sub-sample of participants; and d) peer review (i.e. having a health professional who works in the area of AD examine the interpretation and comment on its applicably to her own clinical work experiences) (Kuzel and Like, 1991).

In the next section, we report only the perspectives of the daughters due to the caregiving focus of this book. Although the perspectives of the mothers receiving care were sought in this study, more than half of the mothers (n=14) received a SMMSE score of less than 17/30, which prevented them from actively participating in an interview. However, once the second round of interviews are completed in nine months time, a full account of both perspectives of the mother-daughter relationship will be published elsewhere at a later date.

FINDINGS

The primary goal of this qualitative study was to better understand mother-daughter relationships within the care process of dementia. Study findings revealed that the mother-daughter dyad journeyed together within an interactive process that progressed through five phases: "recognition", "negotiation", "regulation", "compensation", and "isolation". Within each phase, mothers and their adult daughters held different, yet complementary perspectives of the care process. As mentioned above, the daughters' caregiving experiences and the contextual factors that shaped these experiences will be the focus of this chapter, with particular attention on the impact caregiving had on the daughters' health and well-being.

Building on the metaphor of a journey, a number of interrelated themes emerged from the daughters' transcripts: becoming aware/stepping in, finding the balance, leading the way, carrying the load and holding on/letting go. The following section will more fully describe the complexities of each theme, accompanied by illustrative quotes.

Becoming Aware/Stepping in

The first of the themes identified was that of "becoming aware". Similar to Wuest, Ericson and Stern's (1994) study findings of the "dawning", the current study illuminated how daughters slowly recognized that some of the changes in their mothers' behaviour were part of a pattern, not isolated incidents. This realization had a direct impact on the quality of the mother-daughter relationship. For the daughter who had an emotionally close relationship, she began to notice that her mother and she were no longer "in step together"; there was conflict and tension when none existed before. Amy, who was an only child and described her relationship with her mother as "extremely close", recollected:

> We would do a few things and we'd notice little by little my mother repeating things and losing her temper quickly, not being the kind, gracious mother that I remember...Over the period of, I would say the next year and a half, we noticed little by little more changes taking place and the relationship changed, in that it was one of concern now, not one of enjoyment.

Once Noella, a registered nurse, realized that something was wrong with her mother, she offered to accompany and support her mother through the process of diagnosis:

> Like at first we thought she had depression. So I had a nurse friend who is a geriatric nurse talking to her and she was, you know, my mother got kind of like hypochondriac. She was always going to Emerge and she always knew something was wrong but she didn't talk about it. It manifested in things like chest pain and stomach problems. So I was doing a lot of taking her to the doctors, things like that. So it took a while before, and then of course, when they did diagnose her, I guess we did spend more time together.

For some daughters, their relationship with their mothers changed very quickly once they noticed their mothers exhibited disturbing symptoms, such as rage and excessive confusion. According to Ikkink, Van Tilbeg, and Kees (1999), when older mothers are healthy, interactions with adult children typically involve reciprocity. However, the growing need of support imposed by illness often reduces the power of the parents in exchanges with their adult children (Connidis, 2001). Joan, a married, retired teacher with four siblings, explained how her normally reciprocal relationship with her mother changed:

> She was such an independent person, everything was different then. Our conversations were totally different …now she's not making as many decisions, she tries to, but she has to discuss it with somebody, and so our relationship has changed dramatically because she's become very worried and she would discuss this worry and concern, we're very close and we have always talked so I could pick up the things that were happening to her.

In contrast, Heather, an only child, reflected that the changes in her relationship with her mother had been gradual:

> I think sometimes, unless you step back…the changes, they are very gradual, so you've got to really realize, that this is a change in the relationship. Yes, and I think when I see that, I'm more aware of how mom was and this is how she is now.

Although most daughters expressed feelings of sadness when they noticed their mothers' behavioural changes, Sandy, who was one of three children, was particularly upset as her positive relationship with her mother turned into a distrustful one:

> Actually, mom has turned against me, she's more negative…I was always the daughter whom she could trust.

However, for those daughters who did not have a very close relationship with their mother, they did not pick up on the behavioural changes as readily. Tara, who has one sister with a disability, explained:

> For as long as I can remember, I have been the designated one in the family to take care of my mother…she suffers from panic attacks as well as dementia...I noticed some forgetfulness and whatever, but for me, when she was over here, it was more of a gradual recognition. I just thought that was my mother being her demanding self. And it took me awhile to realize that maybe, maybe it's something more than that.

Similarly, Jennifer, who had one brother and one sister (Julia), commented:

> I didn't know what was going on. I just thought mom was a compulsive liar. And throughout our whole life, she's been very dishonest. But it got worse with Alzheimer's. Now I think it's honest dishonesty.

Becoming aware also took the form of reminiscing, thinking about the time before their mothers became ill and how the mother-daughter relationship started to change. For a many daughters, this realization led to regret and sadness. For instance, Jennifer and Tara reported that AD robbed them of their last opportunity to improve their relationships with their mothers.

However, regardless of their previous relationships with their mothers, all daughters recognized that they needed to "step in" and offer assistance to their mothers. As described by Joan, many decisions had to be made during this recognition phase:

> Many family members, not just myself, got concerned, and I just tried to sort it out in my own mind. What was going on? What's happening to her? What does she want me to do about it? What should I do about it? How much should I interfere? How much should you hold back? And where should I get the help?

Finding the Balance

The second predominant theme, "finding the balance", signified a turning point in the journey between the mothers and the daughters. The daughter offered to help her mother with a variety of tasks that she no longer could do easily or safely (e.g. driving, cooking, taking meds). In some situations, the mother accepted the help that was offered by the daughter, but in most situations, the mothers resisted, at least initially. Not unlike other research findings (McCarty, 1996) daughters attempted to follow their mothers' cues and to balance the mothers' need for respect, independence and safety. This was an active phase of the mother-daughter relationship as they negotiated their changing relationship. Similar to Neufeld and Harrison's (1995) study of reciprocity among caregiving daughters, Sarah explained:

> We [mother and daughter] have each got to give and take. I mean, there's not a right or wrong way of doing it. We just have to work it out…she is still the parent…but mom [who lived in a different city than daughter] needs a little more help. Cooking seems to be a struggle...I thought about getting meals on wheels. And I thought about getting full-time help but I thought, she doesn't want anybody living in her house with her. I wouldn't either...so I thought mom needed to come this direction because it just made more sense…and she realized that too…but we try to get back to [city] as often as we can.

Similarly, Joan described how her mother usually took the lead in their social activities while she assumed the "follower" role:

> She just loves to get out and she's the one who directs the day and I am the follower in that…it is a fun time for both of us. She likes to pay the tip. She likes using her visa card and you know, signing i t ...so I kind of take my cue from mom…I follow mom's lead really…it's a long process and probably we're learning together.

Finding the right balance also involved renegotiating what was best for both the mother and daughter. In Sarah's situation, her mother had lived with her and her husband for over a year, but now resided in a retirement home:

> It's nice to be back on our own again. And not that we don't love mom, but you know, you really need your space.

Most of the daughters reported that this phase of the relationship was awkward for them, constantly wondering how much assistance should be offered to their mothers, as described by Amy:

> She lived in her house. She had been there for 55 years and I respected that, although we [she and her husband] had encouraged her to get into a smaller environment....but she wouldn't let me interfere. And I didn't want to take that independence away from her either. I didn't want her to feeling that we thought that she couldn't cope.

For other daughters, this balancing act also took their fathers' needs and opinions into consideration. Joan explained:

> It was very difficult because you were constantly walking a tight rope. I didn't want to interfere with mom and dad's relationship ....but I wanted to be an advocate for mom too. I wanted to see where she wanted to go. So I had to discuss it with him as well. And I wanted him to be part of the team. That was tough but he gave mom and I the opportunity to pursue what we wanted to pursue because he saw mom wasn't happy. And that bothered him...so we were trying to balance mom's enthusiasm for what she was finding out that might help her, with dad's concern and apathy about professional help.

Leading the Way

Leading the way was the third theme identified from the interviews with daughters. Having acknowledged that their mothers had difficulties with carrying out simple directions, problem-solving and remembering important information, the daughters took control of their mothers' affairs (and eventually their lives). Protecting the mother by monitoring, setting limits and structuring the environment was a means of leading the way. The daughter was clearly in the leadership role now. Similar to Horton and Arber's (2004) findings, daughters who assumed controlling behaviours usually resulted in mothers taking on submissive roles. Heather, an only child, explained how she moved from the phase of negotiation to regulation:

> It is difficult... My mom being dependent... and she is not making decisions so it was awkward for me in the beginning. I'd ask her and then she wouldn't want to, now I just go ahead, so I've gotten through that stage. But I still think it's still difficult for my mother because...she says, "you're treating me like a child" ...but I don't think it is a role reversal, it's just a change. So I am more comfortable with that now. .But at first it felt awkward because most of your life it's been the other way. But I am over that now.

Joan commented that "leading the way" was difficult for her because she did not anticipate taking on the role of "parent":

> I sometimes feel that …about taking on the role as parent, at times, because I'm caring for them so much that that scares me, because that's not something you ever think that you are going to have to do. So that is a bit a frightening role.

Margaret, an only child, also explained that assuming the "mother" role was frustrating:

> But things are changing now and I am more of the mother now. I have to keep reminding her, and you can only do that so long before she gets mad at me, because she is my mother and I'm the daughter. So it is very awkward, it's a very awkward place to be. I wish it [dementia] hadn't happened.

Taking the lead generally caused the daughters to feel guilty but rationalized that it was in the best interests of their mothers. This is a common finding among other researchers (Horton and Arber, 2004; Keefe and Fancey, 2002; Pohl et al., 1997). Heather talked about the need to find a retirement home for her mother:

> It's the guilt…thinking that I am doing too little, too much. Should I be here, and then, what about my life? So it's finding the balance, and now the next step is to start looking for a retirement home. But mom doesn't want to and it's easy to sit here and say to my . mother, "it's time to move" and actually doing it. But right now, I've had enough. I think to she's not capable. She needs assisted living.

All daughters expressed deep concern and worry, usually over the desire to maintain their mothers' independence with the need to ensure they were safe. Dana, who was an only child and had contact with her mother every other day for the past two years, explained her dilemma:

> We want to keep her in her own apartment, to keep her as independent as she can be, but it's not so easy for us because I worry about her. At night, it's the last thing I do, I know when she goes to be, so I call, "are you okay?", and you know, "talk to you in the morning". Then I can hardly wait to get up in the morning to call and ask, "Have you had your breakfast?; Are you dressed?; Did you take your pills?"

Finally, many daughters explained that they needed to control their mothers' actions, especially if they were out in public. Dana explained how she reprimanded her mother while they were shopping:

> We were in the grocery store and she wanted 2 litres of chocolate milk. It was on special and they were all gone. So I said to mom," this is probably better anyway. You only have to open a little bit at a time. It will be fresh, it's much easier for you to pick up. Get a smaller one. She said, "I told you I wanted 2 litres." And I said, "But mom, they're all gone…I said take these, and I'll come back in the middle of the week to get you some". And I gave them to her and she fired them into the shopping cart... and before I realized what I had done, I said to her, "You do that again and we're going home!"

Carrying the Load

The fourth theme that illustrated part of the daughters' experiences was "carrying the load". As the mother's disease progressed, the daughter assumed more and more of the care. Daughters employed outside the home had dual demands. At times jobs suffered. At other times, other family relationships were strained. In some situations, siblings shared the responsibilities of care—eventually taking over all responsibilities. Regardless of the sibling network, all daughters felt a strong sense of filial obligation, as described by Melanie, who is unemployed with two siblings:

> I guess I am from the old schooling, she always did stuff for us, so now it's my turn to do stuff for her and no question about it, it was kind of a given.

Julia, sister of Jennifer, explained her feelings of obligation and duty to her mother this way:

> I say to her " we're concerned –you don't seem to understand when you get angry with me for doing this and that, you raised us when we were little. Now it is your turn."

In certain situations, strong feelings of duty and obligation have been described by Guberman, Maheu and Maille (1992) as the "dark side of family ties." In this study, some daughters felt resentful that they had to take on so much responsibility, especially if they perceived that their siblings were not doing their fair share. This is a common complaint according to Matthews (2002). Margaret described this inequity:

> I am overloaded, and you try and talk to the other ones [1 sister and 2 brothers], and they get mad at you. I'm telling them, well when will you put the garbage out, or just and come and have tea with her [mother], or whatever. They are doing their own thing. I feel that they don't care as much as I do. So I'm overloaded, and I am frustrated with the whole thing. I'm hurt about the other ones not wanting to help as much…my life's had to change because of this…I have to worry about her now. I didn't have to worry before. And now I come over and do all the things that my dad did…I worry. I love my mother.

While most of the daughters described the effects of AD as devastating to the mothers and to themselves, a few said that the experience had actually improved their relationship with their mother. Jennifer commented:

> Now that the disease has progressed and I can see it, it's easier for me to deal with it, because we used to fight all the time and argue…which is kind of a blessing because we get along a little better.

A strengthened attachment between caregiving daughters and their mothers have been reported elsewhere in the literature (Pohl et al., 1997). For those daughters who reported a distant or conflictual relationship with their mothers, they reported some improvement in their relationship with their mother, as described by Brenda, an only child of her widowed mother:

> I have a fairly good relationship with my mother but we weren't always close. I would say that her illness has brought us closer. It has helped me to understand certain things about her.

Others claimed that having a mother with AD had drawn the family closer together. Four sisters (Beth, Crystal, Lynn and Faith) who participated in the study all agreed that their sibling relationships were strengthened as a result of sharing the care of their mother. Beth explained:

> I would have to say that the relationships with my sisters-it's always been good...I would say it's strengthened those relationships.

Faith, one of Beth's sisters who worked full time, explained further how family and workplace supports helped her family care for their mother:

> Crystal, Beth, Lynn and I, and it is amazing, because we are very different people, and yet, very accepting of each other's strengths and weaknesses…I mean I was so appreciative that they were able to do so much and …we all got supportive workplaces where we have flexibility in hours and supportive supervisors so that we to have flexibility in our work schedules to accommodate mom's needs. So a combination of getting along well, having multiple members of the family and flexibility and financial resources, they have all been very important components, as well as supportive spouses.

This theme of needing publicly provided services is noted in other research (Aronson, 1991). Sharon, a part time employee, also mentioned the use of formal supports not only helped offset the demands of care, but were costly:

> I would suggest that it is important to have someone come in, and we always thought that because mom was living with us, and mom has a reasonable income that we wouldn't hold back any type of care. But just because she has some money doesn't mean she can afford to keep paying more and more things. Like even getting her to go to the day program, 5 days a week, it costs almost fifty dollars a week. For someone who didn't have an income, it would be a lot harder.

The stress gets to be too much for some daughters, as Tara explained:

> Right now, I don't get anything from her [mother]. I'm not getting anything in return. There are no rewards in this relationship at all and over the two years that she's been here, there have been times I would find myself so stressed and so upset and in tears that I would just say to my husband, "I just wish she was dead. I just wish that she is dead. It's just, this is too hard to handle."

The lack of recognition of the caregiving efforts is described also by Oddone and Aguirre in chapter 3, as the cause of intense stress and pain for caregivers. The daughters used a variety of personal coping strategies to offset the continuously demanding role of caregiver. In some situations, daughters put parts of their lives on hold as expressed by Julia:

> You have to put off what you have planned or things that you have to do, or want to do in order to do what I have to do for her. Right now it's not so bad, but it will get worse. I know that.

In other situations, many daughters complained that their siblings did not do their fair share, especially brothers. Tracey, who is one of five adult children, explained:

> Mom has four children close by, but the daughters are probably the most regular visitors. My one brother works, and the other brother works and travels but I don't' worry, that's what I do and I'm happy I can do it....my mother had forgotten how to cook...that was really why I quit work...but I don't regret that...sometimes I had some minor annoyances, particularly with my brothers because they never really do much. I feel my brother's could manage more time, and I don't agree, that it is women's work. I am one of 5 siblings, not one of two.

Jan, who was the oldest girl of four siblings and currently unemployed, described a similar situation:

> I'm sitting there one day in my care trying to come home.....and I thought to myself, "you have a problem here.... You have to either quit your mom, quit your family, or quit your job. Oh, quit your job" So I did. I have been home with mom over a year. My husband says quit your job, just quit your job...and it's not a hardship to give it up because, you know, you just cut back somewhere else, but still it is a loss of income.

Professional supports used by the mothers and their caregiving daughters also had a direct impact on the daughters' ability to manage their demanding responsibilities. Many times it was difficult to obtain appropriate health care and home care services, such as access to a geriatrician or home support workers. A few daughters commented that some health professionals helped them to better understand AD and to learn new ways of relating to their mothers. However, as illustrated in the following quotes, others reported ageist views held by some health professionals, which resulted in delayed medical treatment for their aging mothers with AD:

> Mom's family doctor was not supportive at alt. He just didn't think it was worth getting any help for mom, you know, due to her age. (Joan)

> My mom's GP said, "Oh no, that's just normal for her age". And I am thinking, "Bullshit, it's not normal aging!" (Bonnie)

Holding On/Letting Go

The final theme, "holding on/letting go" reflected the last phase of the mother-daughter relationship. Although Wuest, Ericson and Stern (1994) reported holding on and letting go as two separate dimensions in the changing family caregiving relationship in AD, our study findings revealed that holding on and letting go were tightly interconnected themes, in which daughters moved back and forth. In addition, in the current study, letting go involved a gradual emotional and physical separation between the daughter and mother with AD, not one that only involved the decision to place a relative in an institution. Similar to other researchers' findings (Fingerman, 2001), we also found that memories of childhood experiences with parents were associated with the quality of relationships and willingness to care for the parent in late life. Sarah described the mother-daughter relationship like a rope:

> I couldn't imagine doing this if you never had a good relationship with your mom… I think that would be really, really difficult .. .if the relationship wasn't strong to begin with, this puts a real strain on what was left. And if the rope is really thin and there are only a few little strings left, I think that it would be gone. But over the years, your relationship is like a rope to me, it thins out sometimes and it gets pretty thin because there's a lot of factors…but if it's thin to begin with, I don't know. I don't envy those people.

Also, "holding on" pertained to holding on to memories, both positive and negative. Canadian author, Carol Shields (1987), eloquently wrote in *Swan:* "The connective twine between us [mothers and daughters] is taut with details (p. 48)." Study findings revealed that negative memories strained the mother-daughter relationship further while positive memories tended to sustain this relationship, even through difficult times. Bonnie, an only child who reported a very close relationship with her mother, explained it this way:

> She knows, even through all the cloudiness in her mind, she knows and she can feel that her child is here… She's still my mother and I will have no other.

Brenda, who is another only child, visited her widowed mother every second day. The following quote illustrates how she was "holding on" to her mother, especially in light of not receiving much affection from her mother as a child:

> I'm not ready to say good bye yet. Yesterday was a good day. She was looking well, and we were outside and she was commenting on how beautiful it was in the garden. She's very affectionate toward me and she never showed me a lot of personal affection when I was young and I always craved more from my mother while I felt smothered by my father.

Letting go involved the painful process of the daughter recognizing that the mother was no longer present on this journey. Jan's comment illustrates how she oscillated between holding on and letting go:

> I miss mom not being here but I am also relieved that she's not here [home]…and our relationship is better now that she's not here too, because it's not like 24 hours a day, 7 days a week, 12 months a year, you know it was hard….it's like she's not the same person, she's a different person. But then you'll go in and she'll be as bright as a penny—almost like the bright light before it goes out.

Similarly, Jennifer complained that she no longer had a "normal" mother-daughter relationship:

> It's almost like mom has forgotten how to be a mom....she doesn't ask how we're doing, she doesn't enjoy our company as much…I miss being able to go to mom, and ask her for help and for her to console me , and understand what I'm going through. It's all about her now.

Noella rationalized that the change in this relationship can be viewed as a "normal" caregiving transition between mothers and daughters:

> Well I mean it really has kind of gone full circle because she used to look after us and our bodily needs and now we're doing it for her. I'm not sure that she knows me anymore. I don't really think she does particularly.... But that doesn't really matter because, you know, she's – it's just sort of full circle. We look after her now the way she looked after us.

In terms of the final phase of her relationship with her mother, Noella commented:

> I think in some ways... you go through different phases. Like in a way you grieve, like you're losing the person. This isn't the most difficult stage. I mean the most difficult stage was probably when she was constantly asking the same thing over and over and she'd get agitated.... But you know, I could still talk to her. She could still talk then. We still felt, you know, she knew who we were so you still felt a bond but now it's like – you know, as time goes by and she stopped talking and now it's like she's not sure who we are. You know, you still feel closeness and tenderness but you just – it's different. It's a different relationship. I can't talk to her about my life or anything like that. So it's really just more non-verbal, you know, holding her hand and doing those things for her. I mean I miss her, the person she was. I have one video of her and I sometimes watch it and, you know, I miss that person.

Tara also reflected on the past few years:

> And I gotten through that and I've gone past that and I understand that's her anxiety and her fears speaking, and whatever bit of dementia, is complicating all that. But that's her and she's not going to improve and she's not going to change, the one who has to change is me....so I react differently to all that now. Acknowledging that and understanding it in my head as well as my heart has helped.

For some, making decisions about institutional placement occurred at this time. For others, the decision to sever the tie was much more difficult than the decision to hold on. Jan, commented:

> I feel that if I don't see her [mother] at least a couple of times a week, that pretty soon, she won't know who I am.

However, others expressed that their mothers were no longer present on their journey as explained by Margaret: "....she's not my mother anymore. I feel like I have lost my mother."

Discussion

The purpose of this chapter was to describe the daughters' perspective of the mother-daughter relationship within the care process of AD. Although preliminary in nature, the study findings reinforce the importance of using a feminist, life-course methodology to achieve new understandings about mother-daughter caring relationships within the context of AD. In particular, findings illuminated how daughters' relationships with their mothers changed over time, and how this care process influenced the daughters' health and well-being. The insights gained from this research are particularly significant for program planners and policy makers. The first insight is that the family network is important within the care process of AD. Second, gender ideologies shaped the types of family interactions and experiences of daughters caring for mothers with AD. Third, more formal supports are required to help families care for members with AD. Study implications associated with each of these insights are outlined below.

Even though the mother-daughter dyad was the unit of analysis in this study, it was apparent that mothers with AD and their caregiving daughters not only belonged to a family network, they relied heavily on its support. What was most striking was the continuity of the intergenerational bonds between mothers and their adult children, especially for those families with multiple siblings who willingly provided care and support to one another. Yet, daughters with few or no siblings also provided many hours of care to their mothers with AD, despite the fact that many experienced other demands, such as employment. Although there is evidence in this study and others (McCarty, 1996) that the availability of other family members is crucial to the caregiving daughters' health and wellbeing, neither the diversity nor the importance of network size and proximity is reflected in the current Canadian programs intended to support caregivers (Fast et al., 2004). Public programs also need to take into account the impact of caregiving on employed caregivers. Employed daughters in this study reported many negative consequences mirrored in previous research (Keefe and Fancey, 2002), such as quitting their jobs. According to Matthews (2002), "the adequacy of social programs that help family members assist one another is one of the hallmarks of a truly civilized nation (p. 216)."

As expected, the gendered nature of caregiving was supported by the study findings. Assumptions about filial obligations and gender relations framed the daughters' perceptions about caring options. Virtually all the daughters emphasized their familial duty and obligation to care for their mother with AD, especially if their mothers had provided loving care to them as a child. In other words, the dominant culture's ideology of women as "natural" caregivers of the family was rarely questioned, despite feeling some resentment toward brothers uninvolved in the family care network. Similar to other research findings (Guberman et al., 1992; Ward-Griffin, 2002), some of the daughters in the current study were also reluctant to consider long-term care placement for their mothers with AD, due to perceptions of inadequate and/or costly institutional care. Consequently, many daughters continued to be the sole caregivers for their mothers.

According to Aronson (1991), for change to occur in the prevailing pattern of care, it is important to openly question taken-for-granted assumptions about caregiving and women. Conditions must be fostered in which women – caregivers and care receivers- can speak about their experiences and challenge prevailing images of "dutiful daughter and undemanding mothers." Furthermore, in the future, social policies and programs must not be organized around the assumption of women's availability and willingness to provide unpaid labour in the home.

Clearly, different ways of caring for old people that do not disadvantage women must be envisioned. In fact, "visioning" strategies were employed with the participants during both the individual and focus group interviews. When study participants were asked the following question: "Imagine the 'ideal' situation for both you and your mother. What would that look like and what needs to change to realize this vision?", participants began to explore and suggest alternative options of caregiving; one that included caregivers but did not exploit them and the care that they provided. Critical reflection is an important component of feminist research methodology because it helps us to see what is working well and what needs to be changed. In addition, the interviewers offered support and information during the interview, which is one of the responsibilities of a feminist researcher (Oakley, 1981). For example, if a participant identified a common concern or problem of caring for their mother with AD, information that others have faced similar concerns would be shared, hoping to reduce her sense of isolation and enable the participant to identify possible solutions. The focus groups were particularly empowering since they provided an opportunity for the daughters to discuss common issues, contribute to the development of ideas, identify gaps in the system and propose strategies for change. Thus this study created opportunities for consciousness-raising and empowerment, both personally and collectively as a group of caregivers.

Finally, study findings revealed that there were limited formal supports for daughters who cared for their mothers with AD, which frequently led to feelings of stress and strained family relations. Many mothers required assistance with their meals and/ or personal care, but daughters usually found such community services were lacking or inadequate. According to Aronson (1991), the interests of women- either as caregivers or receivers of care-are not a central concern of social policies regarding old people. Fast and colleagues (2004) suggest that there is little public policy in Canada that directly supports caregivers. In fact, family care has been viewed by policy makers as a means of reducing public costs. However, failure to provide adequate formal supports to family caregivers could risk increases in health care costs, such as injuries or illnesses of the individual with AD and/or family caregiver.

The first step in making changes in policy is to reconceptualize the care of individuals with AD, not as a "problem" for families to resolve, but as a societal issue that deserves a collective response. For instance, study findings suggest the need for legislation that provides job flexibility and job protection of employed caregivers. In addition, to ensure that family caregivers have real choices about care requires attention to nursing and home support services provided by the government. Given the diversity in family structure and the special needs of individuals with AD, health care and social services must be responsive, comprehensive, and coordinated across all sectors. As one daughter aptly pointed out, "*It is like that old saying 'it takes a village to raise a child'. Well, I think it takes a village to help a senior [with AD].*"

CONCLUSION

This research highlights the importance of examining the current pattern of care between caregiving daughters and their mothers with AD. Five interconnected themes emerged from the daughters' interview transcripts: becoming aware/stepping in, finding a balance, leading the way, carrying the load, holding on/letting go. Study findings suggested: 1) the family network is important within the care process of AD; 2) gender ideologies shaped the types of family interactions and experiences of daughters caring for mothers with AD; and 3) more formal supports are required to help families care for members with AD. Based on these findings, recommendations related to program development and public policies were made.

Ultimately, decision makers in policy, professional and public circles need to collaborate with seniors and their families in the development and evaluation of programs and public policies related to care provision for individuals with AD and other related dementias.

RECOMMENDATIONS

Three study recommendations that focus on building a caring community include the following:

- Each family is unique. Service providers and program developers need to be sensitive to the family diversity, network composition and proximity of its members.
- Social policies need to be organized around the needs of the senior with AD, not around the presumed availability of female family caregivers. New ways of caring for individuals with AD must to be envisioned that do not disadvantage women. It is important that individuals with AD and their families are involved in the development and evaluation of social programs and public policies, including workplace policies that provide job flexibility and protection of employed caregivers.
- Family caregivers must have real choices about their involvement in the care process of AD. Adequate supports, such as funding for home care, and long-term care facilities, are necessary for this to happen. Health care and social services must also be responsive, comprehensive, and coordinated across all sectors.

ACKNOWLEDGEMENT

This study was supported by the Marion and Chester Fish Research Grant from the Alzheimer Society of London and Middlesex. We would also like to thank Abram Oudshoorn and Rebecca Wadsworth for project organization.

REFERENCES

Allen, K. and Walker, A. (1992). A feminist analysis of interviews with elderly mothers and their daughters. In J. Gilgun, K. Daly and G. Handel (Eds.) *Qualitative methods in family research* (pp. 198-214). Newbury Park, California: Sage Publications

Aronson, J. (1991). Dutiful daughters and undemanding mothers: Constraining images of giving and receiving care in midlife and later life. In C. Baines, P, Evans and S. Neysmith (Eds.) *Women's caring: Feminist perspectives on social welfare* (pp. 138-168). Toronto: McLelland and Stewart.

Aronson, J. (1994). Old women and care: Choice or compulsion? In P. Leonard and B. Nichols (Eds.) *Gender, aging and the state* (pp. 17-43). Montreal: Black Rose Books Ltd.

Beeson, R., Horton-Deutsch, S., Farran, C. and Neundorfer, M. (2000). Lonliness and depression in caregivers of persons with Alzheimer's disease or related. *Issues of Mental Health Nurse, 21*(8), 779-806.

Butcher, H., Holkup, P. and Buckwalter, K. (2001). The experience of a family member with Alzheimer's Disease. *Western Journal of Nursing Research, 23*(1), 33-55.

Canadian Mental Health Association (2000). Alzheimer disease: The tough issues facing families. *Network ,15* (4), 9-11.

Carruth, A. (1996). Motivating factors, exchange patterns and reciprocity among caregivers of parents with and without dementia. *Research in Nursing and Health, 19*, 409-419.

Chappell, N. (1999). Editorial: Canadian Association on Gerontology policy statement on home care in Canada. *Canadian Journal on Aging, 18* (3), i-iii

Chenoweth, B. and Spencer, B. (1986). Dementia: The experience of family caregivers. *The Gerontologist, 26* (3), 267-272.

Connidis, I. (2001). *Family Ties and Aging*. Thousand Oaks, California: Sage Publications.

Cotrell, M., and Schulz, R. (1993). The perspective of the patient with Alzheimer's disease: A neglected dimension of dementia research. *The Gerontologist, 33*, 205-211.

Dupuis, S., and Norris, J. (2001). Roles of adult daughters in long-term care facilities: Alternative role manifestations. *Journal of Aging Studies 15* (1), 27-50.

Fast, J., Keating, N., Otfinowski, P., and Derksen, L. (2004). Characteristics of family/friend care networks of frail seniors. *Canadian Journal on Aging, 23* (1), 5-19.

Finch, J. (1987). Family obligations and the life course. In A. Bryman, B. Bytheway, P. Allat, and T. Keil (Eds.), *Rethinking the life cycle* (pp. 155-169). London: MacMillan.

Fingerman, K. (2001). *Aging mothers and their adult daughters: A studying mixed emotions.* Springer Series.

Guberman, N., Maheu, P., and Maille, C. (1992). Women as family caregivers: Why do they care ? *The Gerontologist, 32* (5), 607-617.

Hall, J. M., and Stevens, P.E. (1991). Rigor in feminist research. *Advances in Nursing Science, 13* (3), 16-29.

Hofman, A, Rocca, W.A., and Brayne, C. (1991). The prevalence of dementia in Europe: A collaborative study of 1980-1990 findings. *International Journal of Epidemiology, 20* (3), 736-748.

Horton, K., and Arber, S. (2004). Gender and the negotiation between people and their carers in the prevention of falls. *Ageing and Society, 24*, 75-94.

Ikkink, K., Van Tilbeg, T., and Kees, C. (1999). Perceived instrumental support exchanges in relationships between elderly parents and their adult children: Normative and structural explanations. *Journal of Marriage and the Family, 61* (4), 831-844.

Keefe, J.M., and Fancey, P.J. (2002). Work and eldercare: Reciprocity between older mothers and their employed daughters. *Canadian Journal on Aging, 21*(2), 229-241.

Krueger, R.A. (1994). *Focus Groups: A Practical Guide for Applied Research.* Thousand Oaks: Sage Publications.

Kuzel, A.J., and Like, R.C. (1991). Standards of trustworthiness for qualitative studies in primary care. In P.G. Norton, M. Stewart, F. Tudiver, M.J. Bass, and E.V. Dunn (eds.), *Primary care research: Traditional and innovative approaches* (pp. 138-158). Newbury Park, Calif.: Sage Publications.

Lincoln, Y. S. (1995). Emerging criteria for quality in qualitative and interpretive research. *Qualitative Inquiry, 1* (3), 275-289.

Lofland, J., and Lofland, L. (1995). *Analyzing social settings: A guide to qualitative observation and analysis* (3rd ed.). Belmont: Wadsworth.

Long, K., Sudha, S., and Mutran, E. (1998). Elder-proxy agreement concerning the functional status and medical history of the older person: the impact of caregiver burden and depressive symptomatology. *Journal of American Geriatrics Society, 46*, 1103-111.

Lyons, K.S., Zarit, S.H., Sayer, A.G., and Whitlach, C.J. (2002). Caregiving as dyadic process perspectives from caregiver and receiver. *Journals of Gerontology, 57* (3), 195-204.

MacRae, H., (2002). The identity maintenance work of family members of persons with Alzheimer's Disease. *Canadian Journal on Aging, 21*(3), 405-415.

Martin Matthews, A. and Keefe, J. (1995). Women, work, and care of the elderly: A Canadian perspective. In J. Phillips (Ed.) *Working carers: International perspectives on working and caring for older people* (pp. 116-138). Aldershot: Avebury.

Matthews, S. (2002). *Sisters and brothers/daughters and sons: Meeting the needs of old parents*. Bloomington, Indiana: Unlimited publishing.

McCarty EF.(1996). Caring for a parent with Alzheimer's disease: process of daughter caregiver stress. *Journal of Advanced Nursing, 23*(4), 792-803.

Merton, R. K., Fiske, M. and Kendall, P. L. (1990). *The focus interview: A manual of problems and procedures.* (2nd ed.). New York: The Free Press.

Miles, M. B. and Huberman, A. M. (1994). *An expanded sourcebook. Qualitative data analysis (2nd ed.)*. Thousand Oaks: Sage Publications.

Molloy, D. W. and Clarnette, R. (1999). Standardized mini-mental state examination: A user's guide. New Grange Press: Troy, Ontario.

Morse, J. M. and Field, P. A. (1995). *Qualitative research methods for health professionals* (2nd ed.). London: Sage Publications.

Mui, A. C. (1995). Caring for frail elderly parents: A comparison of adult sons and daughters. *The Gerontologist*, 35(1), 86-93.

Neufeld, A., and Harrison, M. (1995). Reciprocity and social support in caregivers' relationships: Variations and consequences. *Qualitative Health Research, 5* (3), 348-365.

Pallett, P. (1990). A conceptual framework for studying family caregiver burden in Alzheimer's-type dementia. *Image: Journal of Nursing Scholarship, 22*(1), 52-58.

Parsons, K. (1997). The male experience of caregiving for a family member with Alzheimer's disease. *Qualitative Health Research , 7* (3), 391-408.

Pohl, J.M., Boyd, C., and Given, B.A. (1997). Mother-daughter relationships during the first year of caregiving: A qualitative study. *Journal of Women and Aging, 9*(½), 133-49.

Poirier, S. and Ayers, L. (2002). *Stories of Family Caregiving – Reconsiderations of Theory, Literature, and Life*. Centre for Nursing Research: Sigma Theta Tau International.

Reinharz, S. (1992). Feminist methods in social research. Toronto: Oxford University Press.

Rossi, A. and S. and Rossi, P.H. (1990). Of human bonding: Parent –child relationships across the life span. New York: Walter de Gruyer.

Shields, C. (1987). *Swan: A literary mystery*. Toronto: Stoddart Publishing.

Smith, D.E., (1987). *The everyday world as problematic: A feminist sociology*. Boston: Northeastern University Press.

Stevenson, J.P. (1990). Family stress related to home care of Alzheimer's disease patients and implications for support. *Journal of Neuroscience Nursing, 22* (3), 179-188.

Stoller, E.P. (1993). Gender and the organization of lay health care: A socialist-feminist perspective. *Journal of Aging Studies, 7* (2), 151-170.

Stone, R. , Cafferata, G and Sangle, J. (1987). Caregivers of the frail elderly: A national profile. The *Gerontologist, 27*, 616-626.

Strain, L. and Blandford, A. (2003). Caregiving networks in later life: Does cognitive status make a difference. *Canadian Journal on Aging, 22*(3), 261-273.

Strang, V. and Koop, P. (2002). *Family caregivers waiting placement of cognitively impaired persons*. Unpublished paper.

Talbot, M. (1990). The negative side of the relationship between older widows and their adult children: The mothers' perspective. *The Gerontologist, 30* (5), 595-603.

Uhlenberg, P., and Cooney, T. (1990). Family size and mother-child relations in later life. *The Gerontologist, 30* (5), 618-625.

Ungerson, C. (1990). The language of care. In *Gender and caring* (pp. 8-32). Harlow: Pearson Higher Education.

Walter, C. (1991). Adult daughters and mothers: Stress in the caregiving relationship. *Journal of Women and Aging, 3 (*3), 39-58.

Ward-Griffin, C. (2002). Boundaries and connections between formal and informal caregivers. *Canadian Journal of Nursing Research, 33* (2), 205-216.

Whitlatch, C. J., and Feinberg, L. F. (1999). Making hard choices: Respecting both voices. Paper presented at *the 52th Abnnual Scientific Meeting of the Gerontological Association of America*, San Francsico, CA.

Wuest, J. (1997). Fraying connections of caring women: An exemplar of including difference in the development of explanatory frameworks. *Journal of Nursing Research*, 29(2), 99-116.

Wuest, J. Ericson, P. and Stern, P. (1994). Becoming strangers: The changing family caregiving relationship in Alzheimer's Disease. *Journal of Advanced Nursing, 20*, 437-443.

In: Family Caregiving for Older Disabled People
Editor: Isabella Paoletti, pp. 201-227 ISBN 1-59454-808-0

Chapter 10

LONG-DISTANCE CAREGIVING: TRANSNATIONAL FAMILIES AND THE PROVISION OF AGED CARE

Loretta Baldassar[1], Raelene Wilding[1] and Cora Baldock[2]
[1]Anthropology and Sociology, School of Social and Cultural Studies,
The University of Western Australia, Crawley WA, Australia
[2]Murdoch University, Murdoch, Western Australia

INTRODUCTION AND AIMS

Migration has become a feature of contemporary society and has resulted in a growing number of transnational families. In addition, the greying of the Western world has increased the incidence of migrants needing to care for their ageing parents from a distance. Thus, long-distance care is a growing social phenomenon that is largely unacknowledged and under-researched.

The aim of this chapter is to explore the impact of distance on the experiences of migrants living in Australia who care for ageing, disabled parents in their home countries in Europe. The specific questions we address include: Do they have the capacity and the desire to contribute to the practical, emotional and personal care of their elderly parents back home? Are they in any way able to assist primary care-givers, such as their siblings, who have remained in the home country? What role do their families play in facilitating the provision of care across distance? How do cultural differences in expectations of care and notions of independence influence the delivery of distant care? What are the structural constraints that shape the forms of this type of care-giving?

Our project extends the international research on care-giving based on the intersections of transnational migration studies, family studies and gerontology (cf. Baldassar, Baldock and Wilding, forthcoming 2006). The vast majority of gerontological studies to date assume that care-giving requires proximity and appear to deny the possibility of long distance care (e.g. Lin and Rogerson, 1995; Aldous and Klein, 1991; Rossi and Rossi, 1990). As a result, very little research has been done on the relationships between ageing parents and adult children who live at a distance (Climo, 1992), and the social and policy implications of transnational practices of care have remained largely invisible. The preoccupation with geographic proximity is also evident in family studies research generally and, at the level of theories of the family, it has been explained as due to the reification of the notion of family as a private geographic domain (Gubrium and Holstein, 1990). This reification mirrors the way nations and communities have been theorised as inherently connected to a geographical place.

In response to this literature, our study questions whether proximity is a necessary condition of care-giving, and asks how distance impacts upon the ability of people to provide care. In so doing, we turn to transnational migration studies, which focus on the continuing connections between home and host countries over time and eschew the traditional notion that migration ends with settlement (cf. Basch et. al, 1992). International migration is not seen as a one-off event but rather a life-long process of complex interactions between individuals who often live great distances apart (cf. Baldassar, 2001; Gupta and Ferguson, 1992). This approach to migration led us to conceptualise family relations as transnational sets of processes, and to conceive of the home and host societies as part of the same social field in which geographic distance and national borders do not necessarily prevent transnational care practices or connections to place.

After a brief outline of both the context of our study and our methodology, we respond to the questions raised above by drawing on case study examples taken from qualitative research conducted with Italian, Irish and Dutch families. We examine the interplay of factors that impact on the experience of distant care including, in particular, the arrangement of care in the parent's country, as well as migration histories, types of care, attitudes to care, and gender. Following the case studies, we provide a discussion section that illustrates how the possibilities of distant care are not so much diminished as transformed in the case of parents who are disabled. It also underlines the importance of a family life-cycle approach to understanding transnational family relations. We conclude the chapter with some policy recommendations.

DISTANT CARE: CONTEXT OF THE STUDY

Most of the immediate post war migrants living in Australia, who represent the bulk of immigration to this country, have already lost their parents. However, those whose parents are still alive in the home countries, together with the majority of the post 1970s migrants, face the challenges of 'caring from a distance'.[1] It is important to note, as Ackers (1999) also points out, that the population of the elderly encompasses two generations; those recently retired in their 60s (the 'young-old'), and their parents who are well into their 80s (the 'old-old'). Immigration to Australia is often not an option for either of these groups of elderly kin, not least because current Australian immigration policy reserves very few places for parent migration and the conditions are prohibitively expensive.[2] Further, re-settlement of elderly parents in Australia, while solving the problem of separation from migrant children, often raises many new problems associated with adapting to a different lifestyle, usually without

---

[1] Baldock (1999, pp. 182-192) coined the phrase 'caring from a distance'. See also Baldock (2000); Baldassar & Baldock (2000).

[2] For information about Australian 'parent migration' policies see Crock (1998) and Clothier (1997).

the necessary language skills, and away from familiar routines and supports. It is more common for migrants to rely on siblings, neighbours, paid help and community and government services to provide the day-to-day needs of their elderly relatives in Italy, Ireland and the Netherlands.

The enormous geographic distance that separates some migrants and their kin does not, for the majority, diminish the concern they have for each other. Our research found an extensive pattern of mutual care between transnational family members that is not necessarily impeded by distance and which often increases in intensity in times of crises, including as parents age.[3] Regular telephone calls, letters and, more recently, email and mobile phone text messages are the most common ways by which migrants continue to exchange emotional and practical care with their relatives overseas (Baldassar, Baldock, and Wilding, 2002; Wilding, 2006). Financial assistance is often exchanged. In addition, return visits and parental visits to Australia are important dimensions of providing distant care.

As parents age, perhaps the most significant change in distant care is in the direction of care-giving. When parents are younger and healthier, they are often the main initiators of contact and make the telephone calls, send the emails and write the letters in order to give advice, emotional support or financial assistance. Parents may also be the ones making frequent extended visits. At this stage of the family life cycle, it is the parents who are most heavily engaged in 'distant thinking' (Mason, 1999). However, when parents become disabled, it is their migrant children who tend to initiate contact and provide the majority of support, often with no hope of reciprocation from their incapacitated parents. Financial assistance may also begin to flow in the opposite direction, from migrant to parent or from migrant to parent's primary carer, as a means of participating in care at a distance. With parental disability in older age, it is the migrant child who becomes more heavily engaged in 'distant thinking'.

For the purposes of this chapter we define disabled elderly in very broad terms as people who are not able to live totally independently. They may have some degree of disability — commonly deafness, blindness, dementia, or frailty (decreased mobility). They may also have some level of illness — commonly chronic conditions like hypertension, arthritis, diabetes, cancer, or depression. The disabled elderly, by our definition, require some level of assistance with daily living; from a modest level of intervention, for example, weekly help with shopping, to a high level of intervention, for example, daily help with personal care.

METHODOLOGY

As with all care-giving, transnational care-giving requires both a caregiver and a care recipient, a reality that was particularly important to capture in our methodology. Thus, in order to better document the complexities of transnational care-giving, we conducted ethnographic interviews with both adult migrant caregivers in Australia and their ageing parents in Italy, Ireland and the Netherlands.[4] In a large project funded by the Australia

[3] Other events that result in increased intensity of communication and care practices include illness, divorce, births, and weddings.

[4] Although this chapter focuses specifically on migrants in Australia and their parents in Europe, the project encompassed a much larger international sample. We also conducted interviews with migrants in Australia

Research Council, a total of 50 interviews were conducted between 2000 and 2002 with migrants resident in Perth, Western Australia. Subsequently, another 47 interviews were conducted in Italy, Ireland and the Netherlands with the ageing parents of those migrants. Migrant interviewees in Australia were located through snowballing techniques, supplemented by advertisements posted in the newsletters of specific migrant community groups in Perth. Parents of migrants were contacted by telephone with the permission of their migrant children, who usually spoke to their parents about the process before providing consent and contact details. In a small number of cases, it was not possible to interview the migrants' parents because of physical or mental incapacity. In some of these instances, we instead interviewed the primary caregiver of the ageing parent, who was usually a sibling or other relative.

All of the interviews were conducted using a common interview schedule, which interrogated issues such as: reasons for migration; sense of belonging in the host and home country; the type and frequency of contact with family members; sense of obligation to care for family members; and instances of mutual support exchanged between parents and adult children, including personal, practical, financial and emotional or moral support. Interviews varied in length, ranging from one to several hours. In many cases, the initial interview was supplemented by additional contact by email and telephone in the subsequent months, particularly following the visits of the researchers to parents in Europe. All of the interviews in the Netherlands and Italy were conducted in Dutch and Italian respectively, and later translated into English. The full set of English transcripts and translations were then coded using QSR N5 software to assist with the comparison of the range of responses to the common interview questions.

For the purposes of this chapter, we have focused on a small number of case studies in which migrants in Australia faced the particular challenges associated with caring for disabled elderly parents from a distance. Such cases were relatively infrequent in our project sample, accounting for no more than 20 percent of all respondents. Indeed, many aged parents remained very active in their communities and continued to provide support to their adult children, for example, by sending financial assistance or by visiting to care for young grandchildren. However, the prospect of old age was one that both migrants and their parents were aware of to varying degrees, and most agreed that maintaining supportive transnational family relationships was likely to become more difficult as the symptoms of ageing became manifest. The case studies provided below have been selected because they each highlight a different aspect of the distant care experience, and between them cover the main issues that we have identified in the overall sample. These case studies collectively document the range of factors that impact upon the ability and desire of migrants in Australia to care for their ageing parents overseas. We begin with a discussion of the general features of all three samples and then deal specifically with the Italian sample, followed by the Irish and Dutch.

---

from Singapore and New Zealand and refugees in Australia from Afghanistan and Iraq, as well as the parents of these migrants and refugees in Singapore, New Zealand and Iran (Iran being a primary transit country for refugees from Iraq and Afghanistan).

Case Studies and Analysis

The majority of the migrants we interviewed hoped to be able to participate meaningfully in the care of their parents from a distance. As parents become more frail, the migrants in turn become increasingly reliant on the good-will of their siblings in the home country, who ostensibly gain increasing control over access to their parents. We found that migrants are usually included in the decisions made regarding their parents' care needs, and that relations between geographically distant kin, particularly siblings, often become more intense than ever before as contact between migrant children and parents increasingly has to occur through an intermediary. As a result, an important factor in the experience of distant care centres on what might broadly be termed 'migration history', and, in particular, the attitudes that non-migrating kin have towards the migrant's decision to migrate. In the case of children who are not given 'licence to leave', transnational relations might be strained at the best of times and even more fractious during periods of crisis, such as parental ill-health.[5]

In this context, it is important to distinguish between capacity (ability) and desire (willingness) of migrants and their parents to give and receive various types of care (Al-Ali, Black, and Koser, 2001). We cannot assume that the myth of happy families is the norm. What types of resources a family has, how much money they have at their disposal, and how much money they are willing to commit to distant care, are all factors that significantly impact on the capacity to care and the form of engagement in caring from a distance. The desire to care depends to some extent on the 'health' of family relations (e.g. Baldock, 2003). It is also mediated by notions of what is culturally appropriate care, which is in turn affected by available services. Antagonism between family members is a factor influencing the desire of the individual to participate in distant care. Some people choose not to have anything to do with 'distant' kin who they believe have not behaved appropriately. The crucial implication is that the participation of any one individual in distant care is influenced by a combination of both capacity and desire to participate.

The following case study examples explore the impact of different arrangements of care on the distant care-giver. We include a focus on three main 'types' of care: practical (organising support systems, including finance); emotional (psychological support); and personal (hands on) care.[6] Our analysis of different arrangements of care includes, among other factors, a discussion of attitudes to care, structural care provisions, migration histories, type and degree of parental illness or disability, finance, time, and gender.

Living with Children: Italian Patterns of Care

The Italian sample included migrants from two immigration vintages, a group of migrants who arrived in the 1980s and 1990s, primarily from middle-class and professional backgrounds, whose parents can be described as 'young-old', as well as a group who arrived during the massive post-war immigration waves of the 1950s to 1970s, mainly from working-class backgrounds, whose motive for migration generally included a desire to support their

[5] Baldassar (2001) introduced the concept of licence to leave.

[6] This model of care types is an adaptation of the five types of care identified by Finch and Mason (1993).

extended families back home. In a time when the cost of air travel and telecommunications were prohibitive, their regular and frequent remittances were a significant part of their distant care of loved ones in Italy. Of this group, the few whose parents are still alive are 'old-old' and well into their 80s.

The preference for most Italian parents interviewed, regardless of age and health, was to live out their retirement as independently and autonomously as possible, with a focus on participating in the family life of their children and grandchildren. If assisted living were required, most would prefer to be supported by extended 'family care', and the common (and traditional) expectation was that they would move in to live with a child. Any form of 'institutional care' was considered both the least desirable and least available option; Paoletti, in chapter 1, also reports the negative stigma attached to nursing homes. Italy currently has one of the oldest populations in Europe, with census statistics from the end of the last century showing 16.2 percent of people over the age of 65 and 6 percent over 75 (Trifiletti, 1998). Only a small proportion of these individuals are in institutional care facilities, comprising 1.5 percent of those over 65 and 3.6 percent of those over 75. It was not until 1985 that admission into these facilities was opened to the seriously ill, people who previously were cared for at home. Institutional homes had been largely the preserve of old people who were able-bodied and healthy. Even today, the general community perception is that these facilities are for people ('singles') who have no family to care for them. Indeed, the vast majority (96 percent) of people in nursing homes in Italy are widowed and there are many more women than men (Trifiletti, 1998).

Italy has embarked on a progressive project to improve the provision of aged care services in all sectors including institutional care as well as home care (Trifiletti, 1998). Notwithstanding these developments, for many Italians there is a strong sense of family shame associated with the use of institutional care, which is popularly characterised as 'locking' older people away. Older, more traditionally-minded parents were emphatically hostile to these institutions. One woman, clearly mindful of her approaching 'old-old' age, said angrily that people in these institutions became like "pieces of ice" and that she would not place her husband "in the hands of other people, only traitors would do this, people who betray their parents" (Baldassar and Pesman, 2005).

Younger parents tended to have a more philosophical outlook on their older age. While most had themselves nursed their own parents in their own homes, they were unsure whether their children would be able to do the same for them. A number indicated fatalistically that their children might place them in a nursing home, "when their time came", although all emphatically hoped this would not be the case. One couple explained that they had one son in Australia and two daughters living and working in other regions in Italy; "we can't expect them to stop their lives and careers and interrupt their families to look after us". The prospect of moving from their childhood village to live with one of their daughters in a distant city was not an attractive one. However, they conceded that it would be a difficult choice as to whether to go into a home. The wife commented, "now we say we'd prefer a home, but when the time comes, we might prefer to go live with a daughter", to which her husband replied, "Yeah, I think so".

Currently in Italy it is mainly family members, and primarily women, who care for the vast majority of aged people, including the estimated 20 percent who are over 65 and dependent, although there are a growing number of foreign immigrants employed to take care of dependent elderly on behalf of other family members (Andall, 1999). Institutional care is more expensive and, depending on the region, less available and accessible and certainly generally considered to be less attractive than home-help or *la badante*, colloquially referred to as '*avere una donna*' or having a woman (i.e. carer) in the home. The preference for domestic help preserves the traditional practice of 'family care' despite the fact that it disrupts the families of the women employed to provide such care. An increasing number of women from Eastern Europe, south Asia and Africa are employed to assist with domestic help, including caring for elderly people in their homes or the homes of their children.

The most common pattern of informal care provided by the family, made possible by the traditional practice of living in close proximity to kin, is daily visits from daughters or daughters-in-law. This type of informal care is generally considered a normal duty that falls, first and foremost, on adult children, so much so that the care of the elderly is only considered a problem for those who do not have available relatives (Trifiletti, 1998). Older Italians desire a close relationship with their families, especially children and grandchildren, such that their perceptions about their health and well-being have been found to be associated with how close they feel they are to their children (MacKinnon, and Nelli, 1996).

Unaccepted Departure

The pain associated with not having enough contact with children is often especially difficult for widows. The way people experience and understand health and illness is culturally influenced. While recognising that this may be a more universal experience, widowhood, for Italians, often correlates with deterioration in health or a perceived decrease in wellness and, for women especially, with a loss of independence and opportunities to socialise.[7]

This was certainly Angela's[8] experience after her husband passed away. Angela's negative experience of her widowhood was exacerbated, despite having a son living close at hand, by her failure to accept that Monica, her only daughter, had chosen to live in Australia. Monica is probably best described as atypical in both her migration experience and her attitudes towards family. Her family's reaction to what they perceive as her 'differences' clearly highlights the behaviour expected of 'good daughters'. Monica migrated as a single, young professional in the late 1960s, very unusual for a woman at that time, and, not surprisingly, against the wishes of her family. She explained that Italian families are "bound by duty and gratitude … and family ties" and that her decision to migrate was interpreted by her family as a rejection of these values;

> they had a couple of family councils and there were a couple of attempts to 'guilt-trip' me into coming back; 'What will happen to your parents when they grow old and they need their daughter to look after them?'… They always hoped that I would go back to Italy where I belonged, back home to be the dutiful daughter.

---

[7] MacKinnon & Nelli (1996) found that a number of Italian older women saw health and widowhood as mutually exclusive. Many Italian women, especially the elderly, complain about suffering from what they call 'nerves', a generalised feeling of anxiety, non-specific illness and distress.

[8] All personal names in this chapter are pseudonyms, to protect the anonymity of participants in our study.

Family tensions exacerbated when Monica tried to tell them that she was bi-sexual. Despite the significant and constant pressure on her to return to Italy, Monica explained that going back to live with her family was not an option because they would not accept her sexuality; "they actually called the family priest to bless me.... which I found offensive and humiliating".

What is perhaps most noteworthy about this family story is that despite the high degree of tension between Monica and her family, they maintained regular contact in the form of two or three letters every month until the 1990s, when these were replaced with bi-weekly telephone calls to her parents and numerous emails to her brother, as well as at least one visit per year. Although they disagreed with many of her life choices, Monica's parents have always assisted her financially, helping her to buy her own home, a new car, and paying for half the cost of her and her son's visits. While the regular contact and financial support have been constants in her life, Monica described her family as not having provided her with emotional support; "Because in all the crises I've had in my life, they didn't want to know". She cited as examples how her family offered no support during or after the break-down of two significant relationships. Monica felt it was as if her family were pleased about these, what were for her, major crises, because they always hoped they would precipitate her return to Italy. This pressure for her to return to Italy, although it has been constant, was particularly strong at the time of interview because her mother was alone and ageing and, as Monica explained;

> now that I didn't have a partner any longer, [she thinks] I would sooner or later go back to Italy where I belonged, with my son, whom she loves. ... And there was no question of that. I made that clear straight away, that I was [staying in] Australia even without a partner... and I don't think she was happy at all about it so she didn't provide any emotional support.

Migrating against her parents' wishes, that is, without 'licence to leave', influenced Monica's ability to care from a distance, in particular, Monica's sense of her right to "have a say" in the management of her parents' old age. For example, Monica found her brother's decision to hide the truth about their father's terminal illness from both parents very frustrating. She explains that she was not involved in this decision, "I was just informed". Her brother only rang on her birthday and her son's birthday; "he never rings just to chat". So, when Monica received his phone call out of the blue one day, she knew it indicated bad news: "He just said, 'Dad is sick', so I sort of deciphered and I asked, 'is it cancer', and he said yes. Being Italian, they shy away from words like cancer". The practice of hiding the truth about terminal illness from patients is apparently common in Italy and supported by the medical profession. Monica explained, "They [the doctors] even wrote a false letter... that they gave [my father], saying that he had a cyst, and they wrote a real letter with a real diagnosis to my brother".

Although Monica was unsure it was a good idea not to tell her parents the truth, she felt she could not contest her brother's decision. She felt she had forfeited her right to intervene because of her absence; "I live in Australia... I'm the one who only turns up for three weeks every year". The result was that the father's death came as a terrible shock to her mother and left her in a state of total dependence; "[My parents] had this division of labour. My mother looked after the cleaning and the cooking. My father paid the bills, he looked after the house. So when he died, my mother didn't know how much was in the bank account". Angela cannot drive and had relied on her husband to take her everywhere. His death left her totally at a loss and she had to learn how to become independent.

Despite the tensions in their relationship, it is clear that Monica felt a sense of duty to her mother. She believed that her 'unorthodox' behaviour placed the burden of care squarely on her brother, who visits their mother at least three times a week;

> She's self-sufficient but she's very, very difficult and basically, all the day-to-day hassles are my brother's because my sister-in-law has an elderly mother who's [demented] and so they've divided the responsibilities; she looks after her mother and my brother looks after my mother. But I think they both resent me a bit because they think, 'ha ha, there she is happily in [Australia] without all the daily phone calls and the daily hassles.' So I think the least I can do is spend three weeks there or so to [give them a real break].

Monica continues to resist the 'guilt-trips' to return to Italy and plans not to tell her mother that she will soon retire because, "she will start expecting that I move back to Italy... This is her dream, that I would move back to look after her'. Monica anticipates that when the time comes, her brother will organise live-in domestic support to care for their mother full-time; "they have a *donna in casa* to look after my sister-in-law's mother... so when my mother becomes either physically or mentally unable to look after herself, my brother and his wife will very easily find some reliable woman who will look after her".

Maintaining Ties

Monica's ability to care from a distance was clearly affected by her migration history and the impact this had on her relationship with her parents. Even in cases where relations with parents are good, much depends also on the maintenance of those relationships, as is evident in Federica's case. Like Monica, Federica's decision to follow her husband to Australia in the 1970s was hard for her family to understand. Unlike Monica, Federica's parents eventually accepted her choice. Their change in perspective was greatly assisted by their visits to Australia, which enabled them to verify that their daughter was well and happy. They offered significant financial support, helping Federica and her husband to buy a house and financing many of Federica's visits to Italy. The help she has received from her family in Italy and the fact that Federica is the only daughter (she has three brothers) and is her father's favourite, has increased her desire to return to care for her parents in their old age.

Federica and her family have generally maintained close and regular contact, although there have been what Federica describes as "dark periods" when she did not feel as emotionally supported as she wished; "I've felt that well, I might as well be dead for them because you know, I'm so far away". The sense of isolation was exacerbated by contact being primarily by letter and infrequent phone calls, which gave Federica an unsatisfying level of detail about daily events; "I want to know exactly what's happening and like during the visit home, I used to find out that this happened ... that happened, and I was reproaching my dad for not telling me, also the negative things like somebody died." These dark periods diminished as phone calls became more affordable:

> At first it was really expensive so you couldn't say much. But then when the price reduced – that was very, very important I think because, I mean you can pick up the phone more or less any time and check how things are going when something worries you.

Federica's early experience of isolation left her deeply aware of the need for constant and regular contact and of the importance of visiting regularly. During the first decade in Australia, she says she "only" visited three times due to the cost of travel and the stage in her family's life cycle, "the children were young". It was during this time, before her parents had visited, that Federica felt she was losing touch with her family; "My mum would say things like, 'You made your choice, you know, now [you] take the consequences". Since the 1990s, however, Federica travels to Italy every year, and the constant and regular physical contact has significantly improved family relations;

> The visiting, the physical presence is very important to maintain. To see, to observe the changes, for instance, I could see the changes, like my mum getting older ... In fact, I don't know which one is more important my travelling more often [or] the telephone. They help each other – the more you visit, the better quality the calls.

Federica chooses to visit for at least three months at a time to ensure an adequate level of intimate contact is established. She has chosen part-time employment to ensure she can visit regularly for extended periods, and also, to ensure she can leave at short notice. These extended visits explain why Federica says she has no trouble fitting back into life in Italy, something other migrants, who do not visit as frequently, find very difficult. The decision to return regularly for extended visits has required support from her husband; "because the money is used for visiting parents and family, when it could have been spent in another way, you know, for the other family".

Support from her spouse and financial means are not, however, always enough to ensure her visits can be as long as she would like. The last time Federica visited, she had to limit her visit to 60 days due to social security regulations. She receives a carer's pension to look after her sick husband and this would have been cut off if she had remained out of the country for longer;

> If I stay 61 days, I don't get paid for any of the two months, which is ridiculous really because I've thought, 'Oh, maybe I can stay an extra two weeks and if I don't get paid for [those] two weeks, it doesn't matter. But not being paid for two months is too much, so I had to reduce my time there.

Federica described her family as very close, "You know, there are plenty of arguments, there's plenty of everything but it doesn't matter. In the end, the whole family sticks together". It is the closeness, this sticking by you that Federica believed underlined the significant emotional support she received during a period of personal illness, "they were ringing me at least once a week, and not just Dad but everyone ... I think migrating is a very negative thing but if the family stays close, it can be OK". Between visits, Federica stays in close contact with her father, but for information about the health of her parents and other potentially negative news she relies on her eldest brother, "he feels he's responsible for the family – for the whole family, extended family. But often I also check with my youngest one, just to make sure that things are, you know, not too much on one side."

Federica's mother is slowly becoming more and more dependent; "we all would like her to stay at home but we know that somebody has to be there and well, I'm the available one. I'm the one that wants to be available … because first duty is to your parents. They did whatever they could for us and so you have to give back." Federica is planning to return to Italy to live for part of each year; "Dad always wants me to go back and stay there and you know, when he rings up, 'So when are you coming here?'. Two months after I come back here, he starts asking 'When are you coming?'".

While it is possible to provide practical and emotional support from a distance, the provision of personal care requires proximity. Traditionally, adult children married and settled very close to their parents, in the same town. Even today, especially among rural people, finding a suitable job close to one's parents' home is generally considered highly desirable. In the past, it was often the case that one child remained in the parental home to eventually inherit it, and so also cared for the parents as they aged.

The loss of the parental home not only has an impact on the autonomy of the parents, who now must surrender governance of the household to the child they are living with, it also has a significant impact on the migrant child, who no longer has direct access to their parents' home. In *Visits Home*, Baldassar (2001) discusses the rights that migrants enjoy to their ancestral home, when this home is governed by their parents. Once the governance of a household is transferred from parent to child, as when parents move in to live with a child, the migrant no longer enjoys direct access to that home, but rather their access is now dependent on their relationship with their sibling. The sibling, in whose home the parents are living, theoretically has complete control over access between the parents and the migrant child. This can significantly impede the ability of the migrant child to care for their parents from a distance.

For example, in a rather extreme case, one mother, Sabrina, nurtured an 'ideal daughter' identity for her favourite child, Lidia, who migrated to Australia in the mid-70s to marry an Australian. Sabrina wrote daily letters for the first few months of their separation, kept Lidia's bedroom locked and untouched for more than two decades (even when the room was much needed by her other daughter whose family moved in to live for a period of time), and generally fuelled a great amount of jealousy on the part of her two Italy-based children who could never be as good in their roles as daughters. Lidia's regular visits, during which she was able to give her mother her undivided attention, reinforced her 'ideal-type' status. When Sabrina became frail and disabled, Lidia felt significant guilt at not being able to provide proximate care and experienced torment at not being able to participate in her mother's care via her sisters due to the strained relations between them. She had to rebuild her relationship with the sister who took charge of her mother's care. This sister chose to move Sabrina to her home in another region, giving her greater governance over her mother. Lidia finally restored relations with her sister by spending an extended visit in Italy taking over personal 'hands-on' care of Sabrina, thus giving her sister much needed respite.

Given the importance of visiting in Italian culture and the lack of institutional support, migrant children do feel enormous pressure to make extended visits to assist with day-to-day personal care and to provide respite to siblings and other carers. Their ability to assist in this way is largely dependent on good relations with siblings in whose home they will have to reside during their visit. Alternatively, the migrant needs to move back to Italy with their family to live for an extended period to take over the primary care of their parents. This is not uncommon when the migrant is the only child. For example, one young man, an only child, returned with his Polish-Australian wife and their small daughter, they took over residence and governance of the mother's home and total responsibility for her care. They intend to return to Australia when the mother dies; at the time of writing this chapter, they had been in Italy for 5 years. Returning to care for elderly parents was also an experience of some of the Irish migrants we interviewed, whose patterns of care are examined in the next section.

The Family Home: Irish Patterns of Care

The interviewees from Ireland who participated in this study had migrated to Australia in the 1970s, 1980s and 1990s. The more recent arrivals had relatively young parents, who were often still active in the community and the workforce. However, several of those who arrived in Australia in the 1970s and early 1980s, in particular, were keenly aware of the difficulties of caring for their ageing parents from a distance. The deteriorating mental and physical health of parents posed difficult questions for migrants and their Irish-resident siblings, and required the negotiation of shifting norms of aged care. All of the interviewees were aware of past expectations of aged care, whereby parents would be cared for in the family home by one of the adult children. Indeed, several were able to recount childhoods characterised by multigenerational households, and discussed the daily care provided by their mothers to their grandparents. However, recent trends in the professionalisation of health care, declining household sizes, changing gender norms and new expectations regarding desirable standards of living were mentioned by interviewees as shifting the contexts and expectations of care to such an extent that the form of care their grandparents experienced would almost certainly have disappeared completely by the time of their own old age (see also Daly, 1998; Curry, 1998; Giarchi, 1996; Leane, 1995; Larragy, 1993a, 1993b; Kennedy, 1986).

The social, economic and cultural transformations within Ireland in recent decades have resulted in the building of more accommodation specifically designed for the needs of older people, including nursing homes, hostels and secure independent accommodation (Larragy, 1993b; Daly, 1998). In 2000, it was estimated that 4.5 percent of people aged 65 and over resided in institutional care facilities in Ireland, the vast majority of which were aged 80 and over (O'Shea, 2002). However, expectations regarding aged care provision are in flux, and the children of ageing parents, as well as ageing parents themselves, frequently expressed ambivalence about the increasing availability of institutional support. For example, one Irish mother in her 80s expressed her sense of relief that she had four daughters, two of whom were living in her immediate neighbourhood. She was the envy of many of her local friends, who had no children living locally and were on waiting lists for the limited places available in newly constructed aged care accommodation. At the same time, she expressed a sense of frustration at her remote rural location. One advantage of aged-specific accommodation, she suggested, was that it was usually located close to urban centres. She yearned for the opportunity to make independent visits into the shops and tearooms of the town without relying on one of her daughters or resorting to the one bus a day that travelled past her home in and out of town.

It is in this context of transforming expectations regarding desirable aged care and living arrangements for the elderly that the following two case studies need to be interpreted. It appears that there is no single correct answer for Irish adult children, either in Ireland or abroad, when it comes to deciding on appropriate care arrangements for their parents. Rather, what is appropriate is being negotiated against constantly shifting circumstances and expectations. Yet these shifts must themselves be understood in the context of a strong tradition of inheritance and residence patterns that have previously seen Irish parents prefer to die in their own homes under the care of their children and in the company of their grandchildren. An ideal type of ageing that has existed for multiple generations is difficult to ignore, even in the face of new imperatives and a changing global scene.

Akin to Death

Joe and Jean were forced to face the issue of ageing when they made one of their three-yearly visits to Ireland to visit their families. Not long before this visit, Joe had learned through a telephone call with his sister that his widowed mother was experiencing the onset of dementia. Joe had two sisters living in the same town as his mother, who both offered to have their mother move in with them. However, she steadfastly refused to move out of her own home. In spite of their concerns about a mother living on her own, both of the daughters made significant efforts to fulfil their mother's wishes. The strength of the ideal of dying in the family home is clear in a heartfelt statement made by one of the daughters, Brenda, that:

> [my mother] wouldn't want to go in a home, and we wouldn't want to have her in a home. She's always been very good to us all, so it would be good to return that, she was always there for all of us, you know.

Unwilling to force their mother to move, and unable to move their own large families into their mother's small house, the two daughters cared for their mother by making regular visits. One daughter visited every morning, to ensure that her mother took her daily medications and had a breakfast and lunch prepared. The other daughter visited every afternoon on her way home from work, when she organised her mother's evening meal and medications. They would each complete household chores during their visits, and would take it in turns to have their mother stay in their own family homes over the weekend. Their husbands played a role, too, by mending or maintaining the house, and an unmarried son who lived locally would visit on most weeknights.

According to Brenda, the arrangement was working quite well and their mother was happy. However, the family was worried that their mother might come to some harm if she continued to live on her own, and would prefer that she moved into the home of one of her daughters. Brenda was satisfied that everyone in the family was contributing to the care of their mother in the best way they could, and that the responsibility was being shared evenly. No doubt this perception was in part because the family, including their mother, shared strong expectations regarding the gendered nature of appropriate care (see also Cecil et. al., 1987). For example, although the local son performed little in the way of daily care requirements on his visits, his contribution of regular company was considered to be above and beyond what might be expected from a son. Also, when their mother occasionally complained about the lack of care she received, it was usually in reference to a daughter missing a regular visit, not the desire for more assistance from a son.

This gendered assumption regarding appropriate care-giving may in part explain why Joe was perceived as such a good son, in spite of his inability to provide significant levels of care from Australia. According to Brenda, Joe made important contributions to his mother's care by maintaining contact with his sisters in Ireland. He occasionally provided advice about the situation, but his real contribution was to listen to his sisters and provide them with emotional support. Brenda explained: "the life that we have is much more kind of a burden with my mother and she takes up much more of our time and everything now, and he [Joe] really realises that as well, and he's always very grateful for that".

Gender is not the only factor; distance, too, plays its role in releasing Joe from any sense of obligation to provide more substantive care to his mother. One way in which Joe acknowledged this reduced capacity to care was by relinquishing his rights to the family's inheritance.[9] Upon their mother's death, it is intended that the house will be sold and the proceeds distributed amongst the siblings. This fits the expectations of a reciprocal exchange, embodied in the value of the family house, which appears to be essential for the ageing Irish parent to maintain their sense of independence and dignity while receiving aged care services from their family (James et. al., 1984). However, Joe has made it clear that he does not expect his share, saying: "I'm away from home for so long now, I don't think I should be included in that".

Joe also played the role of the good migrant son by providing greater levels of care and support when he visited family in Ireland. On one visit he completed a large renovation job in his mother's house, and on another visit he took her out on frequent day trips, reducing the need for his siblings to visit their mother. Joe has also made regular telephone calls, sent letters and otherwise maintained contact with the entire family. While Brenda talked about the difficulties that she and her sister faced in maintaining their mother's care on a daily basis, she also expressed a strong sense of how difficult the situation must be for Joe. As their mother's mental capacity diminished, Joe found it increasingly difficult to have any communication with his mother, saying:

> I found the phone calls weren't much good any more, because she felt she'd just have to talk all the time to get the worth from the phone call, so she'd just talk and it would all be rubbish. ... Plus I would ring her and she wouldn't tell them [my sisters] I would have rang either, so it was kind of pointless really.

As Joe transferred his contact from his mother to his sisters, they, too, noticed changes in their mother's behaviour. While their mother would often refer to the family members in Ireland, she rarely mentioned her son in Australia and would even occasionally deny having another son or ever having visited Australia. At first Brenda wondered if this was some sort of unconscious punishment for Joe having gone away, recalling how upset her mother had been when Joe announced his intention to migrate to Australia. But it was understood that this was merely the progress of the illness, and their mother's awareness and memory of a social world was gradually reducing in size to only those people she saw on a daily basis. According

[9] This is also evident in the Italian case. Baldassar (2001) has documented instances in which a migrant's rights to inheritance have been relinquished to their siblings in exchange for the care of their parents and a place to stay during visits home to Italy.

to Brenda, this was particularly hard on Joe, who no longer existed for his mother. However, Joe was less concerned, and had a strong sense of having said his final goodbye to his mother when he left Ireland on his last visit. Indeed, Joe struggled with a different sense of regret and guilt, saying:

> I suppose you would call it guilt, but I think … she's now going to become a burden on them, you know, [and] I say to myself, maybe it would be good if she was to go now, and she wouldn't have to be a burden on anybody then; … it was a strange feeling to think about that, someone you love, to say I wish they could go now really, so that they wouldn't be a burden any more.

Joe's sense of guilt about wishing his mother was physically gone is reinforced by a sense that, for him, she has already gone. The lack of an ability to communicate across distance is akin to death, in that he is unable to have any continuing relationship with his mother. Indeed, Joe feels that he is the lucky one in this situation:

> you get away with a lot when you're not living with your elderly parents, you know what I mean, you get away with it a lot, you don't have to do anything, really, I mean just call on the phone, you know, so I do get away with a fair bit as well, that's right, but we always say we're very lucky coming from large families, because there's always someone there. We get away with murder.

Reducing the Distance

In the case of dementia, distance presents an immense challenge for maintaining relationships at a distance. Terminal illness, too, presents enormous challenges for providing support across distance. When Anne was informed by telephone that her mother in Ireland had been diagnosed with a particularly virulent cancer, she arranged to be on a plane to Ireland within 36 hours. Anne's decision to return to Ireland was made swiftly, but not easily. Her own husband and children were left without her support for a long and indefinite period of time. Her visit was initially intended to be short, to evaluate the situation. However, when a surgeon explained that her mother's life expectancy was no longer than four months, Anne resolved to remain for the duration and contribute to her mother's nursing care. Anne spent the following four months in Ireland caring for her mother with her sisters, returning to Australia only after her mother's death.

By remaining in Ireland as one of her mother's two primary carers, Anne was fulfilling a promise to her mother. When she first migrated from Ireland to England, and later to Australia, her mother was very unhappy and resentful. One of her mother's concerns was that her oldest daughter, Anne, would not be available to care for her in the case of sickness in her old age. This fear became particularly apparent on the last visit before her mother's death. Anne's mother was depressed about saying goodbye and worried that this would be the last time she would see her daughter. Anne did her best to assuage this fear in a long letter, expressing her commitment to her mother's care and reassuring her that the entire family would do everything possible to make sure that she was cared for at home if necessary. To meet this promise, Anne established a savings account in Australia to pay for an emergency airfare to Ireland and maintained only part time and casual employment positions that could be dropped at short notice if necessary. Anne acknowledged that her husband's financial and emotional support was essential to the success of this strategy.

After her mother's diagnosis, Anne's swift return to Ireland and her decision to remain for the duration of the illness were critical to maintaining her mother at home. The local daughters were unable to provide the technical support that Anne's nursing expertise provided, and their own balance of employment, childcare and other responsibilities precluded them from taking on the full time care required to keep their mother in her own home. Indeed, Anne spent some time convincing her sisters that their mother should not be placed into full time professional care in a nursing home. For Anne, this intensive period of caring for her mother was ultimately satisfying, but it did have its challenges.

One of the difficulties that Anne faced was her own lack of support. With her husband, children and close friends in Australia she was geographically distanced from the sorts of emotional and other support on which her locally resident sisters were able to call. But possibly more difficult were the consequences of her migration for her relationship with her mother. Anne's time away from Ireland had been characterised by constant letter writing and telephone calls with her mother. She had also made numerous visits to Ireland, and had her mother visit her in Australia several times. However, this was insufficient to support an unchallenged intimacy between herself and her mother. Anne was aware of a tension that existed in their relationship, which was often expressed in painful ways. For example, Anne was conscious of having limited rights in deciding what care was best for her mother, saying "I had to be really rather careful, you know, breezing in from overseas, and sort of telling them what was best". Even the battle to keep her mother out of a nursing home and to care for her in her own home was fought and won only because she had the support of one of her sisters. Anne was unable to assert her mother's wishes alone, in spite of the fact that her mother "always said she wanted to die in her own home, and she'd always said that she wanted to go out of here in a box".

Anne was also very aware that her decision to live overseas had affected her place in her mother's emotional life. Anne described feeling that her mother preferred the company of her other, locally resident, daughters and could not easily identify with 'that Aussie', as she was sometimes labelled. But it was after her mother's death that Anne was forced to face the full reality of what she had lost by migrating to Australia. In the days following the funeral, the family reminisced about things that her mother used to say or do, and places she would frequent. Anne was left with a relatively small set of memories, and found herself saying on a frequent basis, "I didn't know that", or "I don't remember that". Nonetheless, Anne was able to take great satisfaction in the fact that she had played a large role in ensuring that her mother's preferred means of dying was fulfilled. In the final days of her life, almost the entire family returned to their mother's home from around Ireland and the world to gather at the bedside. It was only at this moment that Anne felt her mother was truly happy. However, Anne's participation in this moment, and her proximity at this last stage of her mother's life, in many ways served to highlight the distance that had characterised the past 20 years of their relationship. While Anne was happy with her life in Australia, and would not want to return to Ireland to live, she was also more conscious of the gradual loss of family and collective memories that her migration had incurred.

NOT LIVING WITH CHILDREN: DUTCH PATTERNS OF CARE

There are two important features that distinguish care for the elderly in the Netherlands from eldercare in Italy and Ireland. First, the Netherlands is a very regulated society, where the government maintains strict control over standards and practices. This means that paid care services must be of high standard, and the government prevails if people cannot afford to pay themselves for institutionalised care in 'verzorgingshuizen' (hostels) or 'verpleeghuizen' (nursing homes). *Hostels* are homes for the aged where residents have their own separate apartments with their own belongings, and live as if in their own home, whilst able to access nursing care and cooked meals. Only severely disabled or chronically ill elderly reside in *nursing homes*. These are generally divided into two separate wards, one for physically disabled people (wheelchair, or permanently bedridden), the other for psycho-geriatric patients (some of whom may of course also have physical ailments). Most are non-profit institutions provided by various church organisations. All Dutch citizens receive a generous old age pension. They pay for hostel and nursing care from their own resources until these run out; subsequently they hand over their pension and the government pays for any remaining costs (Timmermans, 1996).

Secondly, there is a strong sense that older people need to retain their independence from their families. This appears a general attitude in northern European countries; Pyysiäinen pointed out in chapter 6 that, in Finnish culture, there has been an emphasis on elderly people maintaining their own independence from their adult children. Similarly Sand, in chapter 14, says that elderly people in Norway prefer an independent and friendly relationship with their children. This attitude is exemplified in the Netherlands by government policies and practices of ensuring that older people remain in their own homes, or in independent dwellings especially designed for seniors. These include flats for seniors; clusters of homes for people over the age of 55; 'aanleunwoningen' (flats built adjacent to hostels); and service flats. In these dwellings, older people retain their independence but can avail themselves of some services, including an evening meal. Only well-to-do seniors can afford a service flat – all services provided there have to be purchased.

Importantly, though, this need for independence is also felt strongly by elderly people themselves, and their definition of independence appears significantly different from that of Italian or Irish elderly. Dutch surveys have shown that when given a choice between paid care and informal care by children, other relatives or neighbours (so-called 'mantelzorg'[10]) the overwhelming proportion of elderly indicate they prefer *paid* professional care. Older people do not wish to be beholden to their children, do not wish to live with them, or be dependent on their children's care (Timmermans et al., 1997). This means that most people in the Netherlands will not move in with their children when they require care, nor will their children move in with them. They will try to live close to, but not with their adult children.[11] Movement to a hostel is seen as a positive choice. The design of hostels reinforces this sense of independence: all residents have separate apartments with kitchenettes and en suite bathrooms; such apartments have their own front door, with nameplate and letterbox

---

10 *Mantelzorg*: Informal domiciliary care by adult children, other relatives or neighbours

11 As noted by Timmermans (1996) the percentage of older people living in intergenerational households declined between 1976 and 1993 from 16% to 9%; they are now mainly found in rural areas away from the major cities.

(Bijsterveld, 1996). Nursing homes, however, are feared for what they indeed are – places to die in.

The parents of migrants interviewed in the Netherlands expressed the need to be independent, as described above, in very strong terms. When asked about their needs for care, most parents, regardless of age and level of disability, would reiterate that "children are people you are given in loan"; "they have to go their own way". This meant to them that you should not be a burden to your children, and that you should learn to distance yourself from them, not upsetting them with your problems. None expressed any desire to live with their children. As in the Irish case, most parents (about two-thirds) were 'young-old', only recently retired and in good health. Their migrant children were young people with small children who had departed in the late 1980s and 1990s, and their parents were not preoccupied with their own care needs, but with those of their migrant children. On the other hand, there were five instances of people who were 'old-old'. These were parents of transnational migrants who left the Netherlands in the 1960s-1970s; they were in their 80s or older and suffered from physical ailments and/or dementia. These old-old parents did require care and received some of this care from their children. However, even these 'old-old' parents emphasized the importance of independence, and did not expect all care-giving to come from their children.

It is important to stress though that notwithstanding the need for independence felt by elderly people, and their wish not to be a burden, adult children in the Netherlands do carry considerable responsibilities towards their ageing parents. In fact, older people who are not institutionalized (the overwhelming majority of seniors) rely mainly on their children (as well as neighbours) for assistance with things they cannot readily carry out themselves. Approximately 8 percent of the Dutch elderly live in hostels or nursing homes (Timmermans, 1996). Most families are fairly close-knit, and it is common practice for adult children to visit regularly, assist their elderly parent(s) with shopping, accompany them on visits to doctors and take care of household repairs where needed. Their care continues when parents become institutionalized, in that they are often consulted by the staff of the institution about their parents' needs, continue their regular visits, and may even get involved in personal care duties during such visits, although the latter would be a matter of personal choice as paid staff are always on call. The following cases explore the role of transnational migrants in this context.

Distant Care of a Carer

The first case concerns Johanna, a female professional migrant who left the Netherlands in 1964 to take up a position as an academic in New Zealand, leaving both her parents and one older sister behind in her home country. In New Zealand she married an Englishman, moved with him to a number of other academic sites, and finally settled as a family with two children in Western Australia. At the time of interview, she was 61 years old, and a divorcee. Her father had died six years earlier, and her sister Beth, an unmarried professional woman, acted as primary carer for their 92 year-old mother, who was living in a hostel.

Johanna had always maintained very close contact with her parents back home, through correspondence and return visits, the latter made possible by the fact that her academic work allowed her opportunities for travel. Through such communications she had been able to give her parents a measure of emotional support, particularly by ensuring that they had frequent news about and visits from their grandchildren. At the same time, she kept her marital problems a guarded secret so as not to upset her parents emotionally. Any practical care that her parents needed was the province of her older sister Beth. For example, Beth visited their parents fortnightly or weekly when they were still living independently in another city, mainly to do the shopping and assist with any heavy chores. When the mother could no longer cope with cooking the evening meal, Beth found a hostel for their parents near her own residence and took care of the removal of their furniture and personal belongings. Once they were established in the hostel, she continued her weekly visits, took them on outings, chauffeured them to any medical appointments, and provided both practical and emotional care during the mother's rehabilitation after a hip replacement, and when the father was hospitalised with pneumonia. She kept her migrant sister well informed about these matters, and sought some advice on the issue of their parents' move to hostel care, but beyond this Johanna was not involved in any aspects of practical care-giving.

After the sudden death of their father, subtle changes occurred in the care-giving patterns and family relationships. Johanna returned for her father's funeral, and immediately became involved in a number of practical issues, such as the selection of a stone for her father's grave, the sorting and discarding of his clothes, and financial arrangements regarding his will and testament. Upon her return to Western Australia she started weekly telephone calls to her mother, and she increased the number of her return visits, especially as the mother's physical and mental health deteriorated. The decline in her mother's mental health meant she could no longer remain in hostel care and during one of Johanna's return visits, the two sisters visited several nursing homes to decide which would be the most suitable. They also sorted clothes and household items in anticipation of their mother's move to an institution where she would no longer be able to keep her own belongings, beyond the absolute minimum.

As their mother's health deteriorated further, and with the onset of severe dementia, Beth began a process of extensive personal care-giving. This included giving a weekly shower (a nurturing ritual which mother and daughter both enjoyed), helping her mother to the toilet during her visits, and changing her mother's colostomy bag, which had been fitted after a major intestinal operation. The latter was something that otherwise would be done by trained nurses in the hostel, but Beth had taught herself how to do it, so she would not need to rely on nurses when she visited. She also frequently took her mother's dresses home with her to give them a thorough wash. In fact, what she took upon herself was a very demanding and emotionally draining task, and it was at this stage that Johanna began to focus on giving her sister Beth emotional support. Beth began to write long letters in which she detailed everything that was taking place, and phone calls between the sisters also increased in volume and intensity, eventually replacing the weekly long-distance phone calls with mother – no longer possible because of her dementia.

As said, Johanna had begun to visit more often, and during such return visits (usually of about two to three weeks duration) she was able to provide some respite for her sister Beth, by taking over some of the regular visiting to their mother. However, she was never quite able to assist with personal care. Their mother felt uncomfortable and confused when her eldest daughter, who had been her primary carer for so long, was not there to take her to the toilet or help her shower. Also, Johanna admitted in interview that she herself felt uneasy carrying out such personal care tasks, leaving them with a great sense of relief to her sister.

Control and Communication

The next case concerns another female transnational migrant with an entirely different care-giving and family history. Rachel migrated by herself in the 1970s, a young woman escaping from a difficult family where she was always seen as the 'black sheep', and compared negatively with her younger brother. When she told her parents that she was going to emigrate, her father would not speak to her for several months prior to her departure. Nonetheless she tried to stay in close touch with her parents through letters and phone calls, and remained very involved in her parents' well being. This was not always easy for her, because her father was a domineering man, who amongst other things closely monitored the length of any telephone calls between his wife and overseas daughter. This meant that in order to find out how her parents were, she sometimes had to rely on information provided to her by cousins, or by her sister-in-law; she did not receive any of this information from her brother. Rachel also made several return visits (as many as her financial situation allowed) - it appears from her comments mainly to try to gain her parents' approval.

In the mid-1990s Rachel heard from a cousin that her father's health was deteriorating. As she said in interview, she then did a bit of detective work in order to find out what medication he was taking. This made her realise that this medicine had nasty side effects. On her next visit home, she accompanied her father to his doctor to discuss his treatment. The outcome was a change in his medication and an improvement in his health that gave her great satisfaction. Some time later, her father began to show signs of dementia. Rachel visited again, this time with her husband, expecting again to provide assistance. However, her father threatened her physically, used abusive language and forced her out of the family home. Rachel said in interview that after her return to Perth from that visit she could not stop crying for weeks. She suffered from depression and physical ill health for some time. Her father's behaviour – although due to his dementia – was for her a kind of confirmation of his dismissive and critical stance towards her even before she migrated.

During the last period of his life, her father was cared for by his wife, and when he became increasingly aggressive and hard to cope with, moved to a nursing home. After his death, mother and daughter were able to re-establish what Rachel saw as a good relationship. They phoned each other weekly and at length, and the daughter increased the number of her return visits to one a year. Her mother remained in the family home, which had been modified to accommodate her increasing physical frailty. This included a lift chair to her upstairs bedroom, and safety rails in the bathroom. During interview with the mother, then in her late 80s, she indicated that she was on the waiting list to move to a hostel. In the meantime, she said, her son took care of all her needs. He clearly remained the favourite child, seen by his mother as a great support, always willing to help, this notwithstanding the fact that this son and his family lived at a considerable distance and her day-to-day support came from a young couple next door. The mother mentioned Rachel's attempts at caring when her father was suffering from dementia (on the occasion that he threw her out of the house), but dismissed these efforts because her father's care was "none of her business". Rachel, then, had made efforts over a period of about thirty years to give emotional and practical care to her parents, without receiving any acknowledgment for her commitment and sense of responsibility towards them.

These two interviewees each had unique experiences and care-giving histories. Both women had a strong sense of transnational identity: in Mason's (1999) terms they might be said to have been "distance thinkers". Johanna always had considerable opportunities for transnational care-giving (she had the resources to travel) but her desire to give care only became apparent after her father's death, when her mother became increasingly dependent on support and her sister Beth took on more of a burden of responsibility. Rachel had a strong desire to give care to her parents, but was not given the opportunity – her parents rejected her efforts.

In the Italian and Irish case, transnational migrants were often dependent on the good will of their siblings for access to their ailing parents, because these were being cared for by their adult children in their own homes. As we have described, in the Netherlands none of the parents were living with their children. It is clear, though, that Dutch migrants were also dependent on the goodwill of their family back home, especially for information about their parents' well-being at a time when it became more difficult to communicate directly with them. During return visits, the situation may well have been different to the Italian and Irish ones. As their parents did not live with other children, Dutch migrants were able to visit them without having to rely on their siblings' good will. This was illustrated most poignantly by the situation of one migrant daughter who went to visit her father in hospital without her mother's knowledge and against her wishes. On the other hand, parental independence can also bring about the kind of situation Rachel encountered: her father, already severely demented and in need of care, simply refused her entry to the house.

Discussion

A growing concern for many affluent countries is the ageing of their populations and the associated health care issues. The changing population structure and increased longevity of the population, often referred to as the 'greying' of Western societies, has made age care a priority concern. The vast majority of elderly in each of the countries under discussion do not live in institutional care settings. These countries all prioritise 'community care', whereby elderly people are cared for in their own homes as long as possible. In line with this philosophy of care, our research found an overwhelming desire, on the part of elderly people, for independence as an ideal in old age and preferably throughout the remainder of their lives, regardless of cultural background or country of origin. However, there appeared to be clear cultural differences regarding what it means to be 'independent'. There were also apparent differences in cultural perceptions of what were considered by the elderly to be 'preferred' care scenarios. These notions of independence and preferred care were influenced by historical patterns of care, the structural constraints on that care, as well as family circumstance, including the specificities of kin relations. In terms of the impact on distant carers, we found that notwithstanding the cultural differences between sample groups, there was some commonality of experience as well as some general differences.

Notions of 'Independence' and Preferred Care

The elderly in all three samples became dependent only at the point of becoming frail or disabled and it was this decline in ability that resulted in changes in care arrangements. Up until this point, all of the parents in our study were living in their own homes, either with a spouse or alone. While a variety of care arrangements are found in each country of study, there were some key differences in the preferred arrangement of care, often deriving from established historical patterns of care, reflecting differences in notions of acceptable care as well as culturally constructed notions of independence.

One clear context in which these different forms of care and notions of independence became apparent was in terms of the requirement for personal care in old age, and particularly those more intimate forms of care such as washing, dressing and feeding. The Italian and Irish parents tended to prefer all forms of care, including personal care, to be provided by family, or by live-in (family-like) paid help, while the Dutch showed a preference for paid personal care.

The Netherlands has the most developed system of institutional and community care, including hostels, retirement homes and a plethora of personal-care services that support the elderly in their homes. 'Independence' for the Dutch parents tended to mean being supported in their own homes or in care facilities. There was a clear preference in the Dutch sample for personal care not to be conducted by family members but by service providers. The relatively long-standing and well-developed systems of aged care in the Netherlands make this kind of preferred care arrangement possible. In this sense, independence for the Dutch meant not being dependent on family. Indeed, a common refrain in interviews was the desire not to be 'a burden' on children. This was also the case in the Irish sample, but the understanding of what constituted a 'burden' appeared to mean something different.

In Ireland, the most commonly discussed preferred arrangement of care was for the children to support their parents to live in their own home. In this context, 'independence' means being able to live in your own home with minimal interference from people outside of the family. If disability increases to such an extent that constant personal care is required, the preference is for an unmarried child or a daughter to move in with the parent, reflecting the historical pattern of leaving the family farm or home to a resident care-giving child. The intimate care-giving that is provided by adult children to their dying parents is understood as an expected and normal part of the family life cycle, in which the child returns the care they have received throughout their life. There is also the added incentive of the inheritance of the house, which might be seen as a form of fair exchange for the provision of care services. It is arguably this exchange of 'care for care', and of 'the family house for care', that usually operates to remove any sense of the parent being 'a burden' on their care-giving child.

In Italy, which has the least developed institutional and community care structures of the three nations in question, the preferred arrangement of care, particularly for the 'old-old', is for the ageing parent to be supported in an extended family setting, with the parent moving in to live permanently with a child. There is really no alternative in a country which, not unlike Ireland, traditionally relied on the family and the Church (a non-Government sector) for all social services. The preferred arrangement of care is to be able to rely on children for all necessary support. There is a clear tendency for the elderly to believe that if they need to procure support services from outside, their family is not caring for them adequately. There is a corresponding acute sense of duty on the part of children to provide for all the care needs of their parents in order to feel that they have behaved appropriately as 'good children'. 'Independence' for the elderly in this context might mean not requiring outside support, although perhaps the notion is not as culturally relevant to the Italians. Certainly, none of the parents interviewed strove to be independent of their children. Like the Irish, there is also a sense that caring for parents is returning the care received from them as children, including any share in the inheritance.

Social changes in Italian life in recent years, in particular the increase in dual income families and women in the workforce, as well as the significant decline in the birth-rate (Italy has the lowest in Europe), has meant that the traditional preference for extended family living is less feasible. As a result, older people struggle with a strong desire to be in close contact with their families and with the realisation that their children have a range of responsibilities that make it difficult for them to provide the longed for level of support. Adult children also struggle to reconcile the sense of obligation to care for their parents with the various other demands on their time. The growing prevalence over this period for a live-in carer reflects not only the absence of alternative support services, including institutional care facilities, but also is in keeping with the preference for family care in the home (or, in this instance, 'family-like' care) and the cultural construction of independence defined in opposition to the need for outside help. The 'young-old' tended to be more open, at least in their aspirations, to increased community and institutional forms of care, although they also displayed a keen preference for their children to support them and, failing that, for '*una donna*' - live-in home-help.

Impact on the Distant Carer

The different constructs of independence in old age and of preferred care arrangements, in particular, the type of personal care that is desired by disabled parents, have important implications for the migrant wishing to provide care from a distance. The most significant difference in these three samples was in the visit trajectories of migrants. When a parent becomes frail and/or disabled, the type of distant care that migrant children can provide is affected. The increased need for personal, 'hands-on' care often triggers an increase in the frequency and duration of visits, particularly by women. Migrant children can only provide this kind of care when they are visiting their parents. In the case of severely disabled or dementing parents, the objective of the visit is often to provide respite to siblings and other carers, as much as it is to have contact with parents.

Women in the Italian and Irish samples were more likely to participate in long-term visits for the purpose of providing personal care to their parents and respite to their siblings. When this was not feasible, Italian and Irish migrant children often surrendered their rights to inheritance in recognition of the burden of care taken on by their home-land based kin. In the Dutch case, the availability and preference for support services provided outside the family resulted in this form of care not being required or provided by Dutch migrants. The emotional support sought by Dutch parents is possibly more easily given across distance than is the intimately physical support sought by the Irish and Italian parents. Occasional visits home and regular communications may continue to meet the expectations of Dutch parents, but were often perceived as insufficient in the traditional expectations of Irish and Italian parents. Thus, there was a prevalence of cases in the Irish and Italian samples in which the migrants felt it necessary to return home to provide care in the final stages of their parents' life.

Despite this difference in visit trajectories, all migrant carers, across all samples, were similarly dependent on the goodwill of their spouses, siblings and other primary carers for access to their ailing parents. The relevance of migration histories and their impact on family relations is clearly evident in the experience of distant care. In particular, the existence or otherwise of 'licence to leave' can have a significant impact on the migrant's ability to provide any kind of support. While the issue of access was particularly apparent in the Italian case, where parents were often cared for in the home of one of their adult children, it was an issue of equal importance in the Irish case. None of the parents in the Netherlands were living with their children. Dutch migrants were not dependent on the goodwill of their family back home for access, but they did rely on them for information about their parents' well-being when it became more difficult to communicate directly with them.

Further, people in all three sample groups talked about the importance of visiting as the only way to find out for certain how parents are. This indicates a concern about the amount of information or level of truth that their siblings or other carers might share with them by phone, letter or email. All interviewees talked about trying to read between the lines and interpret silences and, especially, trying to 'hear' the truth in the voices at the end of the phone line, something not possible to do when parents are no longer capable of speaking on the phone. These concerns might reflect the common custom of hiding the truth from family members in order to protect them.

A number of factors complicate the picture. Dementia, for example, limits the ability to provide any care across distance to the suffering parent. Indeed, dementia to some extent removes the ability for the parent to express a need for care. Instead, it is clear that in the case of dementia migrants tend to turn their attention to the needs of the local caregiver sibling. The availability of care local to the parent also appears to be significant in determining the sense of obligation of the migrant, regardless of country of origin. Some migrants decide to return to the home country because, either there are no siblings, or it is clear that none of their siblings are able to provide the care necessary to meet their parent's care preferences. For other migrants, such a decision is not necessary due to the extensive support networks already in place. Of course, the presence of such networks can create its own problems for the migrant in terms of access, as already discussed.

Gender is an important factor in the decision to participate in the kinds of visits which make 'hands-on' and respite care possible. Women are more likely to be in a position to find the time needed for these visits; they are usually earning less than their spouses and many choose to take part-time and casual work specifically to enable visits at short notice. They are also more likely to feel confident that they have the necessary care-giving skills. Arguably, there is greater cultural expectation for women to assume this role than for men. Other interrelated factors include birth order (with older children often assuming more responsibility); gender of homeland siblings (if there are no sisters back home then the migrant daughter may feel more obliged to provide 'hands-on' care); and the marital status of siblings (with unmarried siblings often considered more available to provide care).

CONCLUSION

Our research on transnational caring relations also raises some important implications for migration theory. It highlights how mobility is often triggered by the need to give or receive care, rather than any 'rational economic', profit maximisation motive commonly assumed in much migration literature. As Ackers (2002, p.153) has argued, the dynamic of work and economic imperatives are emphasised over and above all other factors, 'rarely if ever examining life course and caring as components of migration decisions'. Similarly, our work confirms the growing recognition that all migrants (including refugees) move for mixed motivations, that it can be hard to disentangle political, social and economic reasons to move, and that migrants are involved in a wide range of what we might term 'transnational' activities (cf. Al-Ali, Black, and Koser, 2001). Migratory movements are not discrete, unilateral or linear: in charting people's care histories we often found multiple moves, in many directions, that may not make the best economic sense. The mobility of care is thus located in the realm of the economies of kinship, including but not limited to the exchange of economic resources within families.

In conclusion, while cultural background is a significant factor in providing appropriate aged care, it is important to note that many of the issues associated with intergenerational responsibilities and 'distant' care of the elderly are not easily differentiated according to national or ethnic group identity (Manderson, 1990). The more or less global factors of increased mobility, changing gender and work patterns and resultant family fragmentation are as important to debates about aged care everywhere as are specific cultural characteristics. It is reasonable to assume that the experiences and needs of older parents are largely the same across the globe. However, differences do exist, and they are just as likely to result from gender, socio-economic, class and educational background, as from any factors relating to country of residence. This said, our research shows that historical patterns in the common arrangement of care in the home-country, closely related to the level and provision of relevant services provided by the state, and reflected in culturally constructed notions of independence and preferred arrangements of care, have a significant impact on the experience of caring of the distant care-giver.

Policy Recommendations and Theoretical Implications: Making Long-Distance Care Visible

Based on our research, we make the following policy recommendations:

- Recognition on the part of employers, government agencies and service providers that immigrants may have a role as secondary carers for parents overseas. Tangible outcomes of this should be:
    1. Flexibility in leave arrangements, allowing immigrants to travel overseas at short notice in emergency situations.
    2. Provision of special bereavement leave of more than 5 days duration for employees who need to attend funerals overseas.
    3. Workplace-based workshops for carers to include sessions with immigrants as secondary carers.
    4. Recognition of the financial and emotional burdens on immigrants as secondary carers in marriage and financial counselling.
    5. Information packages for, and counselling sessions with, prospective immigrants to prepare them for the emotional and financial stress they may face as secondary carers for parents overseas.

- Financial and other support for immigrant carers, for example:
  1. Concession rates for telephone calls to family members overseas.
  2. Emergency relief provision to help with payment of large telephone bills (usually only run up in crisis situations).
  3. Community-based arrangements for interest-free loans to pay for emergency travel.
  4. Special bereavement support by airlines and travel agencies for immigrants needing to return to their country of birth for funerals and other emergencies. This could take the form of both priority seating and discount ticketing.

REFERENCES

Ackers, L. (1999). *Shifting Spaces: Women, Citizenship and Migration Within the European Union*. Bristol: Policy Press.

Ackers, L. and Dwyer, P. (2002). *Senior Citizenship? Retirement, Migration and Welfare in the European Union*. Bristol: Policy Press.

Al-Ali, N., Black, R., Koser, K. (2001). Refugees and transnationalism: the experience of Bosnians and Eritreans in Europe, *Journal of Ethnic and Migration Studies*, 27(4), 615-634.

Aldous, J. and Klein, D.M. (1991). Sentiments and services: Models of intergenerational relationships in mid-life. *Journal of Marriage and Family*, 53, 595-608.

Andall, J. (1999). Cape Verdean women on the move: 'Immigration shopping' in Italy and Europe, *Modern Italy*, 4(2), 241-257.

Baldassar, L. (2001). *Visits Home: Migration Experiences between Italy and Australia*, Melbourne: Melbourne University Press.

Baldassar, L., and Baldock, C. V. (2000). Linking migration and family studies: Transnational migrants and the care of ageing parents. In B. Agozino (Ed.), *Theoretical and Methodological Issues in Migration Research*, (pp. 61–89). Aldershot: Ashgate.

Baldassar, L., Baldock, C. V. and Wilding, R. (forthcoming, 2006). *Families Caring Across Borders: migration, ageing and transnational caregiving.* London: Palgrave MacMillan.

Baldassar, L., Baldock, C. V., and Wilding, R. (2002). Transnational Families and Caring for Elderly Parents. Paper presented at the International Sociological Association Congress, Family Research Committee (RC06), Transnational Families session, 7-12 July, Brisbane.

Baldassar, L., and Pesman, R. (2005). *From Paesani to Global Italians: Veneto Migrants in Australia.* Crawley: University of Western Australia Press.

Baldock, C. V. (1999). The ache of frequent farewells. In M. Poole, and S. Feldman (Eds.), *A Certain Age, Women Growing Older*, (pp 182-192). Sydney: Allen and Unwin.

Baldock, C. V. (2000). Migrants and their parents: Care-giving from a distance, *Journal of Family Issues,* 21(2), 205-224.

Baldock, C. V. (2003). Long-distance migrants and family support: A Dutch case-study, *Health Sociology Review*, 12(1), 45-54.

Basch, L., N. Glick-Schiller and C. Blanc-Szanton (Eds) (1992). *Towards a Transnational Perspective on Migration.* New York: New York Academy of Sciences.

Bijsterveld, K. (1996). *Geen kwestie van Leeftijd: Verzorgingsstaat, wetenschap en discussies rond ouderen in Nederland, 1945-1882*. Amsterdam: Van Gennep.

Cecil, R., Offer, J., and St. Leger, F. (1987). *Informal Welfare: A Sociological Study of Care in Northern Ireland.* Aldershot: Gower.

Climo, J. (1992). *Distant Parents*. New Brunswick: Rutgers University Press.

Clothier, M. (1997). Family Migration Program. *Immigration Law* P97(26), 2.1-2.10.

Crock, M. E. (1998). *Immigration and Refugee Law in Australia.* Leichhardt: Federation Press.

Curry, J. (1998). *Irish Social Services*. Dublin: Institute of Public Administration.

Daly, M. (1998). A more caring state? The implications of welfare state restructuring for social care in the Republic of Ireland. In J. Lewis, (Ed.) *Gender, Social Care and Welfare State Restructuring in Europe*, (pp 25-50). Aldershot: Ashgate.

Finch, J and Mason, J. (1993). *Negotiating Family Responsibilities.* London: Tavistock.

Giarchi, G. (1996). *Caring for Older Europeans: Comparative Studies in 29 Countries*. Aldershot: Ashgate.

Gubrium, J.F. and Holstein, J.A. (1990). *What is Family*. Mountain View, CA: Mayfield.

Gupta, A. and J. Ferguson (1992). Beyond 'culture': Space, identity, and the politics of difference. *Cultural Anthropology* 7(1), 6-23.

James, A., James, William L., and Smith, H. (1984). Reciprocity as a coping strategy for the elderly: A rural Irish perspective. *The Gerontologist*, 24(5), 483-489.

Kennedy, F. (1986). The family in transition. In K. Kennedy, (Ed.), *Ireland in Transition: Economic and Social Change Since 1960*, (pp. 91-100). Cork: Mercier.

Larragy, J. (1993a). Views and perceptions of older Irish people. *Social Policy and Administration*, 27(3), 235-247.

Larragy, J. (1993b). Formal service provision and the care of the elderly at home in Ireland. *Journal of Cross-Cultural Gerontology* 8, 361-374.

Leane, M. (1995). Female carers for elderly people: Implications for women's labour market participation in Ireland. In J. Phillips, (Ed.) *Working Carers: Avebury Studies of Care in the Community,* (pp 58-72). Avebury, Aldershot: Ashgate.

Lin, G. and Rogerson, P.A. (1995). Elderly parents and the geographic availability of their adult children. *Research on Aging*, 17, 303-331.

MacKinnon, V. and Nelli, A. (1996). *Now We Are in Paradise, Everything is Missing*. Footscray: Department of Nursing, Victoria University of Technology.

Manderson, L. (1990). Introduction; Does culture matter? In J. Reid and P. Trompf (Eds), *The Health of Immigrant Australia: A Social Perspective*, (pp. xi-xvii). Sydney: Harcourt Brace Jovanovich.

Mason, Jennifer (1999). Living away from kin: Kinship and geographical reasoning. In S. McRae, (Ed.), *Changing Britain*, (pp 156-175). Oxford University Press.

O'Shea, E. (2002). *Review of the Nursing Home Subvention Scheme*. Dublin: Government of Ireland.

Rossi, A.S. and Rossi, P.H. (1990). *On Human Bonding: Parent-Child Relations in the Life Course*. New York: Aldine.

Timmermans, J.M. (Ed.) (1996). *Rapportage Ouderen 1996*. Rijswijk: Sociaal en Cultureel Planbureau.

Timmermans, J. M., Heide, F., de Klerk, M. M. Y., Kooiker, S. E., Ras, M., and van Dugteren, F. A. (1997). *Vraagverkenning wonen en zorg voor ouderen*. Rijswijk: Sociaal en Cultureel Planbureau.

Trifiletti, R. (1998). Restructuring social care in Italy. In J. Lewis (Ed.), *Gender, Social Care and Welfare State Restructuring in Europe*, (pp 175-206). Aldershot: Ashgate.

Wilding, R. (2006). Virtual intimacies: Family communications across transnational borders. *Global Networks*, 6(2).

In: Family Caregiving for Older Disabled People
Editor: Isabella Paoletti, pp. 229-249
ISBN 1-59454-808-0

Chapter 11

THE RECONSTITUTION OF NEED FOR HOME CARE SERVICES IN THE WAKE OF CANADIAN HEALTH CARE RESTRUCTURING

Diana L. Gustafson
Department of Social Sciences and Health, Division of Community Health, Memorial University, St. John's, Newfoundland, Canada

INTRODUCTION: THE RECONSTITUTION OF NEED

This chapter explores the reconstitution of individual need for home care services following a time of sweeping health care restructuring in Ontario, Canada in the mid-1990s. Ontario Ministry of Health (1992; 1993; 1994) documents claimed that reforms were necessary to create a more accessible, client-focussed, community-based health care system. However, critics of health sector restructuring argued that public funding for home care support[1] was inadequate and created barriers to accessing home care. For instance, individuals and their families reported that the hours of publicly funded home care for which they qualified, were insufficient (Morris et al., 1999). The elderly disabled who are among Canada's largest home care users are often impoverished because of inadequate income support programs, and therefore, less able to fill the gaps in care by paying for private care services (Masuda, 1998). Typically, women family members are expected to supplement home care services at great personal and financial cost to their own health, wellbeing, and career development (Armstrong and Armstrong, 2003). The disjuncture between government funding for home care, institutional assessments of client need, and the subjective experiences of need for publicly funded home care services reflect two parallel ways of knowing about family caregiving and the needs of elderly persons living with disabilities:

The first of these ways of knowing is discoverable in the expressions of embodied subjects and the family members who care for them. Across Canada, the frail elderly and

[1] Home care support refers to a range of health care and homemaker services provided to persons in their home with all or part of the costs covered by a publicly funded provincial health insurance plan.

persons living with disabilities and their families are expressing concern about the political, economic, and moral push toward home-based care (Aronson and Neysmith, 1997; Aronson, 1998; Masuda, 1998; Morris et al., 1999). Families bring this experiential knowledge of increased financial and human costs with them when seeking home care support from community agencies. This subjective knowledge is connected to, but sometimes at odds with, a second way of knowing about family caregiving.

That way of knowing is discoverable in and mediated through the apparently neutral bureaucratic processes that coordinate the activities of health care providers. *Local texts* such as intake and assessment forms and eligibility procedures are interconnected with a wide range of translocal texts. *Translocal texts* such as government home care policy documents are external to but have a regulating effect on the local context. These translocal texts "pass through" local settings organizing in powerful ways the everyday work activities of people on a large scale (DeVault and McCoy, 2002, p. 752). Dorothy Smith (1999) refers to these processes of coordination, administration, and governance as "relations of ruling." *Ruling relations* are "the forms in which power is generated and held in contemporary societies" (Smith, 1999, p. 79). Ruling relations are "those forms that we know as bureaucracy, administration, management, professional organization, and the media. They include also the complex of discourses, scientific, technical and cultural, that intersect, interpenetrate, and coordinate the multiple sites of ruling" (Smith, 1990, p. 6).

The next section looks at the generalizing effects of ruling relations in health care on two local contexts: 1) the everyday activities of home care workers in assessing need and delivering home care services; and 2) the families seeking support services to supplement their care work in the home.

Literature Review: The Discourse of Cost Containment Organizing Health Sector Restructuring

Changes in home care policies and programs were part of an overall health restructuring strategy initiated in Ontario and across Canada in the early 1990s. The federal and provincial governments claimed that sweeping health sector reordering was necessary to respond to profound structural and global changes in the economy. Ontario Ministry of Health documents (1992; 1993; 1994) characterized reform as a necessary response to overspending and inefficiency. Cost cutting strategies included hospital downsizing, amalgamations and closures, job displacement and work redesign, and the privatization of health care services. Two significant changes aimed at achieving the government's vision of a more accessible, client-focussed system moved health care "closer to home" (Armstrong et al., 1994, p. 95).

The Change in Program Structures

The first of these changes came when the Ontario government merged two distinct community-based agencies, the Home Care Program and the Placement Program. The mandate of the Home Care Program was to assist an individual to return home from hospital, or remain in their home, with appropriate home care support. The Placement Program assisted individuals and their families to access a suitable level of care in tertiary community facilities such as nursing homes, homes for the aged, and daycare programs for seniors. Both programs had offices in Regional Health Departments across Ontario that coordinated the delivery of insurable health care services provided in their respective communities.

In the early 1990s, an Ontario government review determined that there was considerable overlap in the populations served by these two programs. Subsequently, the two programs were merged into 43 Community Care Access Centres. Staff positions were cut, work processes restructured, and physical plants eliminated. The government promised that the merger would improve continuity of care while eliminating costly duplication of administrative functions, resources, and services (Armstrong and Armstrong, 2003).

Three years after the merger, however, a community health framework was still in the early stages of development. Although the Ontario Ministry of Health (1994) promised that monies saved through hospital restructuring would be channelled into community-based care, the promised infusion of dollars did not materialize. With less instead of more money at their disposal, overall spending in this sector actually declined between 1992 and 1994 (Ontario Council of Hospital Unions/Canadian Union of Public Employees, 1995).[2] Community Care Access Centres were not prepared for the steadily increasing demand for services brought about by hospital restructuring. More and sicker people needing more complex levels of care were being discharged from hospital into the community (Armstrong and Armstrong, 2003; Morris et al., 1999). At the same time, the Centres were expected to operate a more accessible service, over longer hours, more efficiently, more cost effectively, and with fewer staff. The resulting gap between demand and supply of home care support further supported the government's claim that cost containment was necessary to save the publicly-funded health care system.

The Change in Funding Structures

The second significant change came when the Canadian federal government changed the way that health care, welfare, and social assistance were funded. For decades, the federal and provincial governments shared the health care costs. To qualify for federal transfer payments, provincial health insurance plans had to meet the five principles of universality, accessibility, comprehensiveness, portability, and public administration enshrined in the 1984 Canada Health Act.[3] The aim of the Canada Health Act is to ensure that all Canadian residents have reasonable access to all medically necessary health services provided without direct charge to the individual at the point of delivery. The Canada Assistance Plan was a similar

---

[2] Alberta, another Canadian province, experienced similar problems as only 1/7 of the monies cut from health care were re-channeled into community-based care services (Morris et al., 1999: 22).

[3] The *universality* principle requires that all insured residents are entitled to the services covered by the provincial insurance plan. The *accessibility* criterion stipulates that residents must have reasonable physical availability of services unimpeded by extra billing or other means such as discrimination. To be eligible for transfer payments, provinces must demonstrate the insurance plan is *comprehensive* meaning the plan covers the costs of all insured services provided by hospitals, physicians and a select group of health professionals. *Portability* of health insurance means that insured residents are covered while temporarily out of province and during the waiting period required to establish residency in a new province. The *public administration* criterion requires that the provincial health insurance plan is administered and operated on a non-profit basis by a public authority and accountable to the provincial government.

federal/provincial cost-sharing program that guaranteed the right for social assistance to everyone in need. These pieces of federal legislation were a testament to Canada's commitment to social responsibility for health and welfare.

That legislated commitment was eroded in 1996 when the Canada Assistance Plan was eliminated and the Canada Health and Social Transfer Act was passed. These changes altered the way that monies for health and social services were transferred from the federal government to the provinces and territories. Under the new act, these monies were consolidated into a single block of funding.[4] The federal government claimed that block funding would limit federal spending and add predictability to federal budgeting (Masuda, 1998). For the provinces, however, the Canada Health and Social Transfer Act signalled a 30% drop in revenue that amounted to $4.3 billion for the years 1996-97 and 1997-98.

Unlike other health care services which are federally regulated under the Canada Health Act, home care is under provincial control. There is no comparable federal legislation with principles regulating how provinces must allocate dollars for home care services. As Sheila Neysmith (1998) explains, without the "power of the purse… the financial incentive for provinces to maintain and develop services now disappears because [federal-provincial] cost-sharing has been replaced by a fixed 'megatransfer' " (p. 235). When vying for a share of the reduced resources, home care did not fare well against "the powerful interests that represent acute care" (p. 235).

The Human Impact of Changes to Program and Funding Structures

The drop in the amount of federal transfer payments for health and social services meant there was even less money to go around for families needing social assistance and home care services. Especially hard hit were poor, elderly, unattached women living with disabilities who are among the largest users of home care services (Wilkins and Park, 1998). Women make up more than half the Canadian population and have one of the longest life expectancies in the world (Health Canada, 1999). As a woman ages, she is more likely than a man to spend her later years unattached and living with long-term activity limitations associated with chronic pain, degenerative diseases, and chronic physical and psychiatric conditions (Statistics Canada, 2000). A woman living in poverty is more likely than her wealthier counterpart to be disabled. Conversely, a disabled woman is more likely to be poor with some reports suggesting that as many as 60% of such women live below the poverty line (Masuda, 1998; Morris et al., 1999). Not surprisingly, unattached woman over 65 years of age and those from Aboriginal and other minoritized communities tend to be among Canada's poorest and these groups make up a disproportionate number of the elderly living with disabilities (Health Canada, 1999).

These data suggest that persons living with disabilities are more likely to depend, in whole or in part, on the welfare system for basic needs such as food, shelter, and homemaking services. Moreover, persons living with disabilities depend heavily on the home care system to carry out activities of daily living such as bathing and toileting as well as managing

[4] Monies for public education were also rolled into this block of funding supporting critics concerns that the social welfare state was under attack under the Canada Health and Social Transfer Act.

medical problems such as recurrent bladder infections that may result from living with some chronic physical disabilities (Masuda, 1998).

Prior to the two previously described changes in the structure and funding of home care, many seniors with disabilities moved into formal care settings as their care needs increased. Since block funding cut monies for beds, staff, and services, and impeded reasonable access to health and welfare benefits, more frail elderly and those living with disabilities remain in home-based care for longer time frames (Masuda, 1998; Morris et al., 1999).

Individuals and families identify a disjuncture between their self-reported need for home care services and how their needs are assessed by community agencies mandated to provide publicly funded services (Gustafson, 2000; Simpson and Porte, 2000). Many women living with chronic conditions and disabilities do not ask for help because they fear they cannot demonstrate sufficient need. In a climate of fiscal constraint, some aging women *feel* disentitled to receive home care services (Drozdow-St. Christian, 2000). As Jane Aronson (1998) found in her study of mothers and daughters, it was not only the disadvantaged who felt less entitled to receive publicly funded home care services. She quotes potential home care recipients who say, "We can't expect much"; "There are so many of us now"; and "They just don't have the money, you see" (Aronson, 1998, p. 125).

The generalizing consequence of the discourse of cost containment recasts elderly disabled persons as an "expensive burden on society" (Aronson, 1998, p. 125) rather than a group who should have guaranteed access to health care services. Another generalizing consequence of this disjuncture is that family members, usually women, are left to assume individual responsibility for providing caring labour traditionally considered a social responsibility. A comparison of institutional action[5] before and after restructuring illustrates how the dominant discourse of cost containment that accompanied health sector restructuring in the 1990s had a generalizing effect on the way that agency workers reconstituted individual need for home care services.

PURPOSE OF THE STUDY AND OVERVIEW OF CHAPTER

The aim of the study was to examine how the discourse of cost containment central to the Canadian government agenda of health care restructuring converged with and penetrated the work of home care agency workers who decided who was eligible for home care support. Using a method of social inquiry called institutional ethnography, this retrospective investigation compared the documentary practices used in assessing an elderly disabled person's home care needs at two distinct historical moments. The study illustrates how client need is reconstituted in ways that contain costs by limiting eligibility for home care services and downloading care work onto household members.

The study compared two intake forms that initiated assessment of client need, determine eligibility, and coordinated delivery of services: a) the Home Care Program Medical Referral form used by health care providers in one Ontario Regional Health Department prior to home care restructuring; and b) the Community Care Access Centre Client Assessment form used

[5] Institutional action, as explained later in this chapter, does not refer to a specific organization or context but rather to those textually-mediated processes that are organized around a specific ruling function which, in this case, is health care.

after the introduction of block funding in the Canada Health and Social Transfer Act. These frontline documents regulated what kinds of patient or client information health care personnel entered into the textually-mediated communication process, how that information was taken up and acted upon by others, and ultimately, how much, if any, home care support was provided to those elderly persons with disabilities and their families.

The comparison of documentary practices focused two questions: First, how do the discourses of family caregiving and cost containment converge and penetrate the everyday activities of health care providers who decide who is eligible for home care support and under what conditions? Second, how do post-restructuring documentary practices reconstitute the concept of need in ways that achieve the government's goal of cost containment and justify downloading the human and material costs of caring labour from governments and paid workers onto unpaid family members, usually women?

Each intake and assessment form and the process it initiated differently organized how need was constituted to determine eligibility for home care services. The analysis revealed that pre-restructuring documentary practices centred the subjective experience of need known to embodied subjects alongside the biomedical model of health care. This concept of need is displaced in the post-restructuring intake, assessment, and eligibility process by the penetration of the discourses of family caregiving and cost containment. These two discourses operating at and beyond the local setting reconstituted the concept of need in apparently neutral ways that limited eligibility for publicly funded home care support by first exhausting family support and private health coverage. The chapter concludes with recommendations for restoring governance processes that encourage social responsibility for health and welfare.

The next section introduces institutional ethnography as a method of social inquiry. This is followed by an overview of the method of data collection and a presentation and discussion of research findings.

Institutional Ethnography as a Method of Social Inquiry

Institutional ethnography is a research strategy that facilitates the exploration of the connections and disjunctures between individuals' subjective expressions of need and the ruling relations that organize the "everyday world" or the work activities of those who decide if and how these needs are met (Smith, 1987). This method of inquiry involves investigating the "ways in which people are actually involved in the production of their everyday work, examined with respect to how that world is organized by and sustains the institutional process" (Smith, 1987, p. 166). Unlike other methods, institutional ethnography does not focus on subjective states but rather traces the complex of textually-mediated communication involved in a particular institutional action. As DeVault and McCoy (2002) point out, "a central feature of ruling practice in contemporary society is its reliance on text-based discourse and forms of knowledge" (p. 753).

Institutional action is coordinated and linked to the exercise of power both at and beyond the local setting in which the work activities occur. Ruling relations are neither an "abstraction" nor are they readily recognized as concrete by individuals engaged in their daily work (Gustafson, 2000). Instead ruling practices may be experienced by individuals as bureaucratic red tape that must be negotiated to achieve an end that may seem disconnected from the knowledge or experience that workers bring to that activity.

Institutional action cannot be mapped in its totality (DeVault and McCoy, 2002). The interconnectedness of local and translocal texts is too messy and complex for that. In chapter 15, Nikander takes a similar methodological approach analysing specific institutional practices, interprofessional meetings, as a practical site for decision making over service and help allocation to elderly people and their carer providers. Nikander is interested in showing how decisions on various agreed upon policies and principles of elderly care are turned into practice. In both chapters institutions are shown in their making.

Institutional ethnographic studies tend to focus on a single strand of action which, in this case, is a process that begins with an intake and assessment form. This form is a single component in a complex, textually-mediated communication process that moves patient or client information from one health care provider or text reader to the next. The form mobilizes the activities of health workers in performing a client assessment in a concrete social and historical context. The form organizes what client information is included and centred in the process, and what information is excluded or marginalized. Only the information included in the record becomes eligible for discussion and action further along the communication process. Information that is not included in the text is rendered unavailable for interpretation or action.

As the worker generates a completed form, that form constitutes the "textual reality" or the institutional facts about the elderly person with disabilities and her or his health care needs (Smith, 1990, p. 79). The power of this objectified knowledge lies both in its concreteness as text and in the ruling relations that give authority to documented accounts over oral histories (DeVault and McCoy, 2002, p. 762). Thus, the intake record and the work process it organizes, produce an image of need that comes to represent and be disconnected from the subjective knowledge and experience of the individual needing home care services. And as this analysis shows, the institutional facts of the case disqualify or displace the subjective knowledge and experience of the health care personnel enacting the work processes.

Comparing how the intake form coordinated the delivery of home care services at two historical moments illustrates how the concept of need is constituted in and by the text itself and by other bureaucratic practices internal and external to the organization. That is to say, translocal texts external to community agencies such as government legislation together with local texts such as administrative policies and procedures regulate and standardize the kinds of information that are collected, communicated, interpreted, and acted upon as the intake record is passed from one health care worker to the next. In this way, these local strands of action become understandable within and connected to the discourses of cost containment and family caregiving operating in the larger ruling relations of health care.

Data Collection

As a health care insider working in an Ontario hospital in the 1990s, I was familiar with the Home Care Program intake and assessment process that existed prior to health sector restructuring. Drawing on my network of contacts in health care institutions, medical and nursing faculties, and professional associations, I recruited nurses from one southern Ontario hospital, two community-based provider agencies, and three Community Care Access Centres. The conventional rules about a "sample" group that govern positivist research do not apply here (DeVault and McCoy, 2002, p. 764). This method of social inquiry is not concerned with collecting data about subjective experiences of participants or developing descriptive categories about a given population. Instead, participants were selected based on their intimate familiarity with one or both intake processes. Rigour comes from building a map of the social relations that is faithful and consistent across multiple accounts and sites (p. 764).

In a series of face-to-face and telephone interviews conducted over four months with six participants operating in different settings, the nurses described their work activities in relation to one or both texts. Interviews lasted from 10-90 minutes with the shorter communications concerned with clarifying details described in longer communications. Interviews were not tape recorded because some participants expressed fear of reprisals.[6] Instead the data were detailed in handwritten notes and a series of hand drawn schematic diagrams that depicted the actual sequence of work activities.

In institutional ethnographic studies, interviews are open-ended with a view to learning "how things work" (DeVault and McCoy, 2002, p. 757). Rather than exploring a particular client case, the focus was on mapping and analyzing "the institutional nexus that shapes the local" (Grahame, 1999, p. 7). In this case, the focus was on understanding how information about the patient or client's needs were communicated from one person to the next in both textually-mediated processes. The participants and I had copies of the intake forms to guide our discussions and develop an account of how an individual who needed home support hooked into community agencies who delivered those services.

To analyze the data, I began by comparing the content and format of the intake and assessment forms. This research strategy does not, however, treat the intake record as an independent document whose meaning is located solely in the words and tick boxes printed on the page. Nor is the intake form static. Therefore, I also compared and analyzed the communication processes initiated by the intake records to establish how local and translocal texts organized the everyday work actions of health care providers and their interactions with clients. The analysis revealed how each process differently constructed an image of individual need for home care support, accomplished the functional and ideological work of the agency, and mediated the ruling relations of health care. The next section describes the research findings beginning with the intake form and the assessment procedure used prior to health sector restructuring.

[6] As I discuss in detail elsewhere, my difficulties recruiting participants and gathering texts and information from the employees at Community Care Access Centres were strongly suggestive of "a dynamic of consolidating and concealing authority that was systemic rather than agency specific" (Gustafson, 2000, p. 187).

Research Findings

The Assessment of Need Prior to Health Sector Restructuring

In the early 1990s, the intake process for the assessment of patient need began when a physician completed a Home Care Program Medical Referral form. Only physicians had the legislated authority to initiate a request for publicly funded home care services. In most instances, individuals or families in need approached their family doctor with whom they had an established relationship. Usually, the family doctor was familiar with documentation on, or had participated in, the bulk of physician-patient interactions. The physician operating from a biomedical model of care assessed the individual's health and level of need. The health assessment included the individual's subjective experience of need alongside objective means of health assessment such as a physical examination, and biochemical and imaging tests. Brief but relevant details of that medical history and prognosis were documented on the medical referral form.

The intake form was a one-page form with a rectangular space in the upper right hand corner used for imprinting the person's vital statistics including Ontario Health Insurance Plan[7] number. Six data fields at the top and bottom of the form were for fixed responses. These tick boxes prompt the text reader to add information about the individual's prognosis (i.e., improve, remain stable, deteriorate), if the diagnosis is known the person and their family (yes/no), and the type of home care services requested (e.g., nursing, physiotherapy, homemaking, and so on).

Four free-text fields take up the remainder of the form. These fields are entitled, "Diagnosis," "History," "Medications," and "Specific Orders". The free-text design allowed the physician more latitude than fixed-response fields for creating a narrative account of the individual's health status. This, in turn, enabled the text reader to enter more subjective and objective data about the individual's needs and treatment goals into the communication and decision-making process. At the bottom of the form are lines and spaces for dates and signatures of the physician and subsequent text readers such as the Home Care Case Manager. The physician dated and signed the Home Care Program Medical Referral form before sending it on to the next text reader in the process.

The next text reader was the Home Care Case Manager. Although this nurse worked out of the local hospital, she was employed by the Home Care Program in her local Regional Health Department. The Case Manager reviewed the facts of the case as documented on medical referral form. If the individual was hospitalized or in another care setting, the Case Manager familiarized herself with the documentation created in those local settings about the individual's medical history and level of cognitive and physical functioning. In order to complete the intake form, the Case Manager also met face-to-face with the individual to assess their level of need. If the individual was in hospital at the time of the referral, the Case Manager met formally with nurses and other care providers. The Case Manager also visited the patient's home to assess the setting and meet with family members who knew the individual and their care needs. Using her nursing knowledge, the Case Manager interpreted all these data. In narrative form, she wrote salient details of her assessment of need and listed

[7] Ontario Health Insurance Plan (OHIP) is the provincial health care plan that pre-pays at the point of delivery a wide range of medically necessary services for all eligible Ontario residents.

recommendations for the range of professional and non-professional services in the "Specific Orders" field.

If, for example, the physician ordered nursing care, the Case Manager may have recommended such treatments as catheter care or dressing changes. When a physician ordered a professional service, the individual was also entitled to receive non-professional services such as homemaking support and meals-on-wheels. Therefore, patients in need of professional services did not have to pay out-of-pocket for non-professional services. The Case Manager's recommendations contributed to the assessment of need and the institutional facts of the case. After dating and signing the medical referral form, the Case Manager passed the form along to the next text reader.

The next text reader in the communication process was the Home Care Program Coordinator who was also employed by the Regional Health Department in her community. Upon receiving, reviewing, and interpreting the facts of the case documented on the medical referral form, the coordinator communicated with community-based agencies to organize the date and time to begin delivering services in the home. The coordinator then called the individual or the individual's family to tell them when services would commence.

To summarize the process in place prior to health care restructuring, an individual with a health need hooked into agencies that provided home care services when a physician initiated a Home Care Program Medical Referral form. The form commenced a textually-mediated process of assessing need and coordinating the delivery of appropriate home care support. The predominantly free-text design allowed health care providers to use their professional knowledge and experience when entering patient data and constituting individual need. The subjective experience of need known to embodied subjects entered into the communication process on at least two occasions. Eligibility was based on documentation of an individual's expressed need and on the clinical observations of the physician and other health care workers. The textual reality of a patient's need was made legitimate by the authority of the very process that constituted that image of need. In this way, each text reader acting in relation to the text accomplished both the functional work (the coordination of home care services) and the ideological work (the maintenance and support of individual health and wellbeing) of the Home Care Program. The next two subsections compare and contrast these findings with the intake form and process used in the post-restructuring era.

The Intake Form Used after Health Sector Restructuring

The Client Assessment Form was a two-page form used in a Community Care Access Centre to initiate the assessment of an individual's need for home care support. Note the word 'client' replaced the word 'patient' as a way of referring to the individual requesting home care services. While 'patient' continues to be the term used in common everyday language, the term 'client' is seen with increasing regularity in Ontario Ministry of Health documents, professional standards of practice, and health professional educational curriculum (Gustafson, 2000). The change in the title of the form is an indicator of the procedural and ideological shift away from a medically driven referral for supportive care toward a fiscally driven assessment of individual need for a service. This text-based change reflected and reinforced the wider social discourse that reconstituted the individual from a patient needing care to a client seeking a service.

While the first page of the Client Assessment Form consists entirely of fixed response fields, the second page had both fixed response and free-text fields. Like the earlier text, there were fields on the first page for the client's vital statistics including the Ontario Health Insurance Plan number. Unlike the earlier text, there were also spaces for the client's social insurance number, the physician's billing number, and the expected dates of discharge from hospital and from home care services. Like the earlier text, there was a field for home care services requested. Unlike the earlier text, there were eleven tick boxes as well as spaces for the names of therapists were or had been providing a particular health service.

Information about the client's diagnosis was no longer a large free-text field but was limited to three spaces: one for each of the primary and secondary diagnoses, and another for the name and date of any relevant surgical procedure. Data about treatment goals that were previously documented in a free-text field had to be organized by the text reader to fit into one of ten tick boxes. These tick boxes included "assess level of care required", "teach treatment protocol", "reintegration into community", "adjustment to altered functional status", and "return to total self-care." Another fixed response field listed support services including drugs, dressings, equipment, diagnostic/laboratory services, transportation and oxygen, each with a space for the name of the supplier. There was also a field entitled "Admission Status" where the text reader was prompted to indicate the disposition of the file. There were four tick boxes to choose from: "Admitted", "Service Delay", "Not Admitted", and "Transferred in."

One-third of the second page was devoted to fixed response fields listing various aspects of a client's physical and functional status. Each had a tick box for either "independent" or "dependent." There were three options from which the text reader could choose for describing a client's mental status: "lucid", "forgetfulness", and "confusion." Data about the client's mobility and place of residence were similarly condensed. The remainder of the second page was divided among six free-text fields for present health and social history, past history, medications, treatment orders, treatment goal, and plan. The agency worker could use these spaces to add narrative data about the client's health status.

In addition to health data, the Client Assessment form also contained fields for non-health data. One field was entitled "Client lives with" and another "Next of kin/Support." These fields included tick boxes and spaces where the text reader recorded the name, age, relationship, and phone number of persons who may participate in the client's care. Another field called, "Financial Information" prompted the text reader to tick boxes indicating the type of subsidy, if any; whether or not the client was employed; the kind of private coverage, if any; the names of other agencies involved with the client such as Department of Veteran's Affairs, Public Health Nurse, and so on.

While the form provided approximately the same amount of space for the health care worker to include information about the client's health needs, an equivalent amount of space was devoted to space for non-health related data about family and kin support, private insurance coverage, and other financial information. The predominance of fixed fields over free-text fields standardized much of the data collected. The next section looks at how the Client Assessment form organized the work of constituting client need and determining eligibility for home care support.

The Assessment of Client Need after Health Sector Restructuring

Unlike the process in place prior to health sector restructuring, a post-restructuring request for home care support could be initiated by anyone – the elderly person with a disability, a family member, a concerned neighbour, a nurse, or a physician. Widening the portal of entry to home care services was in keeping with the government vision of a more accessible health care system. This change appeared to advance the right of individuals to be advocates for their own care or that of a family member (Gustafson, 2000). Widening the portal of entry also appeared to recognize the competence of all health professionals to negotiate care options with a client without speaking through the voice and authority of the physician (Gustafson, 2000). According to the coordinator of one Community Care Access Centre, however, physicians continued to make most of the home care referrals. Moreover, information about who might initiate a home care referral and how to successfully negotiate the process was not widely known to the public. Together, these factors limited the likelihood that non-physicians would initiate a request for care (Gustafson, 2000; Masuda, 1998).

If an individual or a family member was aware of this change and needed home care support, they would call a Community Care Access Centre in their area. The caller was greeted by a receptionist who documented the numbers and types of incoming calls. After screening the call, the receptionist transferred the caller to an intake worker. The intake worker was usually a nurse although other health professionals such as a social worker, occupational therapist, or physiotherapist were hired and trained to perform this job function. The intake worker collected and documented as much health and non-health related data as the caller was able to provide. Based on her knowledge and experience, the intake worker determined if the request merited further consideration. She might close the file at that time or pass it along to the District Case Manager.

The District Case Manager who was usually a nurse, reviewed, interpreted, added to, and acted upon the form. She completed the field indicating who initiated the request: physician or other. Completing this tick box indicated whether or not a physician was aware of all treatments ordered by other health professionals. According to one Case Manager, the rationale for keeping the physician informed was to ensure that non-physician recommended treatments were not contraindicated.[8] Similarly, if the client did not initiate the referral, the Case Manager, in accordance with provincial legislation, was required to obtain client consent for treatment. This meant discussing home care support with the individual before ticking off the appropriate field indicating whether or not a client gave consent. Consent was discussed when the District Case Manager arranged to meet and assess the client's needs either in the home or the hospital. If the client did not initiate the referral, this would be the first time the client's subjective experience entered into the process.

When compared to the previous process, there were fewer opportunities for these expressions of need to enter into the assessment process. Moreover, it was not the client's subjective experience of need that was centred in the process. Nor was it medical or nursing knowledge and experience that organized the decision-making. The key difference in this

---

[8] As I explain elsewhere (Gustafson, 2000), the tick box encourages agency workers to inform the physician of a referral thus reinforcing the power of the physician as a gate keeper in the process. Virtually all non-physician recommended treatments were regarded as requiring physician review. This is at odds with the intent to widen the portal of entry.

post-restructuring process was the documentation of non-health client information that was privileged alongside health information in the assessment of client need and eligibility for support.

The section entitled “Reasons for Non-Admission” had eleven tick boxes or criteria of non-eligibility. Three of these were “no OHIP[9] coverage,” “needs can be met as an outpatient,” and “condition inappropriate.” Another criterion for non-eligibility was if the applicant’s home was “not suitable.” Given that the frail elderly and persons living with disabilities are more likely to live in poverty and in unsuitable housing (Health Canada, 1999), this criterion could be used to limit eligibility for members of these groups. Morris and colleagues (1999) report that homeless and transient populations as well as those living in poverty and in rural and isolated areas have limited or no home care support when compared with other Canadian populations.

Other tick boxes prompted the text reader to deny home care services if a potential client’s condition was not expected to improve, or if the family is not available to participate in care. In the case of an elderly person with a disability, the presence of these criteria would seem to make a person’s need for home care services especially acute. Yet these criteria could be considered conditions for denying or reducing services.

If the facts of a case revealed one or more reasons for non-admission, the District Case Manager could close a file at that time. If none of the conditions for non-admission existed, the District Case Manager called one of the service provider agencies with whom the Community Care Access Centre had a contract. The textual facts of the case were communicated to the agency coordinator. The agency coordinator acted upon the documented facts by scheduling an appropriate caregiver. According to two women employed by service provider agencies, the “appropriate” caregiver was the one able to provide the necessary care (as stipulated on the Client Assessment form) at the least cost to the agency in the shortest period of time. This observation was supported by other research that reports variable continuity and quality of care, inadequate number of provider hours, and care providers with minimal levels of knowledge, skill, and institutional support (Masuda, 1998; Morris et al., 1999; Neysmith, 1998)

To summarize the process in place post-restructuring, anyone could contact their local Community Care Access Centre to initiate a request for home care services. The process began when a Client Assessment form was initiated. Non-health data about family and kin support and private insurance coverage was privileged alongside health data. Identifying other sources of home care support meant that these sources could be exhausted before drawing on the public system. This strategy contained agency expenditures by shifting the demand and cost of services from paid workers to unpaid family members. Thus, the discourses of family caregiving and cost containment converged to disqualify or reduce the amount of services provided to those who required more costly, more intensive, and longer term home care support such as that required by the frail elderly and those living with disabilities. In this way, each text reader acting in relation to the text accomplished both the functional work (the coordination of home care services) and the ideological work (cost containment of insurable home care services) of the Community Care Access Centres.

---

[9] OHIP is the acronym for the Ontario Health Insurance Plan.

DISCUSSION

The Convergence of Cost Containment and Family Caregiving in Institutional Action

In the 1990s, the Ontario government expanded the meaning of a home care service. A home care service is any service that supports a client remaining in the home, and that can reasonably be provided in the home by a health care provider. This policy change was consistent with the government's vision of a shift from hospital-based to community-based care, from physician-driven to client-focussed care, and from costly to a fiscally responsible system. The assumptions underpinning this policy change were that individuals prefer to stay in the home, that community-based care is better than institutional care, and that there is a family ready, willing, and able to support an individual being cared for at home.

Unlike the Home Care Program Medical Referral form used prior to health sector restructuring, the Community Care Access Centre client assessment form collects data about health coverage and other financial data as well as information about members of a presumed family unit who could potentially meet the needs of an elderly person with disabilities. Collecting data about kin support is consistent with Ontario Ministry of Health guidelines requiring that individuals first exhaust the support of friends and family before turning to publicly funded support (Aronson, 1998). Collecting data about private health coverage suggests that the individual must first exhaust these sources also before being eligible for publicly funded services. Thus, translocal texts such as the Canada Health and Social Transfer Act "pass through" local settings reorganizing in powerful ways the everyday work activities of Community Care Access Centre workers. The concept of individual need is reconstituted in and through local texts that coordinate the delivery of home care support on a large scale. A process that had been governed primarily by subjective expressions and biomedical assessment of need has been transformed by the fiscal imperative to ration public resources. This transformation is part of the shift from social responsibility to individual responsibility for health and welfare, from government to private sector interests, and from paid health care professionals to household members as wageless workers.

The reconstitution of need has several generalizing effects that are well documented. Transferring the direct financial costs of caring for the elderly disabled from public facilities into the home transforms in powerful ways the everyday activities in both workplaces. First, the medical and nursing knowledge and experience of those health care providers who enact the institutional process are no longer central to decision-making. Rather, the converging discourses of cost containment and family caregiving reorganize workers' decision-making (Armstrong and Armstrong, 2003; Gustafson, 2000). There is a reduction in the amount of publicly funded home support provided by community agencies to elderly persons with disabilities and the families who care for them (Masuda, 1998; Morris et al., 1999). The labour processes begun by paid workers in hospitals and community agencies is completed by the unpaid labour of mothers, wives, and daughters in the home (Aronson, 1998; Neysmith and Aronson, 1997; Morris et al., 1999). Women's unpaid home care work reduces labour costs incurred by Community Care Access Centres, increases revenues in the private service economy, and contributes directly to the well-being of the economy. Thus, the direct costs of labour are not eliminated but are transferred, together with less visible financial and psychological costs, to women in the home (Armstrong and Armstrong, 2003).

The remainder of this discussion looks at the problems with the concept of family caregiving that is assumed and mediated by the restructured institutional action.

Family Caregiving and the Myth of Universal Structure and Function

Embedded in the current documentary process is a false belief about the universality of structure and function across family groupings (Eichler, 2001). This bias does not reflect the material context of people's lives in Canada. The traditional family – the legally and continuously married, heterosexual couple with one or more children – constitutes only a small percentage of contemporary family units (Eichler, 2001; Statistics Canada, 2000). Numerous demographic and other social trends have contributed to the growth of other family constellations.

One trend is the high rate of union dissolution affecting both married and cohabiting couples. This increases the number of lone-parent families and one- or two-person households. Many couples postpone legal marriage, and the rate of non-marital cohabitation is increasing among opposite sex and same sex partners. There are fewer extended families, that is to say, families that include non-nuclear relatives. Another trend is the decline in fertility rates to below replacement levels. This trend coincides with an increasing life expectancy (Statistics Canada, 2000). Collectively, these changes have resulted in an overall decrease in the size, structure, and functional capacity of households. Moreover, co-habitation, divorces, and re-marriages result in an incongruity between household membership and family membership. This incongruity blurs the lines of accountability and responsibility for providing care to aging relatives (Eichler, 2001). The next subsection looks at this issue.

Who is the "Family" in Family Caregiving?

Connecting the problematic concept of *family* with the concept of *caregiving* presumes that there exists a family unit whose constituent members contribute more or less equally in care work (Eichler, 2001). Despite the considerable evidence that women, and not the family unit, are the primary care providers, researchers continue to describe home-based care using the term *family* caregiving (Richards et al., 2003, Schofield et al., 1997; White et. al., 2004).

Women more than men care for an aging spouse in the home because of the age differences between married partners and the longer life expectancy of women (Morris et al., 1999). Wives, daughters, and daughters-in-law provide most of the care support for aging parents, the frail elderly, and those who are chronically ill or disabled (Aronson, 1998). In 1996, over one million Canadian women aged 25-54 years (15% of women compared to 9% of men) reported providing unpaid care to a senior and a child (Statistics Canada, 2000). In this way, the discourse of family caregiving renders less visible the unpaid care work provided by the closest available female relative. As the guardians of family health, gender-neutral terms such as family caregiving and "sandwich generation" (Robinson et al., 2003; Statistics Canada, 2000) belie the disproportionate burden of care work assumed by women.

At the same time, women's identification as natural carers within the family remains hidden and unchallenged by processes that assume that the "family" is able and willing to provide care (Baines, Evans, and Neysmith, 1998).

In some situations, the care provider and the care recipient are viewed as a client unit. This re-labelling shifts the focus away from a woman's role in providing unpaid care work and recasts her as a consumer of health care services. On the one hand, women's care work can then be viewed as a women's health issue given the negative impact of home-based care work on a woman's health and well-being (Armstrong and Armstrong, 2003; Aronson, 1998; Morris et al., 1999). On the other hand, re-labelling a care provider as a client ignores the economic value of her contribution to the well-being of the care recipient and to society. Simultaneously, the care provider is reconstituted as a dependent in relation to the health care system. According to Fineman (1995), care providers acquire "a derivative dependency flowing from their roles and the need for resources their caretaking generates" (1995, p.162). Thus, the downloading of household care work onto women can create a paradoxical dependency of women in the discourse of family caregiving.

Family Caregiving and the Multiple Burdens Assumed by Women

For many reasons, women tend to suffer a greater economic burden than their male counterparts when assuming caring duties. A disproportionate number of women, particularly members of minoritized groups are concentrated in low-level service occupations, domestic labour, or part-time employment (Morris et al., 1999; Neysmith and Aronson, 1997). These jobs are characterized by lower wages, long unpaid hours of work, poor job security, rigid work schedules and lack of health benefits. Women tied to an hourly wage are more severely penalized financially for taking time off than women and men in salaried employment. Yet women more than men lose time from their jobs because of personal and family responsibilities (Statistics Canada, 2000). With limited material resources, few women can afford to reduce their time in the paid work force to take on unpaid labour. Those who remain in the paid work force have less time and energy to devote to the rigours of home-based care.

Women as a group tend have less disposable income than men both while married and after union dissolution. This is because women tend to be paid less than men for performing the same labour (Statistics Canada, 2000). Consequently, women caring for an elderly, disabled person generally have less money to pay for respite care or non-insurable or non-professional health services (Aronson, 1998; Morris et al., 1999). While home-based care can be satisfying for some individuals and their family care providers, it can be burdensome for those who lack time, skill, knowledge, or emotional and financial resources (Morris et al., 1999, p. 35).

In addition to problems reconciling paid work and unpaid care work, another problem with the discourse of family caregiving relates to the nature of the labour itself. When examining the health care activities rendered by professional and home-based care providers, there is considerable overlap in the work that cannot be explained solely on the basis of care setting or formal training. In both cases, the worker must assess, plan, implement, and evaluate care. Both are expected to support activities of daily living such as toileting, feeding, preparing meals, dressing, bathing, and ambulating. Both are expected to understand and follow guidelines regarding medication administration, treatment options, nutrition, and safety. Other less tangible activities include maintaining a health history of the care recipient and making decisions about health and illness management and other life activities. The most salient difference between professional and home-based care providers is the presence or absence of compensation for services rendered. Thus, women in the home bear a disproportionate burden of health care restructuring as they become the wageless workers who complete the labour begun by paid health professionals.

The Family as a Safe, Restful Haven

Home-based care is an imperative constituted in the post-restructuring documentary process. That imperative pivots on an idealized image of the family as a safe, restful haven for giving and receiving care. The family home is presumed to be a comfortable and familiar setting with household members who are willing and able to assume care work within the context of functional and loving relationships. This image may be at odds with the economic and social reality of smaller, variable family structures where women work outside the home (Eichler, 2001). Certainly, there are some individuals who experience a greater sense of personal control living at home than they have in institutionalized settings (Morris et al., 1999, p. 34). But for others, the decision to accept home-based care may be the best among poor options when compared to institutional care or "living alone dangerously" (Morris et al., 1999, p. 34).

The romanticized ideal of home-based care glosses over the complexities of caring for the elderly with disabilities while at the same time, sustaining a healthy familial relationship between care provider and care recipient. While family caregiving may be advanced as the "loving choice" made by care recipient and care provider, there is an "element of compulsion" which may create or exacerbate intergenerational conflict, physical, emotional and economic abuse, and safety issues due to care providers' inadequate training and skill (Morris et al., 1999, p. 18).

Women's subjective accounts of their care work convey their ambivalence about caring for elders in the home (Aronson, 1998). They describe the demanding and unending nature of the caring role, the discrepancy between their knowledge and skill and the demands for a safe and competent level of care, and the difficulty retaining an identity as a loving daughter or spouse when some activities may involve inflicting discomfort or pain.[10] These challenges can be (mis)managed with reduced access to skilled technical support and other human and material resources necessary to do care work in the home (Neysmith, 1995; 1998). The moral push toward family caregiving can further victimize economically vulnerable household units and increase the risk of physical, financial, and emotional abuse of elderly disabled. Ironically, downloading responsibility for health care to the home and family is justified on the basis of medical and moral benefit to the individual.

[10] Examples of such activities range from administering injectable medication, disempacting bowels and other toileting activities, caring for decubitus ulcers, and various kinds of movement and physical therapy.

Family Caregiving as Altruism

The *giving* in family caregiving denotes a voluntary, uncompensated act as in the giving of a gift. The reification of caring as a gift emphasizes the relational and emotional aspects of the act rather than the material or instrumental aspects of care work (Baines, Evans, and Neysmith, 1998). Current documentary practices in Ontario require that individuals must exhaust (financially and emotionally) family and kin as care providers in order to be eligible for publicly funded services. At the same time, the discourse of family care*giving* naturalizes the labour performed in a private home setting as an altruistic act offered willingly by a charitable donor to an equally accepting recipient in an intimate and mutually beneficial relationship.

The discourse of family caregiving embedded in the post-restructuring assessment and eligibility processes hides the involuntariness of a relationship that emerges from the moral push to engage in home-based care. Also less eligible for discussion is the ambivalence experienced by both participants in this exchange (Aronson, 1998). Moreover, the discourse of family care*giving* hides the economic benefit accruing to the wider society when the labourer undertakes work that decreases demand for publicly funded health services.

Conclusion

While the detailed review of a single strand of institutional action for assessing client need may appear pedantic, it is these very bureaucratic details that organize the work of health care workers and the outcomes these workers produce. A retrospective comparison of the bureaucratic processes before and after restructuring illuminates an important point of disjuncture between government funding for home care, institutional assessments of client need, and the subjective experiences of need for publicly funded home care services. Put another way, the apparently neutral discourse of need constructed in and through local and translocal texts can be at odds with the subjective and embodied ways of knowing about need that are experienced by an older, disabled person and her or his family care providers. In particular, the comparison reveals how non-health related client information enters into the institutional process that assesses client need and how that information is interpreted and acted upon to achieve functional and ideological goals of the Community Care Access Centres. The medically defined concept of need has been transformed by the introduction of financial considerations into an administrative process for establishing a person's eligibility for a service. Financial and family data compete with medical and nursing assessments as the organizers of a text-based image of client need, and ultimately, the quality and quantity of home care services provided to the client.

Historically, Canada's medicare and social welfare schemes have rested on the principles of social responsibility. Transferring the burden for the elderly disabled to unpaid women in private households is a regressive move toward an individual responsibility model of health and welfare. The move to home-based care is predicated on the existence of the traditional nuclear family and widely justified on the basis of medical and moral benefit to the care recipient and the family. Sheila Neysmith notes, however, that the tension between individual empowerment and user consumerism associated with the move to home-based care is motivated by "an even stronger desire to reduce costs" (1995, p. 793). In the short term, the most cost-effective home care service is one the government does not have to fund. This short-sighted approach to the delivery of home care support is further contributing to the vulnerability of the frail elderly and persons living with disabilities, to the social and economic vulnerability of unpaid female family care providers, and to the erosion of the Canadian model of social responsibility for health and welfare.

RECOMMENDATIONS

The three recommendations that follow support the calls for change made by other researchers concerned with equity and social justice for women, seniors, the disabled and other vulnerable populations (Baines, Evans, and Neysmith, 1998; Masuda, 1998; Morris et al., 1999; Morris, 2002).

- The Canadian government in collaboration with provinces, territories, and stakeholders including those who represent the concerns of the elderly and those living with disabilities would develop Home and Community Care legislation (Masuda, 1998; Morris et al., 1999). That federal legislation would be comparable to the Canada Health Act that governs the provision of acute health care. That means enshrining the principles of universality, accessibility, comprehensiveness, portability, and public administration in the new legislation. This legislation would ensure that all Canadian residents have reasonable access to all medically necessary home care services provided without direct charges at the point of delivery. Moreover, no elderly, disabled person or their family would be denied adequate support because of inability to pay or to participate in care. Health care services delivered in the home, just like services provided in hospital, would be a right under the law.
- Ontario and other provincial and territorial governments would issue directives requiring that Community Care Access Centres (and comparable programs) develop and implement new assessment processes. These processes would determine eligibility for home care support based on medical need alone. The ability of family members, and particularly women, to provide care for no pay would not be assumed.
- Provincial and federal governments would re-establish basic standards of social responsibility for health and welfare (Baines, Evans, and Neysmith, 1998; Morris, 2002). The current practice of block funding contains no monies specifically earmarked for social assistance or poverty reduction. The federal government would reinstate the standards previously set out in the Canada Assistance Program which guaranteed that people in need would be supported. This Act would guarantee social assistance income, and restore funding for group homes for people with disabilities, and a wide range of other services. Doing so would demonstrate commitment to addressing the national problem of poverty in Canada – a burden disproportionately carried by the elderly living with disabilities and those who care for them.

References

Armstrong, P. and H. Armstrong. (2003). *Wasting away: The undermining of Canadian health care.* (2nd ed.). Toronto: Oxford University Press.

Armstrong, P., H. Armstrong, J. Choiniere, G. Feldberg, and J. White. (1994). *Take care: Warning signals for Canada's health system.* Toronto: Garamond.

Aronson, J. (1998). Dutiful daughters and undemanding mothers: Constraining images of giving and receiving care in middle and later life. In C. Baines, P.M. Evans and S. Neysmith (Eds.) (2nd Ed.). *Women's caring: Feminist perspectives on social welfare* (pp. 114-38). Toronto: Oxford University Press.

Aronson, J. and S.M. Neysmith. (1997). The retreat of the state and long-term care provision: Implications for frail elderly people, unpaid family carers and paid home care workers. *Studies in Political Economy*, 53(Summer): 37-66.

Baines, C., P.M. Evans and S. Neysmith (1998). Women's caring: Work expanding, state contracting. In C. Baines, P.M. Evans and S. Neysmith (Eds.) (2nd Ed.). *Women's caring: Feminist perspectives on social welfare* (pp. 3-22). Toronto: Oxford University Press.

DeVault, M.L. and L. McCoy. (2002). Institutional ethnography: Using interviews to investigate ruling relations. In F.J. Gubrium and J.A. Holstein (eds.), *Handbook of Interview Research* (pp. 751-76). London: Sage.

Drozdow-St. Christian, D. (2000). Aging well: Strategies for well-being among older women in a "restructuring" Ontario. In D.L. Gustafson (Ed.). *Care and consequences: The impact of health reform* (pp. 243-54). Halifax, NS: Fernwood Press.

Eichler, M. (2001). Biases in family literature. In M. Baker (Ed.). *Families: Changing trends in Canada.* (4th ed.). (pp. 51-66). Toronto: McGraw Hill Ryerson.

Fineman, M.A. (1995). *The neutered mother, the sexual family, and other twentieth century tragedies.* New York: Routledge.

Grahame, P.R. (1999). Doing qualitative research: Three problematics. *Discourse of Sociological Practice,* 2(1): 4-10.

Gustafson, D.L. (2000). Home care before and after reform: A comparative analysis of two texts-in-action. In D.L. Gustafson (Ed.). *Care and consequences: The impact of health reform* (pp. 177-198). Halifax, NS: Fernwood Press.

Health Canada. (1999). *Toward a healthy future: Second report on the health of Canadians.* (Cat No. H39-468/1999E) Ottawa, ON: Author.

Masuda, S. (1998). *The impact of block funding on women with disabilities.* Ottawa, ON: Status of Women Canada. (Publ. no. 98-S-009). [On-line]. Available: *http://www.swc-cfc.gc.ca/pubs/066263473X/index_e.html*

Morris, M. (2002). *Women and Poverty: A Fact Sheet.* Canadian Research Institute on the Advancement of Women. Posted at: *http://www.criaw-icref.ca*

Morris, M., Robinson, J., Simpson, J., with Galey, S., Kirby, S, Martin, L. and Muzychka, M. (1999). *The changing nature of home care and its impact on women's vulnerability to poverty.* Ottawa, ON: Status of Women Canada. (Cat no. SW21-42/1999E). Available on-line: *http://www.swc-cfc.gc.ca/pubs/0662280857/index_e.html*

Neysmith, S.M. (1995). Better care for dependent people living at home. *Canadian Journal of Aging,* 14(4), 792-95.

Neysmith, S.M. (1998). From home care to social care: The value of a vision. In C. Baines, P.M. Evans and S. Neysmith (Eds.) (2nd Ed.). *Women's caring: Feminist perspectives on social welfare* (pp. 233-49). Toronto: Oxford University Press.

Neysmith, S.M. and J. Aronson. (1997). Working conditions in home care: Negotiating race and class boundaries in gendered work. *International Journal of Health Services, 23*(3), 479-99.

Ontario Council of Hospital Unions/Canadian Union of Public Employees. (1995, March). *When patients don't matter: How government cuts are undermining health care.* Toronto, ON: Author.

Ontario Ministry of Health. (1992, January). Goals and strategic priorities: Working document. Toronto, ON: Author.

Ontario Ministry of Health. (1993). *A healthier Ontario: Progress in the '90s.* Toronto, ON: Author.

Ontario Ministry of Health. (1994). *Managing health care resources: Meeting priorities.* Toronto, ON: Author.

Richard, K., E. Moniz-Cook, P. Duggan, I. Carr and M. Wang. (2003). Defining 'early dementia' and monitoring intervention: What measures are useful in family caregiving? *Aging and Mental Health,* 7(1): 7-14.

Robinson, M.M., A.P. Barbee, M. Martin, T.L. Singer, B. Yegidis. (2003). The organizational costs of caregiving: a call to action. *Administration in Social Work,* 27(1): 83-102.

Schofield, H.L., B. Murphy, H.E. Herrman, S. Bloch, et al. (1997). Defining 'early dementia' and monitoring intervention: What measures are useful in family caregiving? *Psychological Medicine,* 27(3): 647-657.

Simpson, P. and S. Porte. (2000). "And then there were none": An experience in building an integrated heath service among the Chippewas of Georgina Island. In D.L. Gustafson (Ed.). *Care and consequences: The impact of health reform* (pp. 199-221.) Halifax, NS: Fernwood Press.

Smith, D.E. (1999). *Writing the social: Theory, critique, investigations.* Toronto: University of Toronto Press.

Smith, D.E. (1990). *Texts, facts and femininity: Exploring the relations of ruling.* New York: Routledge.

Smith, D.E. (1987). *The everyday world as problematic: A feminist sociology.* Toronto: University of Toronto Press.

Statistics Canada. (2000). *Women in Canada 2000: A gender-based statistical report.* (Cat No. 89-503-XPE), Ottawa, ON: Ministry of Industry.

White, C.L., S. Lauzon, M.J. Yaffe, S. Wood-Dauphinee and C.L. White. (2004). Toward a model of quality of life for family caregivers of stroke survivors. *Quality of Life Research: An International Journal of Quality of Life Aspects of Treatment, Care Rehabilitation,* 13(3): 625-638.

Wilkins, K. and E. Park. (1998). Home care in Canada. *Health Reports,* 10(1), Ottawa, ON: Statistics Canada.

In: Family Caregiving for Older Disabled People
Editor: Isabella Paoletti, pp. 251-272
ISBN 1-59454-808-0

Chapter 12

THROUGH KITH AND KIN: SUPPORTING THE FAMILY CAREGIVER FOR THE ELDERLY

Julie Walters and Connie L. McNeely
Department of Sociology, University of California, Santa Barbara, CA

INTRODUCTION

Elderly citizens who can no longer support and care for themselves are often faced with difficult decisions concerning where to live, how to obtain quality care, and how to finance it all.[1] Accordingly, many elderly find themselves in a situation where they must move into the homes of other family members or where family members must provide them with direct in-home care. In other words, much of the responsibility for eldercare falls on the shoulders of family members, with direct caregiving itself increasingly administered by individuals within the family. While many cultures hold long traditions of caregiving for the elderly by the family, this is a particularly poignant issue in the United States, where there is little systemic public relief or support for the aged, and related problems are not addressed in terms of social rights, nor reflected in any government-sponsored ethic of care. Moreover, those family members responsible for such care face myriad related pressures, and often have little support themselves. With this form of eldercare on the rise, we urgently need to gain a deeper understanding, in very practical terms, of the relationship between the needs of these family caregivers and current and possible sources of support for them and, also, of the policies affecting those sources.

To that end, we look to disentangle crucial aspects of the interrelationship between eldercare and family structure in order to illuminate the complex dynamics associated with the role of family caregiver. We address this issue as a fundamental question of family caregiver wellbeing, considering the needs of family caregivers and the degree and manner in which those needs are met -- or not -- relative to eldercare. In broad terms, this means

---

[1] The term "elderly" can refer to a broad and diverse age group spanning at least 40 years of life (NRC 2001, p. 2). For our purposes here, we refer primarily to a chronological demarcation of persons aged 65 and over, with occasional reference to groups aged 55 and over and to the oldest groups aged 80 and over.

attending to the psychological, physical, and financial aspects of caregiver wellbeing (NRC 2001), which we engage to examine caregiver needs and to delineate sources from which support in various forms might be drawn (e.g., other family members, friends, community, nongovernmental and religious organizations, and governmental sources). Moreover, while examining sources and types of support for family caregivers, we necessarily consider relevant policy initiatives and policy approaches to eldercare in the United States today.

As a policy issue, the first point to understand is that eldercare is a public good. Undertaken primarily within the familial domain -- especially by female family members -- it is, in many ways, a prime example of the public-private character of modern life, to the extent that family wellbeing can translate into an important aspect of societal wellbeing. In the United States (U.S.), more than 80 percent of the caregiving needs of the frail elderly is provided by relatives (Lechner and Sasaki 1999), such that the ability of the family to provide service and support is absolutely crucial to the success of eldercare. The relevance of this situation is even more apparent since responsibilities for elderly family members who cannot care for themselves are framed within a variety of changes in the family structure that have led to increased stress on the family caregiver. These include, for example, rising divorce rates, number of women working outside of the home, the geographic dispersion of offspring, and old persons caring for even older persons (Quinlan 1989, p. 37). More to the point, the wellbeing of the family caregiver is a crucial parameter of home eldercare, ultimately affecting the quality of care to the frail elderly family member.

Here, following this introduction, we provide a brief discussion of the contextual background in which family caregiver needs are determined as a foundation for the more detailed examination of family caregiver wellbeing that follows. Accordingly, after presenting a general conceptual overview, we next offer a more detailed assessment of caregiver wellbeing and needs in terms of the three analytical dimensions mentioned above. First, we attend to the *emotional and psychological needs* of the family caregiver for the elderly, focusing particularly on related feelings and mental health outcomes. Second, we look beyond psychological needs to consider the basic *physical needs* faced by caregivers that explicitly and implicitly affect the family caregiving relationship. Third, we address the *financial needs* that are fundamental to almost every aspect of eldercare, in one way or the other, and can present critical challenges to the provision of care. Indeed, note that, although we engage them as distinct issues for analytical purposes, these three dimensions of caregiver wellbeing are highly interdependent, affecting each other both directly and indirectly. Then, given the psychological, physical, and financial needs determining their wellbeing, we discuss various sources of support available to family caregivers in the U.S. This assessment leads us to a broad examination of relevant policy initiatives, followed by a more focused critique and consideration of policy approaches to family provided eldercare. We end with a delineation of general implications drawn from our assessment, summarizing the main points and offering direction for policy recommendations. Ultimately, we seek to provide insight into how effective, thoughtful policymaking might ensure that family caregivers will be able to maintain healthy, productive lives as they perform duties typically defined relative to paid employees in the eldercare industry.

CONTEXTUAL BACKGROUND

Many families are unable to pay for home healthcare services. Yet, given social (and personal) expectations, this means that they must somehow provide the necessary care themselves -- a responsibility that most often falls on the shoulders of female family members, the majority of whom are already working outside of the home. The elderly in the United States, and in other developed countries, are often depicted as distanced from their children and thrust into institutionalized settings relative to those in less developed areas where elders are more revered and more consistently tend to co-reside with their children (Kwon 2000). However, we argue that such depictions are overly simplified and tend to obscure important variations. For example, such assertions ignore the fact that, while co-residence may be lower overall, "considerable contact, exchange, and personal care assistance takes place between parents and children" (NRC 2001, p. 19). In addition, there is evidence that co-residence is increasing; moreover, even in developed countries, co-residence itself can vary tremendously according to race, ethnicity, and class (Grundy and Harrop 1992; NRC 2001; Tronto 1993).

In any case, the rapidly growing number of frail elders has meant an increase in family caregiving needs. This intensification of family and work duties together has led to something of a family care dilemma, and the relegation of caring for the infirm and elderly most often to women family members accentuates the gendered dimension of family caregiving. In the United States, as elsewhere, women have traditionally held the primary responsibility for eldercare as part of their "normal" role as family caregiver, framed within gender and family ideologies defining women as "nurturing" and "women's work" as restricted to the domestic setting.

However, in reality, by the turn of the century, over 60.1 percent of U.S. women of working age were employed outside of the home, and this rate continues to escalate (U.S. Dept of Labor 2002). While some of this external employment is a matter of choice, it is also an absolute necessity for many families in order to manage financially and make ends meet. Moreover, "if we look at questions of race, class, and gender, we notice that those who are least well off in society are disproportionately those who do the work of caring, and that the best off members of society often use their positions of superiority to pass caring work off to others" (Tronto 1993, p. 113).[2] The provision of care in the family can take an enormous toll on women, especially those who are also externally employed. Women who work outside of the home, and who also face large caring responsibilities at home, are often adversely affected by their situation (Tronto 1993, p. 120). This observation raises, most emphatically, the centrality of caregiver wellbeing and needs as vital considerations in eldercare today.

CAREGIVER WELLBEING AND NEEDS

The population is aging, a fact that translates into more and more long-term care needs. Indeed, "we are headed toward a demographic situation in which a single young worker may

[2] Ironically, when poor women exchange their informal family caregiver roles for paid external employment, the work they find most often involves caring for other people (Hicks-Bartlett 2000, p. 43).

be supporting as many as four elders. We do not understand the full economic, social, and health status impacts on these caregivers of caring for very sick people in the home. Caregivers for frail elders are a major population of concern," and caregiver strain and health effects need to be assessed in relationship to care as a family responsibility (Rubenstein 1989, p. 74). Such responsibility can have profound effects on the lives and wellbeing of caregivers and other family members.[3]

Approaches to wellbeing and life quality include assessments of intrinsic and extrinsic satisfaction with life, health and functional ability, and overall emotional states. Intrinsic satisfaction reflects the degree of satisfaction or enjoyment associated with performing an activity, and extrinsic satisfaction is associated with the outcome of the activity (NRC 2001, p. 268). While these have been used to assess the wellbeing of the elderly, we employ them also to consider the wellbeing of family caregivers to the elderly. In particular, we frame them in terms of the kind of "work" faced by these "informal caregivers" -- so called because they typically are not paid, nor are they professionally trained healthcare providers. As in any kind of work, motivation, stress and its effects, task content, working conditions, social relations and contacts, resources, and rewards, among other things, determine worker satisfaction (NRC 2001, p. 264).

Successful home care relies on a supportive environment in which demands on family caregiver time, living space, and physical and psychological capacities, in addition to finances, can be addressed effectively. While presenting an overall depiction of family caregiving as a special consideration in the broader field of eldercare, we focus particularly on within-family dynamics. Our intent is not to romanticize notions of family caregiving, but rather to highlight the indeed practical necessity of bringing these issues and related ideologies to the fore in addressing basic social concerns, and to address the need for more detailed information on family eldercare and support. Conceptions of care reflect both practice and disposition (Tronto 1993), and we capture the various features of wellbeing and needs within three broad domains -- emotional and psychological, physical, and financial -- of family caregiver practice and disposition. That is, we attend notions of subjective wellbeing as questions of life satisfaction expressed in terms of emotional and psychological, physical, and financial states (cf. NRC 2001, p. 14).[4]

The Study

Within a broader frame of information on kin networks, age transitions, and other factors derived from in-depth surveys and statistical reports to set the analytical frame, we also provide case notes on the daily lives and personal histories of selected caregivers and their families as powerful illustrations of our basic points and to provide insight into family caregiving as a question of the life course and conceptualizing the individual as an element within the wider kinship network. Note that, despite this section designation, we do not

---

[3] "Responsibility" can mean different things depending on perceived gender roles and issues arising from class, culture, and family status. Thus, following Tronto (1993, p. 133), we argue for a flexible approach to responsibility encompassing more than typical assertions of duty and obligation.

[4] Other authors in this volume provide additional detailed discussion of these issues: see Paoletti, chapter 1; Oddone and Aguirre, chapter 3; and Watson, chapter 8.

present an actual study analyzing related cases here.[5] Rather, we draw these illustrative case notes from a larger long-term ethnographic study that we are currently conducting on eldercare in various cities across the U.S., with an emphasis on family, work, and community.[6] We use these case notes, based on a series of in-depth interviews and investigator observations, to illuminate various aspects of family caregiving in keeping with research on wellbeing relying on indicators of external objective conditions and subjective self-reports on satisfaction. External objective conditions include, for example, measures of "personal income, neighborhood characteristics, housing status, longevity, health, and disability. These measures were originally designed to supplement the conventional measures of societal progress reflected by developments in the economic sphere" (e.g., gross national product growth rate, investment and saving, income distribution, consumption, etc.). "To the extent that these supplemental objective conditions have an impact on wellbeing that is not reflected in standard economic variables, they provide a richer and broader picture of societal wellbeing." Subjective wellbeing includes not only satisfaction relative to various aspects of life (e.g., income, neighborhood, relationships to children, spouses, and other family members), but also human development and mental health, contributing to "how people feel about themselves as indicated by scales of self-assessment, personal growth, and relationships with others" (NRC 2001, p. 258),[7] as illustrated in the following example regarding caregiver psychological needs.

Emotional and Psychological Needs

> As usual, Susan arrives home exhausted and stressed after spending the day caring for both of her parents, each of whom suffer from some degree of dementia and myriad physical frailties. Just getting to and from their home, she will have driven for at least an hour-and-a-half. Once there, she will have washed their clothes, coordinated their medications, and if, on that particular day, she did not need to take either of them to a medical appointment, she will have arranged for future ones. She will have searched the house for bills that they have neglected to put in the box designated for them, she will have paid those bills, cleaned their pet bird's cage, gone to the pharmacy to pick up medications, gone grocery shopping, prepared two days worth of meals, helped bathe them, cleaned the kitchen and bathroom, and vacuumed. In addition to performing these tasks and providing emotional support, Susan will also have endured a number of emotionally draining trials and tribulations. It is not uncommon for her mother to angrily lash out at her for not doing a chore exactly as she likes, and, on occasion, her father, who suffers from severe vascular dementia, has accused her of trying to steal his money as she put his newly cleaned and folded clothes away. Her emotional rollercoaster is not limited to issues involving household chores. For example, on the many occasions when she has needed to correct her mother on the date of her next doctor appointment, a typical reply from her mother has been, "Well, just put me away in a mental hospital because clearly I'm insane since you say the date is different than I remember." Susan's visits are often

[5] The section designation was an editorial requirement.

[6] Note that we have changed respondent names for reporting purposes.

[7] While reliance on self-reports on wellbeing have been subjected to various criticisms (Schwarz and Strack 1999), self-perceptions are in fact what we aim to uncover and assess, while being mindful of various sources of bias and mis-reporting. For us, recognition of and sensitivity to vagaries of self-perceptions are part and parcel of the analytical task.

> concluded by a final frustrating comment as her mother smiles and states how thankful she is that she has such loving and attentive children -- this in spite of the fact that Susan's two brothers visit once a year at most and provide no assistance in any way in the care of their parents. This is Susan's routine 4 or 5 days a week; it has been her routine for the past two years and will be for the foreseeable future. Given the circumstances, is it any wonder that this family caregiver is stressed and often feels depressed?

Does the caregiver experience happiness, unhappiness, or neutral feelings about the responsibilities associated with the role and about the recipients of care? What other factors affect caregiver wellbeing? How is it manifested? Love and compassion are powerful motivators for caregivers, but they are not enough to eradicate the effects of stress. The experience of seeing a loved one's physical and/or mental faculties deteriorate can create feelings of frustration, powerlessness, and sorrow. Caring for a dementia sufferer particularly has added stress because the loved one may not be able to articulate needs and feelings clearly, may not be able to follow simple instructions or arrangements, and may verbally or physically lash out at the caregiver. In addition, a dementia sufferer must be watched very closely as he or she may wander or try to engage in regular social conditions with impaired judgment. Preventing a fully-grown adult from getting lost or from becoming victim to the many con artists who prey on the elderly can be truly challenging.

Consequently, it is not surprising that depression is a major problem for family caregivers. Considering that nearly 25 percent of American households provide some assistance to an elderly loved one (NAC and AARP 1997), sustaining the emotional health of family caregivers is not an isolated problem. Indeed, the majority (over 80 percent) of informal caregivers are family members (cf. Alexcih et al. 2002). Informal family care providers often think of their service as a duty or, more, as a loss of leisure time than as work per se and, on the one hand, they can derive satisfaction and feelings of self-worth from caregiving. However, on the other hand, limits on personal life and increased responsibility contribute to stress for the caregiver. Note also that, especially for women, external employment is not necessarily related to the overall amount of caregiving provided in the home (Quinlan 1989, p. 38).

Some people make greater sacrifices (which are also subject to perceptions) than do others, a situation that can reflect a moral problem for those who become enmeshed in a caring process that is "exacerbated by the fact that those who are most likely to be too self-sacrificing are likely to be the relatively powerless in society" (Tronto 1993, p. 141). Also, eldercare can represent ethical and moral constraints that raise fundamental questions about our social values (Hanneman 1997). Familial and social pressure to care for aging family members can wear on the one who shoulders the responsibility -- a state of affairs made even more stressful when it rests on a conflicted relationship. The strain of caregiving can test even the best of relationships, but it can become a particular challenge in the face of difficult relational histories. For example, witness Maria's relatively trying relationship with her mother:

> "My mother and I do not get along, to put it mildly. She's always been mean and she certainly made my life a misery. The happiest day of my life was the day I left that house!" Maria, aged 42 and the mother of twin teenage boys, had been widowed several years prior and was working nights as a bookkeeper, a schedule that she had arranged so that she could attend college part-time during the day to obtain her degree ("Finally!"). When caregiving

> responsibilities fell to her -- other family members, including a sister and male cousin (who had grown up with them), were unable to help for a variety of reasons -- Maria felt particularly resentful. She also felt obligated: "What can I do? Everyone will blame me if I don't take care of her. Why can't one of the others give up their lives to help her? It's not fair that I have to be stuck taking care of her, but somebody's got to do it." Since there was not enough money to hire a formal caregiver, Maria agreed to "give up her life," to forego school, and to move her mother into her home in order to provide care for her during the day. Despite her resentment, this was deemed the best option for the family as a whole. Neither respect nor love for her mother, but the strength of social obligation, family ties, and a sense of familial duty determined her decision.

Clearly, this was not an ideal situation and the emotional, physical, and financial costs -- costs that could be quite high even in a more positive relationship -- could exact a heavy toll on both caregiver and recipient if other sources of support and relief could not be found.

Also, despite the accompanying loss of independence, co-residence is often discussed as a positive "solution" for frail elderly who cannot live on their own and as a deterrent to feelings of isolation and abandonment.[8] However, frankly, subjective assessments of wellbeing or the quality of relationships among co-resident family members should not confuse the form of living arrangements with their function. Indeed, "co-residence of an elderly individual with a child and/or grandchildren may or may not be a positive experience for any of the parties involved" (NRC 2001, p. 180). In a worst case scenario, hostility and resentment can breed neglect, emotional cruelty, and physical abuse -- which often the elder family member feels helpless to address.

Research on the psychological health of caregivers provides striking evidence of the emotional toll exacted by caregiving. When compared with the general population, primary caregivers suffer more incidents of depression and anxiety (Schulz et al. 1995). In fact, research indicates that the vast majority of family caregivers are clinically depressed (Gray 2003; Gallagher et al. 1989), and daughters who care for their ill parents are twice as likely to suffer anxious or depressive symptoms as non-caregivers (Cannuscio et al. 2002). Moreover, this psychological stress can often have physical consequences, as is apparent in the following illustration.

Physical Needs

> Nancy is a 66-year-old woman caring for her two frail parents who suffer from dementia. She herself continually battles fatigue, acid reflux disease, and headaches. Moreover, she has continued her caregiving responsibilities even after a serious bone infection that required months of outpatient intravenous antibiotic therapy, and now delays making doctor appointments for herself and neglects her own care due to caregiving demands on her time, energy, and finances.

Just as a caregiver is at risk for depression, anxiety, and other psychological illnesses and disorders, she is also at risk for physical illness. One fifth of all caregivers report that their physical health has suffered as a result of caregiving (Thompson 2004). Furthermore, high

[8] See references on elderly living arrangements in NRC 2001, p. 180.

rates of depression, as discussed above, also can create a chain reaction of additional serious health problems such as coronary heart disease, diabetes, and cancer (Cannuscio et al. 2002; National Institute of Mental Health 2001). Even more striking is the finding that, of elderly spousal caregivers who report suffering from mental and emotional strain as a result of caregiving, 63 percent are more likely to die than non-caregivers (Schulz and Beach 1999). Consequently, the physical illnesses suffered by caregivers are not simply chronic colds or viruses; they are serious conditions that can lead to premature death.

Also, it is difficult for caregivers to maintain healthy eating and exercise routines (Manson and Bassuk 2003) and, of those caring for elderly individuals, at least 20 percent spend 40 hours or more per week doing so in addition to other family and personal responsibilities (Health and Human Services 1998). The typical caregiver is a 46-year-old married female who works outside the home in a relatively low-earning position (NAC and AARP 1997). Consequently, in trying to maintain their own immediate families and job responsibilities, caregivers are likely put their own needs behind those of others. For example, Eula's case is instructive along these lines:

> Eula works as a night cashier at a grocery market, a job that allows her to attend her children and household chores and to have her husband's supper ready for him when he arrives home from his work as an autobody mechanic -- and to provide in-home care to his parents seven days a week. Eula's husband, recognizing that she is often tired and sleep-deprived, mentions how he helps out by driving his parents (with Eula) to their medical appointments whenever he can. He points out that there is little else he can do in light of his job which is necessary to support the family and that, in any case, Eula is better suited to caregiving tasks: "Like bathing my folks. Eula helps bathe them, but I certainly couldn't do that, especially not my mother." There are other caregiving tasks, but he focuses on the "embarrassment" of bathing and having to clean up after them due to incontinence "accidents." It is not unusual that a child would be disturbed by a parent's encroaching infirmity and other challenges to the image of parent as caregiver, but note also the embedded assumptions about gender roles.

Home care is often both physically and emotionally demanding, a fact that, along with changing family structures and kin availability, assumes increasing importance to eldercare possibilities as the population ages. Women, the primary informal eldercare workers, also constitute the majority of the elderly population in almost every country -- moreover, this "feminization of old age" increases with age (NRC 2001). This situation begs the question: What happens as the caregivers themselves age? What happens when the caregiver develops disabilities associated with chronic conditions reflecting functional limitations, i.e., "limitations in major activities, activities of daily living, and instrumental activities of daily living" (Weaver and Ingman 1997, p. 49). One scenario is exemplified in Terri and Corinne's story:

> Terri is 65 and has for several years been the provider of in-home care to her frail parents, both in their eighties, and to her husband, who is 72 and suffering from crippling arthritis. Now, however, Terri finds herself facing cancer, the treatments for which leave her unable to care for her parents or husband for long periods. Her daughter Corinne, now in her early forties, has taken the responsibility of caring for both her parents and her grandparents, as her mother has become less able. Moreover, she is employed outside of the home, bringing in much needed financial resources. She had returned to school part-time with plans to go full-time to earn a graduate degree, but had to withdraw in order to help the family. (She mentions

> that she still hopes to continue her education -- someday.) While officially middle class, the parents and grandparents are on fixed incomes that do not allow for paid "outside help." There are two other siblings, a brother and sister. The sister will, in an emergency, try to "be there" for her parents and grandparents, but she lives almost two hours away and has her own young family to care for. The brother is single and lives nearby, but is not expected nor does he offer to help -- although, when asked, he has contributed financially on occasion. Corinne indicates that it probably does not occur to him to offer, but then looks embarrassed and quickly insists that he is a good son and brother -- "it's just that he has his own life to live." While a variety of factors can explain this particular family dynamic, note also that the parents (and grandparents) maintained and raised their children in keeping with relatively "traditional" gender roles. Corinne mentions also that, over this last year, she has developed a variety of "small illnesses," "allergies," and "nervous headaches."

This is an example of "overlapping generations" (see discussion in NRC 2001, p. 160), along with spatial, affective, and financial considerations within the kinship network. There is some evidence that caregiving parents have strong claims on caregiving from their own children because of "patterning" (Stark 1995). However, lower fertility rates and an aging population, with mounting health problems to the primary family caregivers, suggests the need to develop alternative sources of support not only for the elderly, but for the caregivers themselves in order to better their quality of life and their ability to perform as eldercare workers. Irrespective of cultural, institutional, and behavioral differences, family support -- including emotional and physical support -- is crucial for successful eldercare (NRC 2001, p. 156).

Financial Needs

Household wealth is obviously a critical component in home eldercare. The economic status of families with older persons clearly affects their ability to balance both internal and external eldercare provision and, just as it is for external caregiving, financing is absolutely pivotal in effecting family caregiving. In the U.S., long-term care costs have doubled during each decade since 1970, and home healthcare costs alone grew 91 percent from 1990 to 1995 (NRC 2001). This situation is especially problematic for family eldercare providers since, in the U.S., there is no comprehensive health insurance or healthcare system. Benefits and services are, at best, "piecemeal, non-coordinated, and uneven," with woefully inadequate long-term care provisions -- which are the most frequently needed by the aged (Lechner and Sasaki 1999, p. 220).

Accordingly, the majority (almost two-thirds) of family caregivers to the elderly in the U.S. also maintain employment outside of the home (NAC and AARP 1997; Commonwealth Fund 1999). To treat external employment and internal family caregiving as separate is to fail to appreciate how intimately bound the two are together. Among those both employed and providing family eldercare, two-thirds have reported that they have had to rearrange their work schedules, decrease their work hours, and/or take an unpaid leave in order to meet their caregiving responsibilities (Pavalko and Artis 1997; HHS 1998; MMMI 1999). Although the negative impact of caregiving on a caregiver's immediate income might seem self-evident, caregivers and others often neglect to anticipate the tremendous effect it has on long-term financial stability. Women in particular, since they are the majority of caregivers, are already at a disadvantage due to gendered pay inequities (U.S. Dept. of Labor 2003). In addition, to their disadvantage, many caregivers have to take employment and pay reductions as a result of necessary accommodations for their caregiving responsibilities. As is apparent, this situation presents something of a trap for the informal caregiver. Taking lower paying jobs, switching to part-time, and leaving the workforce all reduce social security benefits for later in life (Young and Newman 2003).

Similarly, since pension contributions are usually associated with salary, working in low-paying fields or working part-time means the employed caregiver is unlikely to have been able to participate in a employer-sponsored pension program (Young and Newman 2003). Social security and pension programs aside, simply making less money means less money available for savings and, thus, less money available for long-term care options.

The U.S. has been very slow to recognize the cost of family caregiving, not only to the individual caregiver, but also to the economy. Recent estimates value informal caregiving at approximately $257 billion, a figure that eclipses the $32 billion for home health care and the $92 billion of nursing home care combined (Amo 2002). In addition, the annual cost to employers for lost productivity of employee caregivers may be as high as $29 billion (Metropolitan Life Insurance 1997). A few large companies in the U.S. (approximately one-third of companies with 1,000 or more employees) have established eldercare resource and referral programs (Galinsky and Bond 1999). However, such programs, when they exist, typically require employee contributions; they also vary considerably and remain an unreliable source of support for the work population in general.

Moreover, even those benefits that do exist are not available to all; significant disparities in healthcare access, particularly for the poorer members of society, are well documented (e.g., Smedley et al. 2003; Flaskerud and Winslow 1998). Note that by 2002, almost 35 million persons in the U.S. lived in poverty -- and this number is increasing daily (Proctor and Delaker 2003). Low-income workers are particularly disadvantaged by the lack of healthcare assistance. Furthermore, not only can poor families not afford healthcare assistance, even middle-class families often have at best limited access to medical insurance and find it difficult to meet rising healthcare costs. Severe reductions in income resulting in "unaccustomed poverty" can add to "objective deprivation a sense of loss and the unavoidable comparison with an earlier and more prosperous time" (NRC 2001, p. 254).

Money for survival is as necessary as the caregiving itself -- is indeed a crucial determinant of the provision and quality of that caregiving. Socioeconomic gradients among the elderly and their families notwithstanding, long-term care for the frail elderly in general represents a significant drain on familial resources that might otherwise provide financial support for the family caregiver.

Sources of Support

With mounting evidence that depressive and physical illness in informal caregivers is a critical issue, what sources of support exist to address the problem? In general, support for the informal family caregiver in the U.S. is at best spotty. However, beyond professional psychological and medical help, we can point to some available nongovernmental support sources. These typically fall into two broad categories: 1) self-education/self-help and 2) programs sponsored by voluntary citizen or religious groups.[9]

Depending on problem severity and personal coping skills, family caregivers suffering from stress and depression may be able to alleviate their symptoms on the basis of self-help information, without seeking professional assistance. Self-help routines typically combine educating oneself and engaging simple cognitive and behavioral techniques to cope with stress and improve wellbeing. For example, there are series of handbooks, guides, and online resources that can help the caregiver in to identify specific sources of stress, recognize aspects that can and cannot be controlled, learn to meditate, communicate better with physicians, and exercise, among other things.[10] Common advice includes recommendations for physical exercise, such as walking at least 20 minutes a day, three times a week, to reduce stress and physical tension, and benefiting the body as a whole (Family Caregiver Alliance 2004).

Also, studies have revealed that, on the individual level, solitary religious and other spiritual activities have proven beneficial to caregiver health. This does not necessarily refer to formal association with a religious group or institution. Almost 75 percent of caregivers report that they use prayer as a way of coping (Morris 1996). For those without access to other support services (e.g., in rural areas), prayer or other forms of meditation may be viable options. One survey of rural caregivers for individuals with Alzheimer's and related disorders found that two-thirds reported that they relied heavily on prayer for coping with the emotional rollercoaster created by their responsibilities (Stolley 1999). Similarly, reading "sacred texts" served as a common source of stress relief (Stolley 1999). Such activities -- e.g., reading sacred texts and praying -- are self-help methods available to caregivers to use singularly or in combination with other options.

Although self-education, exercise, and solitary spiritual activities can be some of the most easily available and inexpensive sources of support, they also can be insufficient in the long-term and do not offer a remedy for the feeling of isolation so often a part of caregiver depression. Accordingly, a more effective support resource might be found in social interaction, e.g., with friends, other family members, and various organizations.

In fact, reaching out to other family members and friends is another informal strategy of support for mental and physical health. Once a caregiver overcomes her reluctance to ask for help or even discuss her feelings, she can benefit greatly. Studies show that caregivers who have strong social support suffer from fewer bouts of depression, illness, and feelings of being overwhelmed (Morris 1996). If a caregiver does not have a supportive family or friends, taking time to socialize is even more critical. Many experts recommend starting an informal support group where members meet occasionally for lunch or coffee to extend mutual support (Morris 1996). For this option, usually just placing a query in the local paper can be sufficient to gather a few caregivers. For more structured social contact, community support programs and voluntary organizations might be an attractive choice. Online support groups are also becoming more popular, although access to them might be limited and their possible effectiveness in relieving the types of problems discussed here is unclear. However,

---

9 Some support programs, while physically held in churches or other religious institutions, may not have a formal affiliation with the religion. Although some support programs administered by religious organizations receive some government funds, when not wholly funded by it, they are placed in the nongovernmental category.

10 E.g., *The Caregiver Helpbook* (Schmall et al. 2000) and the Family Caregiver Alliance (http://www.caregiver.org).

in any case, reluctance to ask for help in the first place is a major barrier to attaining these types of support and respite (Winslow 2003).

Whether administered in association with a government agency or not, evidence overwhelmingly indicates that services typically provided by community or religious organizations benefit both the caregiver and the recipient. Services that provide counseling, information, and ongoing support, have been shown to deter the institutionalization of care recipients with moderate dementia by nearly a year (Mittelman et al. 1996). Similarly, for caregivers of individuals with dementia, those who use adult day care services for their loved ones experience less stress and better psychological well-being than those who do not (Zarit et al. 1998). Consequently, citizen or religious group support benefit not only the caregiver but also the care recipient.

However, again, availability and access to such services are often limited. That is, community support programs can be helpful, but they are not uniformly available and can sometimes be difficult to access -- and this is most often the case for those in most need. In fact, only 10 to 21 percent of family caregivers use formal services provided by public or private agencies (Brody 1990).

Then, of course, there remains the option of support provided by religious and charitable organizations. Such organizations have a long and vibrant history in the U.S. Indeed, as elsewhere, the first hospitals and shelters in the United States were sponsored by religious organizations. However, note that simply attending a religious organization is not what provides the support; support comes through the active involvement with others.

However, all of these sources of support depend on the caregiver recognizing the problem for what it is and taking action. Yet, when dangerously depressed or feeling overwhelmed, that is when the family caregiver is least likely to be able to take positive action and find support. This is another instance in which kinship networks -- family -- might serve as a vital support resource and intervention. Kinships networks in this sense can be conceived as helping networks and, as such, are especially important among the poorest families with little access to other support resources.

Finally, note that employment itself can be a major source of wellbeing and support, not only because of associated remuneration determining access to other resources (e.g., housing, clothing, transportation, education, entertainment, etc.), but also as a source of more intrinsic satisfactions -- "the opportunity to use valued skills and abilities and to acquire additional ones, the sense of involvement in a larger productive process, and the cooperative and friendly relationships that may develop in the workplace." That is, employment is "of major importance with implications for both the stock and flow of wellbeing" (NRC 2001, pp. 13-14).

However, employment can also be a source of dissatisfaction. As Lechner and Sasaki (1999, p. 218) note, "although caregiving can be meaningful and satisfying, and employment can provide a respite from caregiving tasks, many employed caregivers in the United States indicate that managing the two roles is stressful." Indeed, many caregivers end up quitting their jobs in order to care for their frail relatives -- when they can afford to do so. Also, especially for poorer families, maintaining employment can reflect a different dynamic, with kinship networks again cast as helping networks. "Many who hold jobs have kin willing to defer individual pursuits for the sake of others. Because poor families cannot purchase the care their families need, they must supply it to each other" (Hicks-Bartlett 2000, p. 37). Without such familial support, employed work is difficult and sometimes impossible to sustain. The complicated arrangements these family caregivers must make to work and provide care simultaneously reveal how tenuous these arrangements can be, and any emergency or special need can snowball into a family crisis (cf. Hicks-Bartlett 2000, p. 35). Again, the family caregiver role is marked by the paradox embedded in the complex relationship between needs and support.

POLICY ISSUES AND INITIATIVES

In general, the U.S. lags behind virtually every other developed country in providing eldercare. Yes, acute healthcare coverage is provided for some elders through two major policy programs, Medicare and Medicaid,[11] but the medical conditions of the elderly are most often chronic and long-term care services are grossly lacking. Also, Medicare eligibility requirements for home care strictly limit its accessibility (Weaver and Ingman 1997).

The United States is a federal system with eldercare policy administered at two levels: national and state. The federal government corresponds to the nation as a whole, which is constituted by fifty individual states. Earlier, throughout the 20th century, the national, i.e., federal, government had the primary role in policy agenda setting and formulation, while the individual states took on the secondary role of carrying out federal intent. More recently, however, policy responsibilities have devolved more and more to the states. Consequently, the contemporary environment in which policies affecting eldercare and, in particular, family caregiving are made and implemented involves a complex interplay of federal and state governments, with increasing pressure on states to take an active role in addressing related issues. Accordingly, any consideration of policies concerning family caregiving must speak to both national and state level initiatives.

National Policy Initiatives

Current national caregiver support policies primarily do two things: 1) make federal funds available to the individual states for administration of community support programs, and 2) encourage federal and military personnel to plan for their long-term care.[12] Interestingly, it has only been in the past few years that even these initiatives were established. In his second term, former U.S. President William Clinton presented a long-term care plan that included three components, two of which have become law, the National Family Caregiver Support Program (NCFSP) and the Long-term Care Security Act. These two initiatives are the foundations upon which most current policies rest and, consequently, they merit a closer look.

The National Family Caregiver Support Program was implemented in 2000 under the Older Americans Act Amendments. As background, programs and services under the Older Americans Act are administered via a network that includes the Administration on Aging,

[11] See *http://www.hhs.gov/aging/index.shtml#health for* detailed descriptions of these programs.

[12] Former President Clinton also fathered the Family and Medical Leave Act, which allows employees unpaid job protection should they need to leave to care for a child or a sick relative. However, given that it only applies to a maximum 12-week period, it represents only a short-term aid for caregivers.

Area Agencies on Aging, State Units on Aging, and various service providers. Under the NFCSP, members of the network receive funds to expand and restructure services that provide information and support to caregivers, respite care, counseling, training, and other supplemental services intended to complement current caregiver activities. The national government funded the program's coffers for the first year to the tune of 125 million U.S. dollars, a particularly encouraging sign that caregiver support would be on policymakers' agendas for the foreseeable future. By 2003, funding had reached 149 million U.S. dollars. These funds were intended to be used by the states, as discussed below, to improve and restructure the caregiver programs they operate under Older Americans Act.

The second component of former President Clinton's long-term plan, the Long-Term Security Act, applies only to federal and military personnel and retirees, allowing them to purchase at a relatively low cost long-term care insurance as part of their benefits. Although it was difficult to find good long-term care insurance policies even a decade ago, the industry has come a long way in creating packages to benefit retirees. Consequently, this federal initiative may end up creating a precedent taken up by the states and private businesses.

The federal judicial system also has influenced national policy affecting caregivers. In 1999, a United States Supreme Court ruling, known simply as the *Olmstead* decision, forced the states to improve their community services. The Court did this by holding that a state is in violation of the Americans with Disabilities Act (ADA) if it fails to make "reasonable modifications" in existing services for persons whom their own health professionals have determined capable of living in community residences. The notion of "reasonable modifications" triggers a responsibility on the part of states that hitherto had not been recognized. On the one hand, the policy fallout from *Olmstead* has proven somewhat remarkable. Nearly all states have created commissions or task forces to develop comprehensive plans or recommendations concerning the case's implications (Fox-Grage et al. 2001). However, on the other hand, the actual extent to which these commissions and task forces have implemented or adjusted service programs remains uncertain.

Clinton was unsuccessful in persuading the national legislature to pass the third component of his proposed long-term care plan before he left office. Its latest incarnation, known as the Long-Term Care and Retirement Security Act of 2003, has support by leaders from both the Democratic and Republican parties, the major political parties in the U.S., as well as from organizations such as the National Center for Assisted Living and the American Health Care Association (Feeny 2003). Its passage could potentially revolutionize the way employees plan and provide for long-term care. One version (S 1335) of the act provides for 1) an "above the line" tax deduction for qualified long-term care insurance premiums; 2) incentives for employers to offer long-term care insurance policies to their employees through flexible spending accounts; and 3) a small tax credit for those who are already ill (or their caregivers) to help cover related care expenses.

As previously mentioned, the 2003 version of this act has more bipartisan support than ever before. Consequently, there is some encouragement that federal financial support via this type of structure might finally become available for caregivers and their charges. The tax credit alone, though relatively small, would be a step in the right direction to help alleviate some of the financial pressures created by caregiving. However, at this point, its passage is still not reality.

Lastly, the federal government also supports programs that can aid caregivers by allowing states to issue home- and community-based Medicaid waivers. Waiver programs allow the states to use Medicaid monies to fund home and community programs that offer a variety of services to disabled individuals, thus providing relief to caregivers. Common waiver programs allow states to offer services such as assistance with daily activities, respite care, and adult day care. When combined with other state funds, these programs represent a hybrid of both federal and state efforts and foresee some of the most promising opportunities to date for caregiver support through innovative programming.

The above legislation evidences the national government's current role as the primary sponsor of state and community support programs and caregiver financial relief efforts. However, with the federal government at arm's length, the front-line administration and implementation of community support programs and services are left to the states.

State Policy Initiatives

In addition to federally sponsored support programs, some states have made efforts to fund caregiver support programs through their own funds. One state, California, has even created a tax credit specifically to help taxpayers who either receive or provide long-term care. Other state funding options have evolved since the mid-1990s when settlements with the tobacco industry were negotiated on behalf of all 50 states in relation to lawsuits concerning the dangers of smoking, among other claims. The settlement for 4 of the states, who worked separately from the remaining 46, totaled $40 billion to be paid out over a 25-year period. The other 46 states settled with the industry for a 25-year payout of $286 billion (Fox-Grage et al. 2001). The important point here relative to family caregiving is that these tobacco funds are being used by some states to fund community services and support programs that might otherwise have not been available.

Furthermore, the establishment of the National Family Caregiver Support Program under the Older Americans Act in 2000 has allowed a number of states to expand their caregiver support programs. For example, the state of Washington has included counseling for family caregivers (Fox-Grage et al. 2001). Florida and Maine have been able to expand their support services and extend help to caregivers earlier in the care process (Feinberg et al. 2002). The state of Michigan has target funding from the NFCSP to help older caregivers of elderly relatives through, among other things, training and education (Michigan Commission on Services for the Aging 2003). In addition, Michigan is using funds from the multi-state tobacco settlement to provide additional respite programs to caregivers of adults over the age of 18 who are disabled (Fox-Grage et al. 2001). Georgia has utilized demonstration grant monies from the NFCSP to expand a collaborative network of professional and family caregiver groups known as Care-Nets (Rosalynn Carter Institute 2004). Composed of educational institutions, businesses, and family caregivers, Care-Nets develop service and educational programs to meet the needs of caregivers, oversee research, and provide recognition and support for caregivers (Link 2003).

States do little to directly address the financial needs of caregivers. As previously mentioned, one state, California recently instituted a tax credit for caregivers. However, as a whole, states are waiting for the federal government to take the lead on implementing policy that directly provides financial assistance to caregivers.

In general, until recently, U.S. "public policy" and "support for family caregivers" were two subjects rarely spoken in the same sentence. With the landmark National Family

Caregiver Support Program in 2000, national policy attention was finally turned to this critical issue. While some early indicators suggest that NFCSP initiatives, as well as those made in conjunction with Medicaid waivers, are improving the support options available to caregivers, they still fall far short of effectively meeting caregiver needs (Feinberg et al. 2002). A first evaluation of NFCSP's implementation in the states, published at the end of 2002, summarized the preliminary experiences of 10 states in providing support and services to caregivers following the program's establishment and also addressed issues concerning Medicaid involvement with caregiver support (Feinberg et al. 2002). The report found that

1. Little consensus exists among the states about the recognition of families as a central component of a comprehensive long-term care system.
2. Providing explicit support for family and friends of frail elders represents a paradigm shift for many State Units on Aging.
3. State variations in caregiver support are as diverse as the states.
4. The two main challenges in developing and implementing caregiver support services in the states studied are limited funding and workforce shortages.
5. The NFCSP fills a gap for low to moderate income family caregivers through services and programs not previously available to them.
6. Medicaid officials are limited by stringent rules in their ability to help family caregivers.

These findings are simultaneously encouraging and discouraging. On the one hand, this attempt at using public policy to address caregiver needs appears to be making some positive difference. However, on the other hand, there is wide variability of state efforts in caregiver support, in addition to funding limitations.

Reconsidering Policy Approaches

All in all, institutional arrangements can vary dramatically, with fragmented service provision confounding not only eldercare benefit levels, but also individual and family behaviors. A popular explanation for this situation rests on assertions of U.S. preferences for decentralization (Kamerman 1996). However, we argue that decentralization in and of itself is not the real issue; decentralization in its most fundamental guise is an administrative and organizational response. For example, the successful home and community-based model for eldercare in Norway is organized to emphasize decentralization of care (Hokenstad 1999). The real difference is that of a U.S. system based on an ideology of consumerism and commodification, as opposed to one developed around notions of social rights and an ethic of care (Tronto 1993).

Considerations of cost, rather than concern for improving the quality of life for elders and their caregivers, are the largest influence on policy choices (c.f. Weaver and Ingman 1997). By defining care principally as a commodity, we lose sight of the means by which that care is given. In a society with an overriding concern with material productivity and possession, values of caring and nurturance, of the importance of human relationships, are overlooked -- or even challenged -- as key social goals. Acknowledging that caregivers often lack adequate resources, it is easy to see how care can be a burden in such a culture. "Yet the view that care must be private, and the privatizing of the difficulties women encounter as caregivers, further supports the perception that care is not a social concern, but a problem of idiosyncratic individuals" (Tronto 1993, p. 120).

Especially in light of family caregiving and kinship considerations, we argue that *relationships* need to be explicitly considered in eldercare policy initiatives. After all, people do not make choices in isolation from their life circumstances, their beliefs about the world, or their relationships -- including "the priority that people attach to maintaining them, the resources they provide, and the obligations they impose" (Lin 2000, p. 263). Indeed, the centrality of relationships to the coping strategies of family caregivers "implies that policy initiatives that focus only on the individual will face predictable problems" (Lin 2000, p. 264). In general, now, even if relationships are invoked in policy discussions, they are not grounded in any empirical assessment of the pros and cons or the possible consequences for those involved.

A relational perspective suggests a more integrative approach to questions of family caregiving. Eldercare forces us to think concretely about both family and societal relationships and about people's needs within those relationships, not just for the elderly themselves, but also for those family members who provide them with care and caring. Evaluating how those needs will be met requires a re-assessment of public and private values in terms of an overarching perception of caregiving. This means recognizing a danger in thinking about needs only as a commodity. "Such a commodification or reification of needs, obscures the processes of care necessary to meet needs; instead, the 'needs' themselves appear as entities" -- which would not engage us in thinking about caregiving in a direct sense as part of a process with its own implications (Tronto 1993, p. 138).

Indeed, this tendency has led the U.S. to be described as a "careless" society (c.f. McKnight 1995; Tronto 1993). In the U.S., care is usually conceived as, ideally, a private concern; it is supposed to be provided in the household. Yet, with an increasingly aging population and concomitantly expanding needs for family care options, we need to take seriously, as part of our definition of a good society, values of care, responsibility, and nurturance -- values traditionally constructed within women's roles confined to the private sphere -- relative to public policy initiatives and support (cf. Tronto 1993, p. 3).

This approach does not deny the fact that quality caregiving "depends upon adequate resources: on material goods, on time, and on skills." In fact, a principal policy issue is to determine "which caring needs receive which resources"(Tronto 1993, p. 110). However, current fragmented conceptions of care operate to obscure interactive practical, moral, and political aspects of family care requiring policy action. Relational processes, as reflected in eldercare, have fundamental policy implications. Given this trend, a fitting policy response would be the provision of long-term home care, respite, and adult day care services to buttress the informal family caregivers (Hughes 1989, p. 60). Furthermore, as emphasized in a report on aging by the National Research Council (2001, p.26), "given that gender differences in such areas as life expectancy, work history, asset accumulation, and caregiving pervade most societies, it is imperative that policies regarding the well-being of older individuals account carefully for differential gender impacts."

As Rubenstein (1989, p. 72) observes, policy research focuses on studying the impact of programs composed of multiple components. In this case, a home care program might explicitly include family caregivers, along with visiting nurses and social workers. The kinds of variables considered might be variations in entitlement, financing, or types of services provided, and related research might assess the effectiveness of such services, and the relationships among them. "Ultimately, policy options are grounded in understanding individual and family behaviors and their responsiveness to changing life circumstances" (NRC 2001, p. 17).

Conclusion

In this chapter, we characterized the complex nature of family caregiver wellbeing and eldercare in the United States within the context of three analytical dimensions of need and support: emotional, physical, and financial. We explored the contextual background in which family caregiver needs are determined and also discussed the degree to which such needs have been met or unmet by sources within the caregiver's entire relational sphere of kin and community. In so doing, we addressed the profound effect of caregiving on the emotional and psychological wellbeing of caregivers, highlighting issues of stress, anxiety, and depression. In addition, we discussed the relationship between caregiving responsibilities and deleterious physical consequences. We also spoke to the issue of financial needs, especially in the context of employment and investment ability, highlighting the disproportionate impact on women who make up the majority of family caregivers. In addressing these various needs, we noted their lack of exclusivity and their impact, not only on the caregivers themselves, but also on their families and on society as a whole.

Practical Considerations and Recommendations

- Current sources of support and services for family caregivers in the United States fail to address the interdependent nature of caregiver needs and wellbeing.
- At minimum, a comprehensive assessment is critically needed of the emotional, physical, and financial supports and services available to family caregivers.
- Similarly, focused research on the economic impact of caregiving activities is needed in support of the prioritization of related policies.
- The effect of external employment in particular must be an explicit consideration in the evaluation of family caregiver wellbeing.
- The increased aging of the population requires increased policy efforts to directly address the needs of the family caregiver.
- An in-depth understanding of kinship and community interrelations should be brought to bear in the formulation of eldercare policies.

References

Alexcih, L, Zeruld, S., and Olearczyk, B. (2002). Characteristics of caregivers based on the survey of income and program participation, National Family Caregiver Support Program: Selected issue briefs. Washington, DC: Administration on Aging.

Amo, P. (2002). The economic value of informal caregiving, U.S., 2004. Presented at the Geriatric Psychiatry meeting, Orlando, FL.

Barondess, J., Rogers, D., and Lohr, K. (Eds.). (1989). *Care of the Elderly Patient: Policy Issues and Research Opportunities*. Washington, D.C.: National Academy Press.

Brody, E. (1990). *Women in the middle: Their parent care years*. New York, NY: Springer Publishing Co.

Cannuscio, C., Jones, C., Kawachi, I., Colditz, G., Berkman, L., and Rimm, E. (2002). Reverberations of family illness: A longitudinal assessment of informal caregiving and mental health status in the nurse's health study. *American Journal of Public Health,* 92, 1305-1311.

Commonwealth Fund. (1999, May). *Informal Caregiving*. New York: Commonwealth Fund.

Donabedian, A. (1989). Quality of Care and the Health Needs of the Elderly Patient. In Barondess, et al. (pp. 3-13).

Family Caregiver Alliance. (2004). Fact sheet: Taking care of you: self-care for family caregivers. Available at http://www.caregiver.org.

Feinberg, L., Newman, S., and Van Steenberg, C. (2002). *Family caregiver support: policies, perceptions, and practices in 10 states since passage of the national family caregiver support program*. San Francisco: Family Caregiver Alliance.

Feeny, S. (July, 2003). *Passage of Long-term Care and Retirement Security Act of 2003 called vital to boosting retirees' ability to save, prepare for health needs.* Available at *http://www.acha.org/news*.

Flaskerud, J., and Winslow, E. (1998). Conceptualizing Vulnerable Population's Health-Related Research. *Nursing Research*, 47 (2), 69-76.

Fox-Grage, W., Coleman, B., and Blancato, R. (2001). *Federal and state policy in family caregiving: Recent victories but uncertain future.* San Francisco: Family Caregiver Alliance.

Gallagher, D., Rose, J., Rivera, P., Lovett, S., and Thompson, L. (1989). Prevalence of depression in family caregivers. *The Gerontologist*, 29, 449-456.

Gray, L. (2003). *Caregiver Depression: A Growing mental Health Concern*. San Francisco: Family Caregiver Alliance.

Grundy, E. and Harrop, A. (1992). Co-Residence Between Adult Children and Their Elderly Parents in England and Wales: Informal Parental Support. *Journal of Social Policy*, 21 (3), 325-329.

Gwyther, L. (1990). Clinician and family: A partnership for support. In N.L. Mace (Ed.), *Dementia care: Patient, family, and community*. Baltimore, MD: The Johns Hopkins University Press.

Hanneman, R. (1997). Your Money or Your Life: Access to Medical Care as a Social Problem. In D. Dunn and D.V. Waller (Eds.). *Analyzing Social Problems* (pp. 39-46). Upper Saddle River, NJ: Prentice Hall.

HHS (Health and Human Services). (June, 1998). *Informal caregiving: Compassion in action.* Depart of Health and Human Services, Washington D.C.

Hicks-Bartlett, S. (2000). Between a Rock and a Hard Place: The Labyrinth of Working and Parenting in a Poor Community. In S. Danziger and A.C. Lin (Eds.). *Coping With Poverty* (pp. 27-51). Ann Arbor: University of Michigan Press.

Hokenstad, M.C. (1999). The Elderly at Home in Norway. In R. Heiner (Ed.). *Social Problems and Social Solutions: A Cross-Cultural Perspective* (pp. 228-231). Boston: Allyn and Bacon.

Hounsell, C., Humphlett, P., and Lewis, J. (2002). *Your future paycheck: pay, social security, pensions, savings, and investments.* Washington, DC: Women's Institute for a Secure Retirement.

Hughes, S. (1989). Home and Community Care of the Elderly: System Resources and Constraints. In Barondess, et al. (pp. 55-61).

Kamerman, S. (1996). The new politics of child and family policies. *Social Work*, 55 (3), 453-466.

Kwon, I. (2000). Population will need a quality home-care system. *St. Louis Post-Dispatch*, p. B7.

Lechner, V., and Sasaki, M. (1999). Japan and the United States Struggle with Who Will Care for Our Aging Parents When Caregivers Are Employed. In R. Heiner (Ed.). *Social Problems and Social Solutions: A Cross-Cultural Perspective* (pp. 216-227). Boston: Allyn and Bacon.

Lin, A.C. (2000). Social Contexts in the Making of Public Policy. In S. Danziger and A.C. Lin (Eds.). *Coping With Poverty* (pp. 262-272). Ann Arbor: University of Michigan Press.

Link, G., (2003).The Aging Network implements the National Family Caregiver Support Program. Washington DC: National Association of State Units on Aging

Manson, J. and Bassuk, S. (2003). Obesity in the United States: A Fresh Look at Its High Toll. *Journal of the American Medical Association*, 289, 229-231.

McKnight, J. (1995). *The Careless Society*. New York: Basic Books.

Metropolitan Life Insurance Company. (1997). *The MetLife Study of Employer Costs for Working Caregivers*. Westport, CT: Metropolitan Life Insurance Company.

Michigan Commission on Services for the Aging. (2003). State Plan on Services to Michigan's Older Citizens: Fiscal years 2004-2006. Lansing: Michigan Commission on Services to Aging.

Mittelman, M., Ferris, S., Shulman, E., Steinberg G, Levin B (1996). A Family Intervention to Delay Nursing Home Placement of Patients with Alzheimer's Disease. Journal of the American Medical Association, 276(21):1725-1731.

Morris, V. (1996). *How to care for aging parents.* New York, NY: Workman Publishing.

NAC (National Alliance for Caregiving) and AARP. (1997). *Family caregiving in the U.S.: Findings from a national survey,* Bethesda, MD: National Alliance for Caregiving, and Washington DC: AARP.

National Institute of Mental Health. (2001). *Older adults: Depression and suicide facts.* (Publication No. 01-4593). Rockville, MD: National Institute of Mental Health.

National Research Council (NRC). (2001). *Preparing for an Aging World: The Case for Cross-National Research*, Panel on a Research Agenda and New Data for an Aging World/Committee on Population and Committee on National Statistics/Division of

Behavioral and Social Sciences and Education. Washington, DC: National Academy Press.*Olmstead v. L.C.* (1999). 527 U.S. 581.

Pavalko, E., and Artis, J. (1997). Women's *Caregiving and Paid Work. Journal of Gerontology* 52B (4), 170-179.

Proctor, B., and Delaker, J. (2003). *Poverty in the United States: 2002*. Washington, DC: U.S. Census Bureau.

Quinlan, E. (1989). Special Perspectives on Home and Community Care. In Barondess, et al. (pp. 36-43).

Rosalynn Carter Institute. (2004). Care-Net: Establishing Community Caregiving Networks. http://www.rci.gsw.edu/carenetpages/carenethx.html

Rubenstein, L.V. (1989). Home and Community Care of the Elderly: Research and Policy Issues. In Barondess, et al. (pp. 71-76).

Schulz, R. and Beach, S.R.. (1999). Caregiving as a risk factor for mortality: The Caregiver Health Effects Study, *JAMA* 282, 2215.

Schultz, R., O'Brien, A.T., Bookwals, J., Fleissner, K., (1995). Psychiatric and physical morbidity effects of dementia caregiving: Prevalence, correlates, and causes, *The Gerontologist,* 35, 771-791.

Smedley, B.D., Stith, A.Y., and Nelson, A.R. (Eds.) (2003). *Unequal Treatment: Confronting Racial and Ethnic Disparities in Health Care*. Washington, D.C.: National Academies Press.

Stark, O. (1995). *Altruism and Beyond: An Economic Analysis of Transfers and Exchanges Within Families and Groups*. Cambridge: Cambridge University Press.

Stolley, J. (1999). *Study Report: Prayer and Care*. Chicago: The Park Ridge Center.

Thompson, L. (2004). Long-term care: Support for family caregivers. Issue brief. Georgetown University Long-term Care Financing Project. Washington, DC.: Georgetown University.

Tronto, J. (1993). *Moral Boundaries: A Political Argument for an Ethic of Care*. New York: Routledge.

U.S. Department of Labor, Bureau of Labor Statistics. (2002, January). *Employment and Earnings*. Washington, DC: U.S. Department of Labor.

U.S. Department of Health and Human Services and U.S. Department of Labor (2003). *The future supply of long-term care workers in relation to the baby boom generation: Report to Congress*. Washington, D.C.: U.S. Department of Health and Human Services and U.S. Department of Labor.

U.S. Department of Labor, Bureau of Labor Statistics. (2003). *Highlights of Women's Earnings in 2002*. Washington, DC: U.S. Department of Labor.

Weaver, M., and Ingman, S. (1997). Aging and Health Care. In D. Dunn and D.V. Waller (Eds.). *Analyzing Social Problems* (pp. 47-55). Upper Saddle River, NJ: Prentice Hall.

Winslow, B. (2003). Family Caregivers' experiences with community services: A qualitative analysis. *Public Health Nursing,* 20, 341.

Young, L. and Newman, S. (2003). *Caregiving and retirement planning: what happens to family caregivers who leave the work- force*. San Francisco: Family Caregiver Alliance.

Zarit, S., Stephens, M., Townsend, A., and Greene, R. (1998). Stress reduction for family caregivers: Effects of adult day care use, *Journal of Gerontology*, Series B, 53 (5), S267-276.

In: Family Caregiving for Older Disabled People
Editor: Isabella Paoletti, pp. 273-294
ISBN 1-59454-808-0

Chapter13

EXTRACTING THE ESSENCE OF FORMAL CAREGIVING: A COMPARATIVE STUDY OF FORMAL CAREGIVERS IN ENGLISH AND GERMAN CARE HOMES

Ingrid Eyers
Surrey University, Tizard Centre University Of Kent,
Canterbury, KENT, United Kingdom

INTRODUCTION

This chapter will present the essence of the skills required to undertake formal caregiving within an institutional temporal framework. When the care needs of an older person become such that the provision within the family or by friends is no longer appropriate or feasible, the move into a care home often becomes unavoidable. In fact nursing homes are a topic that is often in the back ground of family caregiving. In various chapter in this book, the topic of care home is discussed by interviewees. Paoletti in Chapter 1, and Baldassar and her colleagues, in chapter 10, show how care home are despised as cagiving solution in Italy. Similarly, Oddone and Aguirre, in chapter 3, point out how care homes are constructed as a negative caring solution in Argentina. Within the context of family caregiving it is therefore important to also consider formal caregivers who become an integral part of the daily life of an older person living in a care home. Moreover, it is noticeable as some aspects of formal caregiving resemble specific issues raised in relation to family caregiving, in particular, care skills.

A comparative study of care staff in English and German care homes aimed to establish how time restricting government policies relate to the use and acquisition of caregiving skills. The findings present how the essence of formal care is extracted and identify how essential invisible, intangible and immeasurable care skills are used in this working environment.

The provision of formal care needs to be seen within the context of the policy framework surrounding the care home industry. This chapter will discuss and compare the English and

German policies that regulate the care home industry and then consider the literature that relates to the issues that impact on caregiving in an institutional environment such as bodywork, emotional labour, communication and time to care. After providing an overview of the mixed methods used to collect data in care homes in both countries, the research findings will be presented and discussed.

Policies Surrounding the Provision of Institutional Care in England And Germany

Formal caregiving in England and Germany takes place within a historically rooted structural framework established by the governments of each country. As representatives of the conservative and liberal welfare system within Europe (Esping-Andersen, 1990), England and Germany have approached the issues that arise from an ageing population in different ways. The key differences relating to the research described in this chapter are based in the funding of a care home placement and the staffing policies.

Funding

In Germany funding of a care home placement is determined by the Sozialesgeseztbuch XI (Social Care Act XI) passed in May 1994. This resulted in the introduction of a state regulated longterm care insurance system that was linked to the well established health-care insurance system. Financial support from the care insurance (Pflegeversicherung) is dependent on a 'care needs' assessment. The amount of funding provided is determined by clearly defined care categories that in turn are linked to the assessed time needed to support someone in their 'activities of daily living'. The categories stated are as follows:

- Category I: 'Erheblich Pflegebeduerftig' [great need of care]. Daily at least 90 minutes of care to be required, of which at least 45 minutes are to be spent on basic care.
- Category II: 'Schwerpflegebeduerftig' [severe need of care]. Daily at least 3 hours of care required, of which at least 2 hours are to be spent on basic care
- Category III: 'Schwerstpflegebeduerftig' [severest need of care] Daily at least 5 hours of care required, of which at least 4 hours are to be spent on basic care. (Source: §15 SGB XI in Beck 1995:10, Klie 1997:113/14)

This 'needs led' system of funding clearly indicates how government policy rations the contact time between caregivers and older people.

The long-term care insurance only covers the care element of the cost of a care home placement in Germany. The 'hotel costs' are met by the individual's personal income. If the personal income is too low then Social Services undertake a 'means test' which, unlike England, includes a financial assessment of relatives who could be called upon by the State to contribute towards the costs. This can be seen to involve German families more directly in the formal care process than their English counterparts.

In England, the state funding available to an older person living in a care home is both 'needs' and 'means' tested. The 'needs test' is related to an individuals medical condition and provided by the National Health Service (NHS). This is intended to meet the cost of Registered Nursing Care Contribution (RNCC). The stated aim is to

> 'meet the cost of registered nursing time spent providing, delegating or supervising care in any setting. It does not cover personal or social care costs or the cost of resident's accommodation' (DH 2001).

The 'means test' relates to the financial circumstances of an individual and is conducted by Local Authority Social Services. These funds are to cover the cost of accommodation and social care needs of an older person with limited financial resources. This system rations qualified nursing in English care homes and results in a high proportion of formal caregivers being care assistants who do not require qualifications to meet the health and social care needs of older people.

Staffing

The staffing levels encountered in an English care home are determined by the Care Standards Act 2000 (DH 2000) and the number of caregivers working in each individual English care home is negotiated between the regulating authorities and the proprietor. Whether or not qualified nurses are employed is dependent on the 'target market' the care home proprietor has chosen. The total number of caregivers employed is primarily determined by the number and dependency of the residents. This consequently determines the ratio of caregivers to residents and impacts on the contact time available in which care is given. However, as the funding system described earlier indicates, the main providers of 'hands-on-care' in an English care home are care assistants.

In Germany legislation states that 50% of the care home staff must be qualified caregivers (Goberg 1997). This ultimately results in qualified staff being involved in the daily provision of 'hands-on-care'. In contrast to England, the German qualified staff are not only qualified nurses who have undergone their training in a hospital environment. Many of the German qualified caregivers have undertaken a formal three-year training programme to become 'Older Peoples Carers' (OPC). This training aims to provide formal caregivers who have a sound knowledge base of the health and social care needs of older people living either at home or in a care home. As the funding system indicates, the number of caregivers working in a care home is linked to the dependency and the number of residents in a care home.

These diverging policies relating to the funding of a care home placement and staffing highlighted the issue of contact time between caregivers and care recipient. In turn this led to focusing on the skills used by formal caregivers working in the institutional temporal framework of a care home. The blend of skills is dominated by the requirement to undertake bodywork which will be discussed in the next section.

Bodywork

Bodywork presents an important aspect of care home work as older people who make the transition into a care home do so because they require assistance with everyday activities such as getting up, washed and dressed in the morning. This involves the intrusion into the personal and private sphere of older people who are also coming to terms with a medical condition that impacts on their everyday lives. Living with a stroke, Parkinson's or dementia, for example, are medical conditions that have an effect on an older person's ability to independently undertake everyday activities that most adults take for granted.

The very personal bodily function of using the toilet to excrete urine and faeces is a situation that often depends on the assistance, guidance or support of a second person. Formal caregiving to older people in their own home is, for example, described by Twigg (2000a), who points out that caregivers recurrently identified dealing with 'shit' (*the term used by Twigg in her article)* to be difficult as the smell was hard to bear and had 'an all pervasive, stomach churning quality that lingered about the person' (Twigg 2000a:396). This part of bodywork may be unpleasant for caregivers but what about the dignity and personal concerns of the older person? As this is an area that is not discussed within 'polite society', it is not an issue that is easily researched from the perspective of an older person. However, such an intrusion into the personal sphere of bodily functions is an aspect of life that every adult can be expected to empathise with, as it relates to a natural bodily function that we all experience. Whilst coping with incontinence may be unpleasant for caregivers it must surely be perceived to be degrading and undignified for an older person.

Much of the bodywork undertaken in care homes is collectively termed as 'basic care' in both England and Germany and involves tasks perceived to be rudimentary such as washing, dressing and toiletting an older person. As stated earlier the staffing levels determined by policy makers in England result in 'basic care' being predominantly provided by care assistants, whereas German policies result in both qualified staff and care assistants performing these tasks. The division of labour between qualified staff and care assistants replicates the division of hospital nursing care identified by Lawler (1991) where nursing is divided into basic nursing and technical nursing.

The 'dirty work' undertaken within care homes has been identified as invisible (Lawler 1991; Lee-Treweek 1997; Twigg 2000b). The fact that it is invisible is not only because it happens behind closed doors or screens but also because it can be seen to be related to society's perception of traditional female roles where 'caring is central but poorly valued' (Lawler 1991:35). The perception that women enjoy care work as it is seen to be an extension of their natural role (Lee Treweek 1997) is further emphasised by the invisibility of the informal 'mothering skills' (Mason 1996; Ribbens 1994; Williams 2002). Within the care home industry, it appears to be assumed that women are naturally equipped to be caregivers and deal with bodily substances encountered in bodywork and that they are always sympathetic and able to provide emotionally for others. However, both evoked and experience emotions are an integral part of caregiving and the literature surrounding emotional labour will be reviewed in the following section.

Emotional Labour

Emotional labour is closely linked to the undertaking of bodywork which unavoidably evokes emotions in a caregiver who is at the same time likely to be using emotional labour tools in the provision of care. This indicates a dichotomy encountered in emotional labour in the provision of care. Emotional labour is discussed by Hochschild (1983) who identifies that in order to survive in a job, such as that of a flight attendant, there is the need to detach oneself mentally from personal feelings that are defined to be similar to the sensory experience of hearing or seeing. In caregiving, emotional labour relates to the fact that whilst trying to detach themselves from personal emotions, caregivers are also using emotional labour tools in order to work within an institutional temporal framework. The daily routine for an older person living in a care home is as described by Valins (2002), who presents a very structured day which is determined by meal times and the shift patterns of care staff. Within this framework, basic care is provided by a limited number of care staff and in both English and German care homes, the contact time between older people and care staff is restricted (Eyers 2000a). In order to meet the care needs of the people they are employed to care for within a tight time schedule, emotional labour skills become a necessity (Eyers 2000a; 2000b; James 1989; Lee-Treweek 1997).

Emotional labour can be seen as demanding skilled work, as it is about 'action and reaction, doing and being' (James 1992:500). James defines it as 'the labour involved in dealing with other people's feelings, a core component of which is the regulation of emotions' (James 1989:15). Within the care home as a work place, emotional labour tools are implemented as a means of manipulating an older person into being co-operative, so that care can be provided in the shortest possible time (Eyers 2000a, 2000b). The 'emotional tools' used in care are identified to be; listening, gentle persuasion, firm direction, discomfort and force (James 1989:24). This represents a further development of Hochschild's (1983) groundbreaking work in emotional labour, where labour is perceived to be better understood and used by women. Hochschild states:

> 'In general, lower-class and working-class people tend to work more with things, and middle-class and upper-class people tend to work more with people. More working women than men deal with people as a job. Thus there are both gender patterns and class patterns to the civic and commercial use of human feelings. That is the social point.' (Hochschild 1983:21)

The established low status of bodywork indicates how the healthcare industry uses gender differences to its advantage but does not acknowledge its the commercial value. Formal caregivers who are able to facilitate and order emotions are seen to be of interest to commerce as such attributes keep customers happy. Emotional labour is an invisible, intangible and immeasurable skill that, as Lee-Treweek (1996) points out, has become a sellable low priced commodity within the public sphere. Within the care home industry, it is a factor that is of great importance in the production of care. However, the 'handle' used to gain a firm grip on the emotional labour tools used by caregivers is connected to communication strategies in the provision of care. This aspect of formal caregiving will now be considered.

COMMUNICATION

Within care homes, the main function of communication is to ensure the smooth execution of care tasks (Sachweh 1999). Throughout the healthcare industry, communication can be seen to be important in service delivery, whether to establish a diagnosis, provide treatment or care. However, Lee-Treweek (1997) indicates that from the perspective of caregivers, communication with the older people is perceived to be 'useless'. In contrast, Davies (2001) acknowledges the importance of empowering older people living in care homes by providing opportunities to make choices and decisions relating to their everyday lives.

Autonomy for an older person living in a care home may not mean they can wash their own face but it should mean that they have the autonomy to ask or indicate that they would like to have their face washed (Davies 2001:85). To indicate that they would like to have their face washed implies the need for communication between caregiver and care recipient. In the interface between an older person living in a care home and caregivers, communication can be seen to be very much part of meeting health and social care needs.

A review of the literature did not identify any publication clearly establishing the link between the use of emotional labour tools and communication skills. However, Sachweh (1999) undertook linguistics-based research in a care home in the Black Forest, Germany. Here communication between caregivers and care recipient were both observed and tape-recorded and the data collection was complemented by interviews with caregivers. The analysis of the communication between formal caregivers and care recipient focused on the selection of words, use of dialect, construction of sentences and tone of voice. In this research, emotional labour was not considered by the researcher. Nonetheless, the report of her findings includes descriptions of communications that can be identified as emotional labour. This is exemplified by Sachweh's (1999:113) statement that 'it is undeniable that the main function of communication in medical institutions is to ensure the smooth execution of a care task'. It is further pointed out that communication strategies are used to ensure effective care and 'routine' and 'ritual' communication patterns are identified. The use of compliments and praise and how this resulted in compliance were identified, thus implicating the use of the emotional labour tools described by James (1989:24).

Sachweh (1999) makes reference to how care staff in the sample home behaved like mothers in both verbal and non-verbal communication with the older people living in the home. 'Baby talk' was observed to be used mostly by women aged around 40 and from interviews with caregivers, it was identified that the use of 'baby talk' was related to their lifecourse experiences, as the majority of female respondents had brought up children before taking up employment in the care home. To be perceived as a 'good mother' by the older people they cared for was one of the greatest compliments caregivers could receive (Sachweh 1999:175). Male caregivers in the sample were seen to be less likely to use 'baby talk' in either their tone of voice or selection of words. The findings further indicate how the tone of voice can be used to be either friendly and supportive or fearful and threatening. Whilst not identified by Sachweh as such, the tone of voice used when communicating with an older person can be linked to the use of the emotional labour tools. The tone of voice can be encouraging or threatening and consequently be part of the emotional labour tools such as gentle persuasion, firm direction, discomfort or force. This is exemplified by Sachweh's

(1999) description of the tone of voice used to communicate with non-compliant older people living in the sample home and highlight how order is established with the use of emotional labour tools. It is the creation of order so that bodywork can be performed efficiently which is crucial to formal caregiving. The following final section completes the circle as it relates back to the issue of time in caregiving initially considered in the policy review.

TIME TO CARE

Time to care has been an issue identified in the provision of domiciliary care by Ungerson (2000) and Twigg (2000b). Ungerson (2000) identifies how the shortage of time results in care tasks being fragmented so they can be performed at speed. This can be seen to reflect Lee-Treweek's (1997) observation that care is provided in the shortest possible time. However, neither Lee-Treweek (1997), Twigg (2000b) nor Ungerson (2000) follow through the issue they have highlighted to relate time to governmental long-term care policies.

The policy framework surrounding the provision of institutional longterm care in England and Germany determines the contact time in which 'hands-on care' can be provided to older people who live in care homes. This calls for time management skills in caregivers. Within the sphere of their family life, formal caregivers are likely to have developed skills that are useful within the care home environment. In their own home, many multi-tasking women are accustomed to managing the household time budget and fragmenting their own time into 'time bites'. Jurczyk (1998:298) describes how women develop into 'time acrobats, negotiating a tightrope, performing risky balancing acts without a safety net'. These balancing acts are a crucial element of care work. In order to maintain their balance on the tightrope, caregivers need to undertake emotional labour. Thereby establishing the link between invisible, intangible and immeasurable emotional labour skills with the measurable factor; time.

The staffing levels encountered in English and German care homes influences the available contact time between older people living in care homes and their caregivers. Ultimately it is government policies surrounding the care home industry in England and Germany that determine the ratio of qualified staff to care assistants on duty throughout the day. The number of caregivers on duty is relative to the number of care recipients and the time of day. The funding available to each individual in a German care home is determined by a care assessment that is then related to the time based care categories described earlier. This can be interpreted to be care rationing, as only basic care needs can be met within the resulting contact time.

Research reported by Wingenfeld and Schnabel (2002) in Germany, indicates that the amount of time needed to provide care is greater than that stipulated within their governments' longterm care policy framework. In the sampled homes they found that 83 minutes per care recipient per day was the average time needed to meet what was seen to be the absolutely necessary care needs. The data further indicated that there was little correlation between the care category an older person had been assessed to be in and the actual amount of time spent on their care, and care needs were described to be 'vast and complex' (Wingenfeld and Schnabel 2002: 26).

In keeping with the quality assurance culture encountered in both countries, procedural guidelines are being established aiming to ensure 'best practice' in care homes. Procedures that are developed within the quality assurance systems provide guidance on performing specific tasks within a given time frame and are exemplified in an article published in a German journal widely read by care home managers (Frosch and Zimmerscheid 1995). In this article, an example of the procedure used to assist a resident at mealtime is given; the task is to be undertaken by a qualified member of staff within an average time of 45 minutes. Considering the time element in German care funding, this could result in nearly half of the daily care time being taken up by a single meal for someone in Category II (minimum of two hours per day for basic care) indicating a procedure that must in reality be difficult for formal caregivers to implement.

The procedure relating to the task of assisting an older person with a meal will incorporate a combination of bodywork, emotional labour, communication and time management skills and would take place in what Davies (1994) describes to be 'process time' as opposed to 'clock time'. Within the context of childcare in Swedish nurseries, Davies (1994:279) argues that 'care requires process time' which she further sees as encapsulating the 'hidden' aspects of care giving. Davies (1994) defines 'process time' by focusing on the task of feeding and draws parallels between the care of an infant and a person who is senile, pointing out that it is difficult to pre-determine how long it will take to complete the task. In this instance, it is acknowledged that an older person's brain and motor skills may co-ordinate less well and that it takes time to chew and swallow food. How long that will take cannot be predetermined and the 'process time' is therefore immeasurable, despite the fact that within an institutional setting, eating is an activity structured by actual clock time. Davies (1994) consequently questions the quality of life experienced in such a situation. The example of quality assurance procedures outlined by Frosch and Zimmerscheid (1995) indicates the conflict between 'process time' and 'clock time' within an institutional environment and indicates the role of time in the provision of care. This indicates the importance of formal caregivers ability to balance 'process time' and 'clock time'.

The skills required to balance time in the provision of formal care was researched in a cross-national study of care home staff in England and Germany. The following sections present the research methods used in the study and provide an insight into the analysis and findings.

RESEARCH METHOD

The research methods used for the study presented in this chapter aimed to establish the skills used by formal caregivers in order to successfully provide care within a policy driven institutional temporal framework encountered in care homes. The study was conducted in purposively selected care homes, four in England and four in Germany (Eyers 2002). To establish if formal caregivers participating in the data collection were meeting the needs of similarly dependent older people, structured interviews were conducted with the care home managers. This interview data provided a profile of the dependency and needs of the residents and also a profile of the formal caregivers employed in the sample care homes.

To extract the blend of skills used by formal caregivers, data was collected by conducting audio-taped interviews lasting approximately 40 minutes with an average of three qualified members of staff and three care assistants in each of the four sample homes in both countries. In one German home four qualified staff and four care assistants were interviewed which lead to a total of 50 interviews. In the interview qualified staff and care assistants were asked to describe the work done on the day of the interview and were asked where they had learnt to care specifically for older people. This was followed by asking the participants to read and respond to text vignettes presenting everyday situations that could be encountered in English and German care homes. The four separate vignettes related to someone who has had a stroke (Edith); someone diagnosed to have Parkinson's disease (Phyllis); someone diagnosed to have Alzheimer's (John) and the fourth relates to Maude, a wheelchair bound amputee and Derrick who is not given a diagnosis but is described to have been doubly incontinent and going to unexpectedly need more time to be cared for. The following example is the vignette relating to Maude and Derrick (see appendix for the other three).

Maude is a mentally alert 78-year-old lady who is wheelchair-bound because she had both legs amputated six months ago. She has been in the home for six weeks and is still coming to terms with her situation. Once she is in her wheelchair she is able to partially wash and dress herself. However, she is unable to dress the lower half of her body. You have helped her onto her wheelchair and left her to wash and dress herself as far as she can. You have gone on to Derrick intending to return back to Maude. This usually works well but to your surprise Derrick has been doubly incontinent, this has caused a lot of mess as Derrick has unsuccessfully tried to cope with the situation himself. You may well have encountered a similar situation, what would you do?

Vignette Maude and Derrick

This vignette presents a situation where the emphasis is on the caregivers time management skills and conflicting responsibilities. Formal caregivers are confronted with a situation where they need to make decisions that can influence not only the well being of the two residents but also the outcome of their morning's work. Maude is described as a mentally alert, semi-independent person who is still coming to terms with the facts that her legs have been amputated and that she is having to live in a care home. No reference is made to Derrick's medical condition or cognitive abilities; the only information provided is that he has been doubly incontinent. Caring for Derrick will be unexpectedly time consuming, yet Maude's needs also have to be met. This vignette also presents a situation where respondents can refer to teamwork and communication with both residents and their colleagues in order to cope with the situation.

The German responses to the vignette and the description of their daily routine was transcribed into English, as having the data in one language facilitated 'open coding' analysis (Strauss and Corbin 1998). This provided the means to 'uncover, name and develop concepts, opening up the text to expose thoughts, ideas, and meanings contained therein' (Strauss and Corbin 1998:102). The interviewees' responses to the vignette were studied closely to establish how respondents for example related to 'time' which in turn created sub-categories such as 'taking time', 'making time', 'spending time' and 'shortage of time'. This process of coding is 'the act of relating categories to subcategories along the lines of their properties and dimensions' (Strauss and Corbin 1998:124) and provides an opportunity to look at how categories relate to one another. Each category relates to an issue that can be defined as being significant to the respondent whilst the subcategories answer questions and contribute towards giving the concept greater explanatory power (Strauss and Corbin 1998).

The combination of the data sets collected in this study provide an opportunity to link policy and practice. The study exemplified how, at 'grass-root' level, policies influenced the production of care and identified the skills used in order to effectively and efficiently provide care to older people living in English and German care homes.

The findings from the study will now be presented and discussed. After exemplifying data from the care home managers the interview data, including the responses to the text vignettes, will demonstrate how the essence of formal caregiving was extracted.

Research Findings

The comparison of the policy framework surrounding the care home industry in England and Germany indicated that contact time would be an important issue in the provision of care. This was confirmed by the data from the care home managers which identified a contrast in the contact time between formal caregivers and residents in England and Germany. The average contact time between resident and care staff during the most labour intensive two hours of the day was established. This was achieved by multiplying the number of care staff on duty by 120 minutes and dividing the resulting figure by the number of residents in the home that day. Consequently, in England, from 8-10am, each resident can on average expect a maximum of 29 minutes contact time with care staff. The staffing includes all qualified staff and care assistants on duty and the time includes any distances staff may need to walk between the nursing station, residents, bathrooms, sluices, laundry and kitchen. In Germany, each resident can on average expect a maximum of 16 minutes contact time with care staff from 6-8am. As in England, this time also includes distances staff may need to walk. However, the purpose build of a German home often means that the distances between all facilities are shorter than those encountered in England. This is because, at the time of data collection, a majority of English care homes were originally built as large family homes purchased specifically to be converted and extended into care homes to meet the needs of older people (Eyers 2002). Identifying the limited period of contact time in both countries indicated the importance of formal caregiving skills.

Key to this study was the interface between caregiver and the care recipient. From the perspective of an older person, the contact with a caregiver is strongly influenced by individual needs whilst from the perspective of caregiver the contact is influenced by their skills and the requirement to accomplish the tasks they are employed to do. The individual needs of an older person are linked to medical condition, care needs, social needs and the desire to maintain autonomy. The ability of caregivers to meet these individual needs within a limited period of time is determined by their care skills and ability to balance time. The data from this study contributed towards identifying a formula of skills that are vital to formal care giving. The elements of this formula will now be presented and discussed.

SKILLS USED TO PROVIDE CARE

The findings from interview data collated for this study indicate that the knowledge, understanding and skills required of care staff can be grouped into five categories: medical; bodywork; emotional sensitivity; communication and time budgeting. Together these categories can be seen to present the essence of caring for older people living in a care home. These individual elements that formulate the essence of caregiving will be presented in the following section of this chapter.

Medical Knowledge and Understanding

A resident's medical condition is a factor that impacts on many of their abilities to undertake daily activities independently. Understanding the medical condition in turn influences the approach care staff take towards the situations they encounter with residents, as their understanding facilitates their ability to effectively and efficiently provide care.

Not surprisingly the qualified staff in both countries generally presented an understanding of the medical conditions described in the vignettes. This was established by looking for specific indicators relating to each medical condition in the responses to the vignettes. However, in both countries there appears to be a greater understanding for residents living with Parkinson's than those living with Alzheimer's or a stroke. Amongst the care assistants in both countries, there was very little understanding of the medical conditions presented in any of the vignettes. Care assistants who did present an understanding of the medical conditions in the vignettes actually related the situation to experiences they had had within their family or with residents they knew to have been living with a stroke, Parkinson's or Alzheimer's. This is exemplified by Tracy, an English care assistant, who in response to the vignette 'John' said:

> **Tracy (English care assitant):** I have actually done some shifts on the MHU [Mental Health Unit] so its not too bad and my Nan had Alzheimer's – I used to care for her as well, so I would … Interview extract from response to vignette 'John'

The qualified staff in both England and Germany can be expected to have knowledge of older people living with medical conditions such as a 'stroke', 'Parkinson's' and 'Alzheimer's'. Whilst this was not always explicit in the responses to the vignettes, it is to be expected that during their training to become a qualified healthcare worker, they will have been taught about neurological and cardio-vascular illnesses that include the medical conditions described in the vignettes. Their occupational qualification implies medical knowledge of such diagnoses. However, in England this does not imply an understanding of the social care needs of an older person who is living in a care home, as opposed to receiving treatment in hospital. In Germany, the qualified staff who trained as general nurses are in a comparable situation, whereas the OPCs can be expected to have knowledge and understanding of older peoples health and social care needs.

Like the English qualified staff, the German qualified general nurses took a task-orientated approach to the situation presented in the vignettes. For instance, completing the task of washing and dressing Derrick, Edith or John took priority over considering or enquiring why they might be incontinent. It also excluded the older person from the planning process and possible opportunity to participate in the completion of the task and redevelop everyday personal care skills. However, the OPCs tended to take a more person-centred approach in their responses, an approach which can be expected to have a more positive impact on the quality of life encountered by the older people for whom they are employed to care.

In contrast, care assistants from both countries, at most, had an understanding of the medical condition based on their personal experience, either within the family or from their work caring for older people. This indicates a need to provide training to both qualified staff and care assistants in order to develop an understanding of the medical conditions prevalent amongst older people living in a care home. Such a knowledge base would, potentially, enable care staff to be more confident in knowing what an individual with a particular medical condition can be expected or encouraged to do independently. It would also provide a better understanding of the frustrations older people living in a care home might be experiencing. Knowledge of a medical condition also informs the care decision making process that forms part of the bodywork conducted by both qualified staff and care assistants. This in itself can result in a care task being completed more effectively and efficiently.

For the qualified staff in both countries, their knowledge and understanding had been measured, as they will have successfully passed exams that permit them to practice in their chosen occupation. However, the care assistants gained their skills invisibly and their knowledge and understanding of the medical conditions encountered in their work is intangible and immeasurable.

Understanding and Knowing How to Provide 'Hands-on-Care'

Understanding and knowing how to provide 'hands-on-care' is key to the undertaking of bodywork for older people in a care home. The provision of care in English and German care homes is task orientated towards providing care within a limited period of time and involves work that is physically heavy, dirty and highly repetitive.

In both England and Germany, the bodywork required to meet the needs of Maude and Derrick involves tasks that are defined to be 'basic care' (Grundpflege) such as washing and dressing. The term 'basic', used spontaneously in both English and German literature and by caregivers participating in the study, implies simplicity and devalues the importance of the task to an individual older person. How a care task is performed could be fundamental to their well-being.

Washing and dressing Edith, who has suffered a stroke, calls for a different knowledge base of bodywork skills from those required to care for Maude, a wheelchair bound amputee or John, living with Alzheimer's. Yet in each case, the initial task to get someone up, washed and dressed can be seen to be the same. For all caregivers, knowledge and understanding of how to provide the required care, especially to somebody who may have physical limitations or be cognitively impaired, is key to efficient caregiving. In the description of their daily work and in response to the vignettes, the participants themselves appeared to take bodywork for granted and expected others to find it unimportant. It is invisible work that takes place behind closed doors and involves the use of invisible, intangible skills that consequently appears not to merit discussion by the participants in this study.

Emotional Sensitivity

The responses to the vignettes indicated that emotional labour tools would be used in the situations described. However, the analysis of the data also identified a dichotomy in the emotions experienced and evoked in the provision of care. In his response to the vignette 'John' (appendix), a qualified member of staff in England indicated a potential revulsion against the smell he might encounter if John were doubly incontinent. A German care assistant, also indicated that she could be fearful of John becoming physically aggressive. These caregivers are experiencing emotions of revulsion and fear which they know they need to overcome. At the same time they will be evoking emotions in John that will make him co-operate with the actions they need to perform in order to undertake the bodywork needed to change his trousers. Experiencing revulsion and fear calls for the use of emotional labour skills to cope with their own emotions. At the same time, they are also using emotional labour tools, such as firm direction, in order to complete a care task as quickly as possible.

The qualified staff in both England and Germany can be expected to have received training that assisted them in developing strategies to cope with the emotions they experience when encountering situations in the conduct of bodywork that are initially unpleasant. An understanding of the medical conditions encountered in care homes can also be expected to provide qualified staff with a knowledge base that will result in the appropriate use of emotional labour tools. However, care assistants in both England and Germany are unlikely to have the support of tutors or mentors whilst they are developing their care skills and will, as the research findings indicated, invisibly learn from their colleagues how to deal with situations that arise.

During the interviews, all participants were asked where they had gained their skills to care for older people. Wiebke, a German care assistant who commenced employment in the care home after leaving school replied:

> **Wiebke (German care assistant):** ... I started on Unit 1 with Frau A [a care assistant] and Sister B who took me round with her and bit by bit she showed me what to do until I started to work alone with the residents....

Interview extract in response to the the question establishing where skills to care for an older person were gained.

Wiebke, indicates how she learnt to care for older people 'on-thejob'. Consequently the use of emotional labour tools such as listening, gentle persuasion, firm direction, force or by causing discomfort to the care recipient, will have been observed and potentially copied. However, the use of emotional labour tools is an essential skill used to provide care within a limited period of time. As much emotional labour takes place in conjunction with bodywork, it also happens behind closed doors and is invisible and immeasurable. However, the findings indicated that emotional labour was closely linked to communication.

Communication as an Instrument of Care

The responses to the vignettes and the description of the daily routine in this study indicate how communication is used as an instrument of care to create order but not to empower older people. In the provision of care, communication can be seen to be pivotal not only to gather information in order to make a care decision but also to implement emotional labour in order to control time. Even the use of the nurses call 'bell' system by older people living in a care home can be seen to be controlled by formal caregivers in order to support the budgeting of a valuable commodity, time. Taking control of the nurse call system is also physically taking control of time to maintain order in the process of providing care.

In the vignettes, asking Edith, Phyllis, John, and Maude and Derrick questions to gain background information about the situation they are confronted with would enable caregivers both to make care decisions and to empower the older person. However, as findings indicated, the decision making process undertaken by the majority of care staff was based on their personal knowledge and understanding of the medical condition and the situation they were confronted with. As the extract from the interview with Dagmar, a German care assistant, indicates, if a task needs doing, it is done without question.

> **Dagmar (German care assistant):** … If she needs to be cleaned up then it goes without saying that's what I do. I make sure she is clean before she has her breakfast. …

Interview extract from response to vignette 'Edith'

This lack of communication indicates the importance of providing care staff with a sound knowledge base of medical conditions encountered in care homes, therefore enabling the skilled completion of bodywork. It further indicates an insufficient understanding and knowledge of the link between health and social care needs of older people living in a care home and how disempowering the lack of communication can be for an older person in this situation. However, the research findings do indicate that communication was clearly used to implement emotional labour tools by care staff in both countries. The use of emotional sensitivity exemplified indicates its role in enabling caregiving within the temporal framework of a care home that will be discussed in the next section.

Balancing Time

The temporal framework of a care home is structured around the shifts of care staff and residents' meal times. Care of the residents' bodily needs is provided within the approximately two hour 'time bites' that these factors create during the day. Within the time bites, caregivers need to balance often conflicting 'process time' with 'clock time'. For example the 'process time' needed to assist Derrick to wash and dress after being doubly incontinent is in conflict with the average 'clock time' of 16 minutes available for his care. In the analysis of the data the concepts 'taking time', 'making time' 'spending time' and 'a shortage of time' indicated how formal caregivers budgeted the time at their disposal will now be exemplified.

Taking Time

In the data analysis, it became clear that 'taking time' literally meant taking away time initially allocated to one resident to meet unexpected needs of another. Within the context of the responses to the vignettes, 'taking time' is a factor that can be observed in the respondent's description of how they would behave in the given situations. 'Taking time' can be seen to mean that someone is creating 'process time' to complete a task thoroughly and to the best of their ability. The use of the term 'take' however also implies gaining possession. This in turn raises the issue of the ownership of time. Does the resident own the time they need for their care because they are paying to receive care? In Germany the funding system is explicitly related to the timing of care. In England, at the time of data collection, in the norm, the cost of a care home placement was not related to the amount of time needed to provide care. However, care is one of the main services a care home is providing and therefore it is justifiable to state that residents pay for time as a commodity in the same way as they do for their meals and other 'hotel services' received in the home. As such the commodity 'time' is then controlled by the care home management and allocated to care staff to use to the best of their ability. They in turn are paid for the work they undertake to provide care. Consequently care staff can be seen to rightfully be in control of time as a commodity that is distributed back to the care recipient as the purchaser.

The responses to the care vignettes exemplify the impact of 'taking time' to perform tasks thoroughly, as they highlight how staff adapt to expected but not regular situations that arise within their daily routine. This is an example of how the balance between process time and clock time is achieved when undertaking care work.

Making Time

A method of accommodating 'process time' is also found in the concept of 'making time'. The interview data indicated that this meant being creative and carefully planning a work schedule and is a concept that can be observed in the responses to the vignettes and in the description of the daily work of the interviewees in both countries. It can be seen as a term that describes forward planning to create anticipated 'process time'. Whilst time is a restricted commodity, care staff in both countries appear to see how they can creatively use and take control of time.

This is exemplified by Meta, a German care assistant, who clearly describes how she made extra time for her morning shift by showering a resident the previous day. Meta also describes how the night staff create extra 'process time' for the day staff by preparing a resident for the day. Meta relates to time in her response to the vignette 'Edith' (appendix) and describes her actual situation as follows:

> **Meta (German care assistant):** ... everybody has to be down in the dining room for breakfast at 8:00. Breakfast is served from 8 to 9 and the residents all feel they have to be down at 8:00 on the dot and that is almost impossible for us to achieve. Yesterday I showered somebody in advance, so they didn't need showering this morning. That way I only needed to give one resident a shower this morning. That made this morning bearable. But if you're on your own and you've got seven people to look after - actually it is only six, because there is

> one who looks after herself. The night staff usually do one, it's a lot of work if you've got to shower, wash and dress the residents in a short period of time. Then there is Mr. N. who has a urine catheter, a colostomy and he's got a gastric tube. I usually take care of him when the others are all down at breakfast, poor man.

Interview extract from response to vignette 'Edith'.

This extract shows how Meta creatively manages her allocated time and how she actually chooses to care for a highly dependent resident when she knows most others residents are preoccupied eating their breakfast and therefore less likely to use their 'bell' and interrupt her while she is caring for him. Whilst Meta did not use the term 'making time' she can none the less be seen to have ownership of her time at work and is able to 'make time' in order to facilitate 'process time'.

Spending Time

The concept 'spending time' identifies time as a valuable resource that has to be controlled and budgeted. Time as a commodity can only be 'spent' if it readily available. In her response to the 'Edith' vignette, Helen talks about 'spending time' whilst making it clear to Edith that, unfortunately, there are times when she might have to be patient and wait for someone to come and assist her. Helen made the following comment after reading the vignette 'Edith':

> **Helen (English care assistant):** You've just got to make sure when you get this lady up, you've got time to make sure she has got her hearing aid in – so you can spend time talking to her and reassuring her that, unfortunately, in a home you can be left for a couple of hours before the next person comes on and does anything, is a normal situation.

Interview extract from response to vignette 'Edith'.

On the one hand, Helen is willing to 'spend time', yet, at the same time, she would be making it clear to Edith that in a care home, time was a rare commodity. This exemplifies how time can impact on the quality of care and how 'spending time' is also part of emotional labour, thereby highlighting how emotional labour and time management are closely linked skills which impact on the care older people experience when living in a care home.

Shortage of Time

Care staff responses from both countries related both overtly and covertly to time. Given the availability of time to English and German care staff, it was to be anticipated that the shortage of time would be an issue. The shortage of time was identified by interviewees to be related to what they perceived to be a shortage of staff. However, all participating care homes had staffing levels in keeping with government policies. In England, Audrey was acutely aware of the lack of time. Her response to the 'Edith' vignette was:

> **Audrey (English care assistant): ...** It's lack of staff - it's terribly stressful - you just cannot do the job properly because you don't have time.

Interview extract from response to vignette 'Edith'.

Joyce, an English qualified nurse, clearly pointed out the shortage of time for all care staff by stating the following:

> **Joyce (English qualified nurse):** Myself - and as I feel the majority of my staff would also like to say they'd give the appropriate care but it would have to be done quickly - we don't have the time to be spending an hour with this lady even though we would like to, and she is frustrated by her condition but we also have the time factor to think of. I would want to help her with her breakfast - make her a fresh cup of tea, perhaps make her fresh toast or a sandwich - to encourage her to have something to eat - not just leave it until the coffee round at ten. ...
>
> **...** - just try to encourage her to eat something at least - and obviously whilst she's doing that, I could be making the bed at the same time - that cuts down the time spent.

Interview extract from response to vignette 'Edith'.

Joyce also exemplifies the use of emotional labour tools and how she would potentially budget the commodity 'time' by multi-tasking and not only talking to Edith but also by making the bed whilst encouraging Edith to eat.

Roswitha, a German OPC (Older Persons Carer), made the statement:

> **Roswitha (OPC)**: ...Breakfast is not important, she's got all day to eat it! Our residents have plenty of time, we don't...

Interview extract from response to vignette 'Edith'.

Whilst Roswitha did not necessarily know there was only an average of 16 minutes available for each care recipient between 6 and 8am she was, like her English colleague Joyce, conscious of the fact that there was an unavoidable shortage of contact time between caregivers and care recipients.

CONCLUSION

The findings from this research indicate that the relationship between caregivers and older people living in a care home is strongly influenced by an amalgam of invisible skills that form the 'care production lubricant'. This lubricant enables caregivers to work within the temporal framework imposed upon them by government policies. It is clear that caregivers in both England and Germany provide care to older people living in care homes with the best intentions and to the best of their ability. As the findings indicate, caring for older people is by no means unskilled work and calls for specialised skills.

This study relates measurable 'clock time' to the invisible, intangible and immeasurable skills used by formal caregivers to facilitate 'process time' within a restrictive temporal framework. The essence of the 'care production lubricant' consists of:

1. Knowledge and understanding of the health and social care needs of older people living in a care home
2. The ability to provide 'hands on care'
3. Emotional sensitivity
4. Using of communication as a care tool
5. The ability to balance time

It is the blend of these components that form the essence of care. A weakness in just one of these components could be detrimental to effective and efficient formal caregiving to older people living in a care home.

All caregivers require an understanding of older people's medical condition. This needs to be accompanied by attributes that include an understanding and knowledge of how to provide care, an accomplished use of emotional labour, the skill to work within 'time bites' and the ability to communicate to enable empowerment. Only if these attributes are acknowledged, enhanced and rewarded by policy makers can older people living in English and German care homes hope to experience a good person centred caregiving that facilitates quality of life.

Recommendations

It has in the past been recognised that formal caregiving is an area of employment that is taken for granted and undervalued (James 1992; Lawler 1991; Lee-Treweek 1996). Having extracted the essence of caregiving it is to be hoped that it will be possible to inform policy makers of the important role these skills have in providing effective and efficient care.

The comparative nature of this study identified the importance of time in the provision of care and the, to date, unacknowledged skills used by formal caregivers in order to provide care within the contact time determined by government policy. The findings from this study result in the following recommendations being made to policy makers:

1. Acknowledge and value the importance of formal caregivers invisible, intangible and immeasurable skills in both countries
   a) Heighten the awareness of the importance and value of the 'care production lubricant'
   b) Ensure these skills are recognised and included in training programmes for all formal caregivers employed to meet the needs of older people
   c) Ensure they are acknowledged and rewarded as highly valuable skills in the employment market.
   d) Ensure funding of a care home placement is such that the care home industry can afford to provide training and financially reward formal caregivers.
2) Improve contact time in the provision of care.
   a) In Germany an increase in the care time stipulated in the funding categories
   b) In England design future care homes to facilitate an efficient working environment.

If policy makers in England and Germany take these recommendations on board it would enhance the lives of formal caregivers and most importantly that of care recipients and their family and friends who continue to care about them.

ACKNOWLEDGEMENT

This chapter was written during my time as an ESRC Postdoctoral Research Fellow (PTA-026-27-290) at the University of Surrey, Department of Sociology. I would like to thank the ESRC for this Fellowship and the studentship (R42200024125*)*, which enabled me to gain my PhD. I would also like to thank Professor Sara Arber for her support and guidance throughout my time as a PhD student and the writing of this chapter.

REFERENCES:

Beck, C.H. (1995) *SGB XI Soziale Pflegeversicherung mit Nebenbestimmungen.* Deutscher Taschenbuch Verlag, Munich, Germany.

Davies, K. (1994) 'The Tensions between Process Time and Clock Time in Care-Work. The example of day nurseries', *Time and Society*, 3(3) 277-303

Davies, S. (2001) 'The care needs of older people and family care givers in continuing care settings' in M., Nolan, S., Davies, and G., Grant (eds.)*Working with older people and their families. Key issues in policy and practice*, (pp75-98)Buckingham, Open Univerity Press

Department of Health (2000) *Care Standards Act,* HMSO, London

Department of Health (2001b) 'Free Nursing Care' [online] *www.doh.gov.uk/jointunit/freenursingcare.htm* (Accessed 14th June2001)

Esping-Andersen G. (1990) *The Three Worlds of Welfare Capitalism*, Princeton, New Jersey, Princeton University Press

Eyers, I. (2000a)'Care assistants overlooked? A cross-national study of care home staff in England and Germany', *Quality in Ageing - Policy, practice and research*, 1(1), 15-26

Eyers, I. (2000b)'Education and Training. Do they really, really want it? A comparative study of care home staff in England and Germany', *Education and Ageing*, 15(2), 159-175

Eyers, I. (2002) 'Die Verwendung von Vignetten in qualitativer, kulturvergleichender Alternsforschung ' (Use of vignettes in qualitative cross cultural in gerontology) in Motel-Klingebiel, A. and Kelle, U. (eds.) *Perspektiven der empirischen Alternssoziologie*. Opladen: Leske und Budrich

Frosch, M. and Zimmerscheid, I. (1995) 'Qualitätsmanagement nach DIN ISO 9000. Umsetzung in die Praxis' *Altenheim*1/95 pp18-27

Goberg O. (1997) *Taschenkommentar zum Heimgesetz und zugehoerige Verordnungen*, Hannover, Vincentz Verlag,

Hochschild, A.R. (1983) *The Managed Heart: Commercialization of Human Feeling.* Berkeley, University of California Press,

James, N. (1989) 'Emotional Labour: skill and work in the social regulation of feelings' *Sociological Review*, 37 (1), 15- 42

James, N. (1992) 'Care = organisation + physical labour + emotional labour.' *Sociology of Health and Illness*, 14(4), 488-509

Jurczyk, K. (1998) 'Time in Women's Everyday Lives. Between self-determination and conflicting demands, *Time and Society* 7(2): 283-308

Klie.T. (1997) *Recht der Altenhilfe. Die wichigsten Gesetze und Vorschriften*, Vincentz Verlag, Hannover, Germany

Lawler, J. (1991) *Behind the screens. Nursing, Somology, and the Problems of the Body.* Churchill, Livingstone,

Lee-Treweek, G. (1996) 'Emotion work, order and emotional power in care assistant work' in V., James and J. Gabe, (eds) *Health and the Sociology of Emotions* (pp. 115-132). Oxford, Blackwell Publishers

Lee-Treweek, G. (1997) 'Women Resistance and Care; An ethnographic study of nursing auxiliary work', *Work, Employment and Society* 11(1), 47-63

Mason, J. (1996) 'Gender, Care and Sensibility in Family and Kin Relationships' in J. Holland, and L., Adkins (eds) *Sex, Sensibility and the Gendered Body*, (pp15-36) Houndsmill, MacMillan,

Ribbens, J (1994) *Mothers and Their Children*, London, Sage, Twigg, J. (2000b) Carework as a form of bodywork , *Ageing and Society* , 20(4) 389-411)

Sachweh, S (1999) *'Schätzle hinsitze!' Kommunikation in der Altenpflege*, Frankfurt am Main, Peter Lang,

Strauss, A. and Corbin, J. (1998) *'Basics of Qualitative Research. Techniques and Procedures for Developing Grounded Theory'* London, Sage

Twigg, J. (2000a) Carework as a form of bodywork , *Ageing and Society* , 20(4) 389-411)

Twigg, J. (2000b) *Bathing – the Body and Community Care*, London, Routledge,

Twigg, J. (2002) The Body in Social Policy; Mapping a Territory, Journal of Social Policy, 31(3) 421-439

Ungerson, C. (2000) 'Thinking About the Production and Consumption of Long-term Care in Britain: Does Gender Still Matter', *Journal of Social Policy*, 29(4) 623-643

Valins, O. (2002) *Facing the Future. The provision of long-term care facilities for older Jewish people in the United Kingdom*, London, Institute for Jewish Policy Research

Wingenfeld, K. and Schnabel, E. (2002) 'An der Grenze zur Überforderung' *Altenheim* 4,pp26-31

Williams, C. (2002) *Mothers, Young People and Chronic Illness*, Aldershot, Ashgate

APPENDIX: TEXT VIGNETTES

1. Edith

Edith is an 87-year-old widow; she had a stroke 6 months ago and was admitted to the home eight weeks ago. The stroke has affected her speech and she is not able to move her right arm. Her right leg has also been affected by the stroke. Edith uses a hearing aid and wears glasses and has dentures. However with help Edith is able to stand and hold onto her frame and with support and guidance she is for example able to transfer from bed to chair. Edith is frustrated by her condition and tends to be grumpy in the morning. Invariably Edith also needs help to go to the toilet. She no longer has a urine catheter. The night-staff sit her on the commode around 6am but then return her to her bed. You have come on duty at 8am and this morning she is in your group of residents. When you go into her room you find she is incontinent and has not touched her breakfast. You probably know someone like Edith – think about that person and tell me how that morning would have been, considering that you also have other residents to care for.

This text vignette establishes a situation whereby the stroke that Edith has suffered impacts on her ability to communicate verbally. She also has dentures and a hearing aid, which are likely to have been part of her daily life for many years and could be seen as a part of Edith before she had the stroke and could therefore be seen as part of her identity. The fact that she had a wet bed could well be related to the stroke, especially as she previously had a urine catheter in situ, which could be a factor that needs to be considered in the provision of care. That she had not eaten breakfast could be approached by care staff from two different angles – she might have lost control of her bladder just after breakfast was served and subsequently lost her appetite. Alternatively breakfast could have been placed in front of her but the effect of the stroke meant that she was not enabled to eat her breakfast independently if it was not positioned correctly or care staff had not yet got round to assisting her and in the meantime she has lost control of her bladder. Edith was described as a person who was 'grumpy', a factor that could either be part of her personality or related to the fact that she was living with a Stroke. However, with help and guidance Edith could maintain a degree of independence. Although she had difficulties speaking, she was able to speak and with her hearing aid in place and dentures in her mouth she should have been able to communicate with the care staff. With support from care staff she was able to transfer from her bed to a chair, this represented something that Edith was able to do. The vignette was placed in the busiest time of day thereby putting the interviewees into a time of day they would relate to as being very busy if not hectic at times. Care staff with an understanding of Edith's medical condition and ability to provide person-centred care could empower Edith to participate in the planning of her care and provide her with choice that could impact on her quality of life. Encouraging Edith to be proactive would also help her towards regaining some independence.

2. Phyllis

Phyllis is 83 and has had Parkinson's for over 10 years. Her family are no longer able to care for her at home and she has now been in the home for a year. You have got to know her well and know her likes and dislikes, abilities and disabilities. Phyllis is one of the residents you care for this morning. Getting her up, washed and dressed went well this morning, however this lunchtime the picture has changed a bit and she is going to need a lot of help to eat her lunch as she can't get a cup or spoon to her mouth. You probably also know someone like Phyllis, considering you also have other residents such as Edith to help, how do you ensure that Phyllis eats her lunch?

This text vignette establishes a situation whereby Phyllis, who had been living with Parkinson's for over 10 years, presents a situation where the care staff know the resident well and are therefore more likely to be able to assess her needs. However, the complexities of someone living with Parkinson's need to be considered in the approach towards assisting her at lunchtime. Here empowerment and independence would play an important factor in the provision of her care.

3. John

John is 76 and has Alzheimer's. His wife could no longer cope with him at home and he has now been in the home for three months. He wanders around the home a great deal and tends to forget to use the toilet. It's mid afternoon and you walk pass him and can smell that he has been incontinent. You probably also know someone like John, how do you go about getting him changed into clean dry clothes when he thinks that he has to go and check the boiler is working properly?

This text vignette establishes a situation whereby John exemplifies many confused older people living in care homes. He was described to be living with Alzheimer's because at present within everyday terminology this appears to be the blanket term used for a confused older person. It would appear to be more socially acceptable than 'dementia' and is a diagnosis all levels of care staff can be expected to be able to relate to. The key element of this vignette was to establish how care staff would cope with having to get him to change his clothes whilst maintaining his dignity and enabling him to be empowered to participate in the decision making process in planning the activity.

In: Family Caregiving for Older Disabled People
Editor: Isabella Paoletti, pp. 295-317 ISBN 1-59454-808-0

Chapter 14

THE VALUE OF THE WORK: ON EMPLOYMENT FOR FAMILY CARE IN SWEDEN

Ann-Britt M. Sand
Umeå University, Department of Social Work, Umeå, Sweden

INTRODUCTION

Most countries in the Western World today face the same phenomena, a growing number of elderly, especially among the oldest old. An older population means an increasing need for care. From a juridical point of view responsibility for care of the old varies depending on country and type of welfare system. In Sweden the municipalities have the utmost responsibility to provide the elderly, ill and disabled with the assistance they need to make living at home possible. Still, as in other countries, relatives do most of the caring (e.g. Johansson 1991; SoS-rapport 1994:22).

Being an informal care provider may affect life in many ways, physically, psychologically and socially. The predicaments of informal care often include the issue of financial support. It may, for instance, prove difficult to combine care of a relative with paid employment. Financial arrangements to support caring for relatives exist in several countries (see e.g. Evers et. al. 1994; Sipilä 1994; Walker 1995; Johansson 1997). These arrangements may be care allowances, disability allowances, cash payments or tax deductions, to mention the more common types of financial support. These allowances are frequently tied directly to the person in need of help, enabling her or him to pay for certain help.

The aim of this chapter is to present and discuss some results of an investigation concerning another type of economic support to family caregivers, namely employment (Mossberg Sand 2000). The principal differences between unpaid care providers, or those with care support allowance on the one hand, and the care providers in this study on the other, are terms of employment and wages. These very conditions were the pivotal point of the study. The relative providing care service is seen as an employed member of the municipality's Home Help Service staff and is to have the same conditions as other employed personnel. Sweden was one of the first countries to introduce this type of support, which has existed since the 1960s. The investigation upon which this chapter is based is to date the only comprehensive investigation and evaluation of employment for relative care in Sweden. The investigation includes four studies, among them a survey study with responses from 1197 persons, representing one-fifth of all those who were employed as relative care providers in the mid 1990s.

Employed relative care providers are a small, yet interesting group since they have experienced the consequences of this type of support. Most research on payment for informal care focuses on care allowances. A care allowance is not comparable to an ordinary wage. In this study of the employed kin care providers I attempt to see their work as comparable to other work in the labor market. *A central question in the chapter is how the work considered here is to be assessed and evaluated compared to professional care work. Another main question concerns the family care providers' own experiences of employment, regarding both financial aspects as well as working conditions.*

Employment provides social security and pension credits for the care provider. Employment furthermore, also means that the person doing the work receives an income. Other kinds of financial support lack the privileges that employment provides and are thus less beneficial to the care provider. I will therefore argue that employment and wages are a better alternative compared to other forms of financial compensation. There are, however, also some difficulties that should be addressed. The chapter deals accordingly with the advantages and problems of being an employed kin care provider.

Even though this chapter dicusses kin care providers in Sweden, the results can be seen as relevant for kin care providers in other countries as well. With a growing number of elderly, questions concerning kin care seem to be more interesting than ever, irrespective of welfare system. That economic problems for the care provider can arise in connection to informal care is a well known risk and payment for informal care is an internationally noted topic (Sipilä and Simon 1993; Evers et al. 1994; Walker 1995; Ungerson 1996). How the work discussed here is to be assessed and evaluated is an open question.

Three circumstances are important to keep in mind when discussing care in the family in Sweden. One is that the *individual is seen as a separate, independent unit in relation to the family in legislation.* The second is that the point of departure is that *both men and women work for wages*. A third circumstance that is closely connected to these two is that *the social security system is based on individuals working for wages.*

In order to understand the comparison between the terms of employment for kin care providers and those of professional care workers it is necessary to place it within the context of Swedish society, which will be done in the subsequent section. I will first present a short overview of background information, focused on demography, legislation and the development of equal rights in Sweden. Secondly, I will describe the concept of employed relative care provider. Following this introduction, methodology and results for the four studies will be presented. In the analysis section I will deal with the following subjects: comparison of working conditions, the question of fair working conditions, division of duties between the kin care providers and others, and advantages of employment. The chapter ends with a discussion, conclusion and some recommendations.

The Swedish Context

There are several reasons to include Sweden in a book about the elderly and family care in an international perspective. Sweden has a long history of an aging population. The age of retirement is 65 years for both men and women. As early as 1975 individuals over 65 years of age constituted 15 percent of the population (SCB 2000). Today the figure is 18 percent which means that 1,5 million individuals are over the age of retirement. The oldest old (80+) total about 430.000 individuals and this group has more than doubled since 1975 (Thorslund and Larsson 2002). Within 25 years it is estimated that the share of retired people will be one fourth of the entire population.

One aspect of the demographic curve is that many newly retired people still have living parents and parents-in-law (about 15-20%, SCB 2000). Another aspect is that the majority of older individuals, about 80 percent, lives at home and cares for themselves or receives help from relatives. Those receiving public home care service have always comprised a minority of the elderly, but as the number of elderly increases more individuals will be in need of help (Sand 2003).

It is unusual that several generations live together in Sweden. Nowadays only a few percent of older people live with their children (Sundström 1994). Most old people live as married or single, but many elderly have at least one child living nearby and about one tenth have children who live in the neighborhood. The web of family surrounding older people is extensive and has been strengthened during the last half century; figures from 1954 and onwards show that personal contacts have increased (ibid.). Interaction between family members from different generations has increased and a survey investigation from the Commission of the European Communities shows that old people in Sweden see themselves as being less alone than old people in other countries (Age and Attitudes 1993). This can be compared to elderly in the countries of southern Europe who feel more alone, despite the fact that they more often live with adult children (Socialstyrelsen 1993:4).

Another characteristic of Sweden is that the state has been perceived as an intermediate of welfare services. The state has taken responsibility for different risks in the lives of individuals, for example by providing universal health insurance, unemployment benefits and pension system. Sweden has a rather large public sector and legislation that places responsibility for the welfare of elderly on society. People in need of assistance are to be provided with the opportunity to continue to live at home, and the task of making it possible lies with the municipalities. This has been a goal since the 1950s. Access to societal assistance is a question of equality and concerns the rights of the individual to receive support regardless of family situation. In Sweden voluntary organizations and the private market do not have the same importance when it comes to the care of older people as they do in countries where the public sectors is less encompassing.

A guiding principle is that the care of old people is a matter of solidarity and should be financed with taxes; need rather than purchasing power should determine access to and level of service (Reg.prop. 1990/91:14; Reg. prop. 1997/98:113). Those who can afford to pay for care do not receive preferential treatment. Nor is public care for the older aimed at the poorest old. Publicly financed care and service is to be attainable for everybody and it should furthermore be of good quality (Sipilä 1997). This does, however, not mean an acceptance of society's interference in private life. Most individuals receiving care are satisfied with the state's involvement and the preferences among old people to obtain such help and care are clear (Svallfors 1996). Especially older women seem to prefer municipal care compared to e.g. help from their own children (Andersson 1993). A common view here is that they are aware of the hard work involved in care work, and that they prefer to have a more independent and friendly relationship with their children, not one bound by obligations.

Sweden is supposed to be the most equal country in the world, at least when it comes to possibilities for women to take part in politics and working life (SOU 1998:6; Stark and Regnér 2001) and legislation aims at promoting gender equality. Women are employed almost to the same extent as men. Swedish women with a lower level of education are more likely to be employed compared to their counterparts in other countries and Sweden is the European Union country with the lowest percentage of housewives. In 1999 only two percent of women of working age were housewives (SCB 2000). This is also true for older women which distinguishes Sweden and other Nordic countries from, for instance, countries in southern Europe (Stark and Regnér 2001).

The possibility of employment for women is due in part to the construction and expansion of a public sector. Through the public sector, which expanded heavily between 1950 and 1970, tasks earlier performed by women at home were moved to the labor market (Axelsson 1992). This is true for health care and care for children and the elderly. The mobilization of female workers was supported by the ideological debate about equality between women and men (Björnberg 1992). An important aspect of this was, among other things, the possibility for women to have their own income. In the beginning of the 1970s changes in taxation rules for married couples made it difficult for a family to live on one income.

The function and role of the family have changed as society has changed. The traditional family of the 1950s, with a male breadwinner and a non-employed woman, has been replaced by the two-earner family (ibid.). This means that both women and men are expected to contribute to supporting the family through work for wages. The family is also more heterogenous than before. Since the 1970s the rate of divorce and separation has increased, as has the number of single person households. Swedish family politics is not directed to the family as such but rather aims at facilitating and supporting individual independency. The Welfare State could thus be regarded as a protector of the individual irrespective of whether the person lives in a family or not.

Keeping in mind that the vast majority of women and men are employed, it is understandable that the need for public care services, including compensation for kin care, is large in Sweden. This fact can also be expected to increase the demand for public help, as it is not expected that anybody should give up working in order to care for a relative, at least not according to the dominant political and ideological goals.

With women in the labor market and a public sector responsible for the elderly, one might believe that care for the elderly and handicapped within the family is marginal in Sweden. However, care in private homes is hardly possible without the efforts of relatives who perform the main part of all such assistance, sometimes at great sacrifice (e.g. Johansson 1991; SoS-rapport 1994:2). Informal care provided by relatives might detrimentally affect their possibility to work outside the home, a risk that politicians are aware of. In the beginning of the 1980s The Committee on Relative Care, appointed by the government, recommended that municipalities provide support and assistance to relatives in their care work and offer suitable forms of employment (Ds S 1981:15, SOU 1983:64). Suggestions were made to introduce a more regulated form of employment, and to give relatives the same conditions as other employed personnel. Later, other governmental inquiries expressed the same notion; relatives' care efforts should be based on voluntary action and the caregiver should receive municipal help and support (e.g. SOU 1994:139). Despite these official recommendations however, informal care was not mentioned in legislation until 1998 and the municipalities are still not required to provide help to relatives through employment or allowances.

The context and history presented above, as well as the growing percentage of older people, constituted an important starting point for the study concerning employed relative care providers which was conducted in the mid 1990s.

The Concept of Employed Relative Care Provider

In the remainder of this text, the person needing/receiving assistence is throughout the text referred to as the care recipient. To refer to a relative's care provided in the home several terms are used: informal care, family care, relative care, kin care etc. In this text I discuss relatives who are employed to provide care. The concept *employed relative care provider* refers then to a person who is employed by the municipalities Home Help Services to assist a relative. This could also include individuals not related to the family such as neighbors and friends. Employment is based on the fact that the individual in need of care applies for municipal help and specifies that he or she wants the relative as helper. It may also be the relative who points out the need for help. The relative must thereafter be judged as suitable for providing care. Regardless of whether personnel of Home Help Service or a relative provide the assistance, the relationship is based on an estimate of the needs of the care recipient. Assistance is given according to the sixth paragraph of the Social Services Act. The care recipient is thereby registered with the Home Help Services and pays a service fee according to municipality regulation. The care provider is then in turn paid a monthly salary, which is based on the amount of care agreed upon. The salary is the same as that of a nurse assistant and covers a maximum of 40 working hours a week. The care provider submits a report showing the care recipient's stay in hospital or nursing home, or that the care provider has been off duty and deductions are made accordingly. The Home Help administrator (in the text also called middle manager) is formally the manager of the nurse assistants as well as of the employed kin care providers.

There are differences between the employed relative care providers and the nurse assistants regarding grounds for employment. A nurse assistant is to have some training in handicap or elderly care. (Practical experience can be counted as the equivalent of training). This is not the case with relatives, even if they sometimes may attend courses on how to handle special disabilities e.g. dementia or schizophrenia. The nurse assistant can, like the kin care provider, have the help of one or two persons. They may also have a close relationship with the care recipient, however, there is no kinship or relation between them. A nurse assistant can be moved to another district, or be assigned to other care recipients. The employed kin care provider cannot be moved or ordered to provide assistence to anyone but the relative.

The Investigation on the Employed Relative Care Providers

The main purpose of the investigation was to study and analyze how life is affected when a relative becomes dependent on long-term assistance, and what employment means in this situation. The municipality is the employee of the kin care providers. The terms of employment call for shared duties between the kin care providers and the municipality. Yet another purpose of the study was to investigate how responsibility and work are distributed between municipalities and kin care providers.

At the outset, nothing was known about employed kin care providers except for the number of them in each municipality. This meant that a rather thorough investigation was considered necessary. The results discussed here are based upon a project containing four studies (Mossberg 1996; Mossberg Sand 2000; Sand 2002). All were of an explorative nature and the studies were to follow each other in order to make use of the knowledge from the previous one(s). *The first study* consisted of telephone interviews with directors of Social Welfare Services and elderly care managers in 50 municipalities and district municipalities, taken from a random sample. Each interview took about 20 minutes. The directors were asked about the situation of formal as well as informal care in the municipality. They were also asked about employment and other kinds of societal help for those who provided help to a relative. The directors provided information about plans for the future concerning care for the handicapped and the elderly, but they had hardly any knowledge at all about informal care or employment for such care.

The second study was a postal survey investigation directed to Home Help Service administrators (middle managers) in the 50 municipalities that were included in the first investigation. Survey responses from 162 middle managers were received. Only persons with experience of employed family care providers were included. As the middle managers are supervisors for the nurse assistants as well as for the family care providers, their responses were of great interest. It is they who decide whether the family care provider will be employed. The middle managers answered questions about the employed family care providers in their district and how they felt about this kind of employment. Being the supervisor for a person who is not a part of the ordinary staff can be difficult. A family care provider does not help other care recipients, and will probably not attend personnel meetings or be interested in other work place related matters. The middle managers may have an interest in elderly care being regarded as a professional job, however this image might be difficult to maintain when untrained family member are involved. They may also feel that family care is a private matter, not to be publicly funded. The investigators' assumptions about middle managers' experiences of problems with employing family care providers proved to be correct. Still, most of the middle managers were concerned about the informal care providers and they wanted to help; however they did not always know how to handle the situation. As their supervisors did not know much about informal care, the middle managers were left on their own to find ways of handling the situation.

For *the third study* an additional random sample of 50 municipalities was made to make a total of 100. A postal survey was sent to all employed relative care providers in these municipalities. Fifteen of the municipalities did not have any employed relative care providers at the time of the investigation. Replies came from 1197 relative care providers in

86 municipalities and district municipalities in Sweden (the response rate was 85 percent). At the time of the investigation, the respondents represented one-fifth of all employed relative care providers in the country.

The questionnaire was very extensive (68 questions) and covered various aspects of the situation for the care provider as well as for the care recipient. There were questions about working situation, economy, how long they had been care providers, how long they had been employed, whether they received help from the municipality, what help they wanted and if they were discontent in any way. Some questions had more of a psychological character: whether there had been any changes in their relationship to the care recipient, was the care responsibility voluntarily or not, how did they deal with the relative's demands, if they could trust other care providers, how they managed to find leisure time and to keep up a social life. Several questions were similar and were meant to, in different ways, seek answers and nuances that might not be as clear if only one question was asked, especially in areas loaded with subjective or moral judgments. The main results from this study will be presented below.

The survey responses of the employed relative care providers were investigated more deeply in *the fourth study* which was an interview study with 40 of the relative care providers who had participated in the third study. In some cases their care recipient also participated. The interviews took place in five different parts of Sweden in order to cover different geographical circumstances. The aim was not to get what is called "theoretical satisfaction" (Glaser and Strauss 1967), rather it was to get deeper insight into the different lives of the employed family care providers. Each interview took about two hours and was tape-recorded.

The collected material was treated in a process involving interaction between data, theory, analysis and interpretation. The two first studies are of a descriptive art and provided background information. In the third study primarily logistic regression was used to seek explanations when many variables were included. The interview (fourth) study provides a deeper understanding by using examples and quotes.

MAIN RESULTS

In the following section I will present some main results from the third study before I return to the questions in focus in this chapter. The results are based on the responses from 1197 between 19 and 86 years of age, with the majority between 45 and 65 (Table 1). The employed relative care providers' relationship to the care reciepient was divided into three groups: children (32%), spouses (27%) and parents (25%). In addition, a smaller group (16%) consists of other types of relations that emerged, namely siblings, daughters-in-law, other relatives and friends. The majority of the kin care providers are women, but 15 percent are men. Women experience greater obligations to perform care work (e.g. Finch and Mason 1993) and the fact that 85 percent of the kin care providers are female is no coincidence. The majority of the men who are kin care providers are in a spousal relationship to the care recipient. However regardless of the relationship, most of the men lived with the person receiving the assistance. The moral obligations created by the dwelling situation and the type of relationship seem to be the most important explanations for why men become care providers. Men seem to provide more kin care than the research in this field estimates. Still, women as providers of kin care are in the majority. Compared to the men, a larger share of women do not live with the care recipient, and have a greater variety of forms of relationships with the care recipient.

Table 1. Employed relative care providers. (Percent)

Age	WOMEN	MEN	TOTAL
-34	8	6	8
35-44	18	16	18
45-54	29	26	28
55-64	32	33	32
65+	13	19	14
Total	100	100	100
N	1020	177	1197

Th care providers in the study would primarily be classified as blue-collar worker or lower civil servant, which is particularly evident when it comes to those who assist their parents or other elderly relatives. When it comes to care for children or spouses, social class is more varied. The kin care providers gave assistence to 1253 persons aged 1-101, of wich 45 percent were younger than 65. As shown in Table 2, among the care recipients there were more men in all age groups except for those 80 years or older. Among the oldest care receipients (80+), there were almost twice as many women as men, which made the proportion between men and women care recipients more even - 49 percent women and 51 percent men. In Sweden there are more women than men with a disability (SCB 2000). There are differences however in how the sexes are handicapped by the disability. It seems for example, that women wait longer than men to admit that they need help at home. This is very likely related to traditional understandings of gender (Sjöberg 1997). The relatively even distribution of men and women care recipients in this study is probably due to the fact that women live longer than men.

Table 2. Care recipients. (Percent)

Age	Women	Men	Total
-16	7	12	10
17-34	10	15	13
35-64	18	26	22
65-79	22	25	23
80+	43	22	32
Total	100	100	100
N	615	634	1249

The care recipients had many different illnesses and disabilities and it was not unusual to note more than one illnes in the same individual. Not including old age related symptoms (vertigo, weakness, impaired motor functions etc.), conditions such as mental retardation, sight disabilities, stroke, heart- and blood diseases, rheumatic diseases and dementia were common diagnoses. Persons with permanent injuries due to accidents were also common. This means that kin care providers assist people suffering from both physical and mental disabilities, and that they may be required to provide both practical and medical care. Very often a more extensive observational care effort is necessary to prevent the care recipient from falling accidents, getting lost and/or similar risks.

The kin care providers had in different ways tried to organize their lives in accordance with the relative's need for assistance. They had for instance decreased their working-hours, altered working schedules and/or stopped working for wages, and it is in connection with these changes that I want to analyze the importance of employment and wages.

It is not unusual that the level of kin care increases over time. One may not consider the assistance as a job until one has to make adjustments in everyday life in order to accommodate the responsibilities of providing the care. In order to become employed as a kin care provider, information about the possibility of employment for this kind of care must reach the relevant group. Providing this information is a municipal task but not all of the respondents in the study had received information this way. The majority (76%) had been unpaid kin care providers before they were employed. The fact that they eventually became employed was primarily due to their knowledge that this was a possibility. Those who were employed as care providers from the beginning were so because a drastic event had changed the situation in terms of how much and what kind of care was necessary for their relative: stroke, traffic accident or a child born with extensive functional disabilities.

To be a kin care provider is seen as self-evident for the employed relative care providers. To be employed and get wages for the care provision was experienced as positive and good, and appreciated. However, issues relating to feelings of moral obligation and money were addressed by the respondents (se e.g. Finch and Mason 1993). Some of the care providers felt that they hade to justify being paid. In the questionnaire, several of them commented (in the space provided) that they would be glad to provide the help for free if the question of what they would live on could be resolved. They also responded that assistance from Home Help Service was insufficient, that the relative would not want to be in an institution or that no other satisfactory alternatives existed. Evidently, a small group of kin providing care for a relative feel that they are more or less forced to do so.

Comparing Working Conditions

In Scandinavian social science and care research a double perspective is prevalent – conditions of work and quality of the care (Eliasson Lappalainen and Nilsson Motevasel 1997). The volume of research in this area has increased parellel with the growth of science of gender studies and feminist research. An important aim has been to make visible and study a phenomenon that is by tradition female and part of female everyday life. A critique of traditional social science in Sweden is that knowledge about and interest for care and care work are absent. A goal of the study of the employed relative care providers has therefore been to make the special conditions of care work visible in comparison with other kinds of work.

The employment situation provides a double connection between society and individuals. Society enters via the care recipient in terms of her/his status as a consumer of public services and via the kin care provider in terms of being employed in the public sector. The wages are subject to taxation and the kin care provider gets access to the social security system, unemployment allowance, health insurance and pension credits. Since employment as a family care provider is described as similar to being a nurse assistant in the municipality's Home Help Service, one aim of the study was to compare their working conditions. Since it can be difficult to combine informal care with full time employment a main issue is how their situation is affected by employment as care provider. Economy is also an important aspect and one that is not only a question of money, but also one of economizing with time and energy. I will analyze and discuss the terms of employment for kin care providers compared with the terms associated with ordinary care work in the light of a governmental recommendation that they should be treated as equals. In this section I use results from all four studies.

The municipalities have been urged to provide the relatives with the same conditions as their own care giving employees. Agains this backdrop, a comparison has been made between the two groups of care givers. As far as terms of employment for nurse assistants are concerned, these are relatively uniform throughout the country. Nurses are paid according to education and number of years of experience. They have regulated working hours and receive extra compensation for working inconvenient working hours (i.e. nights, weekends, holidays). Nurses have the possibility to permanent employment positions with all that thay entail in terms of benefits and job security, and should they be made redundant, they have priority access to other employment (by the same employer i.e. the municipality).

Normally, this is not the case for the kin care providers. Regardless of education (many had relevant training) and number of years in service, the kin care providers are paid the minimum nurse assistant salary and their work does not result in formal job performance evaluations and/or job references, or in permanent employment status. They work all hours and days without compensation for inconvenient working hours. The right to time off and vacations are the same as in the case of hourly employment, i.e. a private problem as opposed to an employer responsibility. The employment period is limited and must be renewed; when and if the need for care ceases to exist, employment is ended and the municipality is not required to provide any other employment.

The terms of employment are thus not equal to those of the nurse assistants more than on a superficial level; the kin care providers have clearly worse conditions. An example is a woman working as nurse assistant in the Home Help Service. When her father's care needs became more extensive she quit her job and took employment as a kin care provider. This change in employment position was her own choice and required that she hand in her notice as nurse assistant which meant that she lost the job security and benefits associated with her previous employment contract. In addition, her income decreased considerably since she received only the minimum salary per hour and received no extra compensation.

However, a few municipalities actively tried to offer kin care providers conditions similar to those who were employed as assistent nurses. There were also Home Help administrators who tried to improve the situation, both generally and in individual cases, yet these efforts were made on their own initiative and not as an explicity and officially formulated strategy on behalf of the municipality. This was true for the group of retired persons among the employed kin care providers (14%). The official retirement age in Sweden is 65. Some of the retired individuals in the study were employed with a very small monthly income. However, some of the respondents had full time employment. There were also individuals who became employed after retirement. These examples of retirees working as employed kin care providers exist only because some Home Help administrators were able to bend (break, would be more accurate) the rules of employment. This illustrates how important middle managers' knowledge about, and attitude towards family care providers and the work they perform, are. If wages are seen as compensation for a work effort there is no reason to stop paying wages merely because the care provider turns 65. There are many elderly in Sweden who perform a great deal of care and the majority of these are not employed and do not receive wages for the care they provide (e.g. Johansson 1991). There is therefore cause to believe that most middle managers do not support the practice of giving elderly care providers any compensation at all.

There do exist other examples of middle managers trying to improve the situation for individual relative care providers. One such example is a woman who had been caring for her handicapped husband full time for several years. At his death she had lost contact with working life but still had 15 years until retirement age. She was then employed as a personal assistant for a young disabled woman. The Home Help administrator was aware of the caring skills this woman had acquired during the years she cared for her husband. Having knowledge of the disabled woman's need for a person with these skills, the Home Help administrator could bring them together. The former kin care provider received better employment conditions as assistant to the disabled women than she had had while caring for her husband. She received a wage based on her working hours, higher income as she was paid for inconvenient working hours, and not least, free time, regular holidays and days off.

Depending on the municipality, the kin care providers may thus have completely different terms, but this may also be the case within the same municipality since there may be differences in how individual civil servants assess the work efforts. The middle managers' responses revealed problems they had experienced with the administration of the employment of kin care providers. They did not always approve of employment and paying wages to kin who provided informal care. Even if elderly care in Sweden is a public responsibility, family care is often seen as a private matter. The worsening finances of many municipalities meant that they often had enough difficulties keeping the assistant nurses employed and finding solutions for those in need of help who did not have relatives.

The discrepancies between the municipalities are also reflected by the fact that 14 of the 100 municipalities originally selected did not have any employed kin care providers at all and were therefore excluded from the study. It is, however, fairly safe to assume that similar kin care efforts existed in these municipalities as well.

In short, it seems to be the kin relationship itself that is the main reason for poorer conditions for kin care providers compared to those of nurse assistants. Had the same care been provid to a non-related person the care providers would have had the same employment conditions as the nurse assistants.

Are Working Conditions Fair?

The formal conditions of employment are not equal to the conditions of other care providers in the public sector. One question is whether wages correspond to the duties performed. The working situations of kin care providers was analyzed in relation to the number of paid working hours and to their work load. The data in this section comes mainly from the third study.

The work load springs from the care recipients' need for assistance and this can vary depending on, among other things, age and illness/disability. Records of the care recipients' illnesses and disabilities exist, however these do not reveal how great the need for assistance is. With the exception of the case of complex illnesses, the need for assistance is rarely stable. It changes over time; sometimes a great deal of help is needed, sometimes less. The need for assistance varies more depending on the individual than on the diagnosis. It is therefore not possible to draw general conclusions regarding the specific physical or mental work load brought about by the various illnesses. Diagnoses are of course important, both from the perspective of understanding the problem and as a background, however they are not to be considered a measure of the work load. Another way of measuring work load is from the responses to the survey questions about the duties carried out by the kin care providers. These vary; some provide help with housekeeping, shopping, and the like while others do "everything". Usually they perform a mix of housekeeping, emotional support, medical care, and more bodily help such as personal hygiene, dressing and undressing, help getting in and out of bed/chair etc. These responses were analyzed in relation to, among other things, paid working hours.

Paid working hours may be a measure of the work load when defined as the number of hours of help that the employed kin care provider will be paid for, as determined by the Home Help administrator's evaluation in relation to the need for assistance. This evaluation is based on a home visit and on an interview in which both amount and type of help is determined by the middle manager. Great needs should be reflected in more hours of assistance being granted. There is no limit for how much help a person might need but there is a maximum for how much one person is allowed to work per day or week. Approximately half of the employed kin care providers have less than 17 hours of paid work per week. Only 12 percent have full time employment. Judged by the number of paid hours one can draw the conclusion that the amount of care work performed does not seem to be very extensive.

The question of whether wages correspond to the amount of care work done can be measured in several ways. In order to understand the work load of the care providers we asked questions about how long one has been a kin care provider and whether working hours were changed or adjusted on account of the care providing. In addition, care providers were asked questions about heavy lifting and/or difficulties sleeping undisturbed on account of care needs of the recipient, and about whether they could leave the care recipient unattended. Most of the employed kin care providers in the study had been so for more than four years, and some for over twenty years. For this reason it is reasonable to talk about long-term assistance. In addition, the need for assistance rarely decreases over time and usually the opposite is the case. However it was not self-evident that increases in the amount of time that care was provided was on account of a new situation. Some of the employed care providers expressed a fear of "rocking the boat" in relation to the middle managers. Most municipalities in Sweden suffered from poor finances during the 1990s which lead to cutbacks on public expenditure. The employed kin care providers were afraid to loose their job and their wages. By keeping quiet they hoped their employment would not be questioned.

The majority of the kin care providers (66%) had been employed in other jobs when their employment as kin care giver began. Some who were not working had quit their job, often on account of the care burden. Amongst those who had been employed, two-thirds made adjustments in their working hours or gave up other work. The reasons for these changes were incompatibility of the hours; providing twenty-four hours assistance left little time or energy to spend on a job. Among all kin care providers, nearly 40 percent perform heavy lifting and 60 percent could never or only briefly leave the care recipient unattended. The responses show that it is not easy to combine care for relatives with a full time job. Despite the fact that most women were working part time, it was sometimes problematic to combine even shorter working hours with providing care. It is thus unlikely that the paid hours for care giving correspond to the care work effort.

Other research has shown clear differences between men and women when it comes to care of close relatives and the tasks performed (Abel and Nelson 1990; Finch and Mason 1993; Graham 1993; Sodei 1995). In this investigation, it is not primarily gender that differentiates the kin care providers, but rather the dwelling conditions and the type of relationship. Nearly 70 percent of the care providers lived with their care recipient and these generally perform more tasks. In addition, the majority of them rarely or never sleep undisturbed the entire night due to their care responsibility. Parents and spouses distinguish themselves by having both physically and mentally heavy work. Spouses, especially the women, experienced fatigue associated with the heavy work and the obvious expectations on them to perform the care. Wives often suffer from lack of appreciation for their work and such appreciation seems to be of great importance to them. I will return to this issue under the sub-heading "Symbolic value of a wage". Especially older wives are often very tired and sometimes depressed. Providing this kind of care for a husband - changing diapers, dressing and undressing, lifting someone much heavier than oneself - in combination with poor sleep, would be heavy work for anyone, and even more so for a person who is old herself.

Judging by the amount of paid work performed by the kin care providers, one would conclude that it is not very extensive. However, if the content and work load are studied, a different picture emerges. Eligability for full inclusion and benefits offered by the Swedish social insurance systems requires that one has paid employment at least 17 hours per week. Since it can be difficult to combine care for a relative with other paid work, and since many kin care providers have few hours in paid employment, many kin care providers are not eligible for full social security benefits. This means that if the care provider has no other employment, she or he will not be fully included in the social security system. Seen in both absolute terms, and in relation to the amount of work done, the number of hours employed kin care givers are compensated for are very low which, in addition to providing a small income to live on, will also have repercussions for their future pension level.

Division of Duties and the Experience of Being Tied Down

A sharing of duties between the kin care providers and the municipality is inherent in the terms of employment, which influences the circumstances of work as well as the possibilities for doing other kinds of work and having free time. Shared duties may in these cases for example be a nurse assistant staying with the care recipient on regular basis. To have a nurse assistant in the home can make other paid work possible and/or can help protect the kin care provider from being over-burdened. Shared duties can also mean the possibility for the care recipient to stay at a nursing home during certain periods, or visit a day care center during the day. A short stay in a nursing home can give the care provider the possibility to get some nights of undisturbed sleep. Shared duties might also be as simple as the knowledge that there is someone to contact in order to get help and relief in a stressed situation. Having someone in the Home Help Service to consult and who can offer concrete advice can help in avoiding worry and anxiousness. The sense of being weighed down, of having everything on one's own shoulders, has been pointed out as the main source of stress for caregivers by Paoletti, in chapter 1. As pointed out by Oddone and Aguirre in chapter 3 in their discussion about a support group for care givers, the most valuable knowledge gained from the support group was that it was okey to take time for themselves and to delegate duties. Moreover, Watson writes in chapter 8 that the existence and availability of support services were described as essential to one's own peace of mind by most of the carers she interviewed.

Two aspects of the employed kin care providers' work stood out. On the one hand care providers often experience a strong sense of being confined, not being able to have control over one´s own time and activities, and on the other hand they experience remarkable joy and gratification in being able to provide assistance. These two sides are associated with the fact that kin care is signified by closeness and continuity. The feeling of being indispensabile, something which caring for a relative very often brings about, could give life new and important content. A responsibility for care sometimes brings about a constant concern about the care recipient: "How is he feeling? How can I make her happy?" This might contribute to feelings of confinement (or involvement) that are not necessarily negative. However, when these feelings of confinement or of being tied down become negative, they ought to be acknowledged.

The sharing of duties between the kin care providers and the municipal Home Help Service as well as between other relatives was also studied. How and between which parties duties are shared may influence the work situation and the possibilities for other kinds of work as well as for free time. The purpose was to analyze the effects of receiving help, or not receiving help from others, on the kin carers' experiences of being tied down (Furåker and Mossberg 1997a). Another question that is addressed is whether the source of the help mattered, i.e. whether the help came from relatives or society. In the next section some reasons contributing to feelings of confinement will be discussed, primarily based on data from the questionnaire answered by the care providers.

TIED DOWN

With the concept "tied down" I mean a physical and a psychological work load that may bring out certain feelings. Sixty percent of the employed care providers could never or only briefly leave the care recipient alone. This can be considered to be a form of physical work load. Another, more psychological burden, is that the possibility to leave the care recipient is accompanied by being worried all the time. Nearly 75 percent of the care providers often felt tied down. Such confinement may bring about feelings of insufficiency leading to greater strain and stress and may bring on frustration, gloominess, anxiousness and guilt (Johansson 1991).

Assistance is not necessarily possible only from society; other sources and combinations of help must be considered as well. For this reason some questions in the questionnaire focused on the kin care providers' possibilities to obtain help from other relatives, friends and neighbors. The informal network of support is important (Qureshi and Walker 1989).

However, despite the fact that many kin care providers receive informal assistance, no co-variation with the lesser experience of being tied down was found in the statistical analysis. The close family unit usually provided assistance which is regarded as an important resource, however it is apparently insufficient to meet the care reciepient's needs. In addition, a relatively large share of the kin care providers did not have any informal assistance at all.

Societal assistance was found to be an important counterweight to the experience of being tied down, which was a significant result. Most of the respondents receiving help in their caring efforts were content and felt that this was necessary for being able to cope. Even if most of the burden is placed on the kin care provider, having someone from the municipality to share the responsibility with offers security and relief. Societal assistance can also be seen as extra security for the person in need of help since violence in situations of care work is a notable risk factor (Tornstam 1989).

Most of the employed kin care providers (62%) did not have regular assistance however, nor did the assistance deal directly with the care tasks. Very few had someone from the municipality to talk to or to ask for help and only seven percent had regular meetings with their supervisor. Moreover, kin care providers were seldom offered help; it was something that the kin care provider had to make an effort towards in order to receive. One example is that of a woman who had a paralyzed husband who was fully dependent on her help. It was not until she eventually had a total physical and mental break down due to exhaustion that her pleas for help were taken seriously.

Sometimes however, help is not adequate. Almost one-fourth of the employed kin care providers stated that they needed more assistance in their work. Nearly three-fourths of the kin care providers experienced feeling of being tied down, which gives rise to the question of why there were not more claims for assistance. It is important to point out that the need for assistance may be much greater than actually stated.

To some extent, the kin care providers had quite modest expectations regarding support and other measures from society. This was in part because they appreciated the wages and had difficulties asking for more. However, another important reason behind the kin care providers not asking for assistance was because the assistance they received was not satisfactory. In some cases, the care recipient's condition had worsened during or after having received institutional care, e.g. they had experienced depression. Another problem was matching Home Help Service nurses to recipients since it was important that they got along. Not all nurse assistants and care recipients get on well together however. But it is also important that the kin care provider and the nurse assistant get along. For some of the employed care providers, especially wives, it was important to have a job outside the home: "A time where I can rest from the care work". This meant that receiving help with household tasks could also be an important way to help the kin care provider. However the nurse assistants were not always willing to help with such tasks. The nurses may look after the care recipient, but not do anything else. Husbands in the same situation however, did not complain about this lack of help with household tasks.

Dwelling situation and time are important; those who live together with their care recipient are more tied down. Those who have been employed for more than two years as a kin care provider claimed to have less freedom than those with shorter spans of employment. This can be interpreted in terms of the process that is involved in bringing about feelings of being tied down. These feelings emerge as a result of the combination of long-term care efforts and insufficient assistance from the Home Help Services.

In this chapter the focus is on the conditions of employment and the finacial conditions for kin care providers. However, since kin care providing also involves close relations, love and care. I will briefly discuss some results regarding these aspects in relation to the work situation and the lack of assistance. The survey directed to the care providers included questions about how the relationship between themselves and the care recipient was affected by the need for help. Half of the kin care providers had not experienced any change in the relationship as a result of the care responsibility. Among those who had experienced changes, the majority stated that they felt that they had become a "nurse" instead of being e.g. a spouse or child. This does not necessarily have to mean a worsening of the relationship. A large group claimed that they had become closer to the recipient. Some however, claimed that they experienced the relationship as poorer. Reasons for this seemed to be changes in the mental state of the recipient and/or a too extensive and lonely care responsibility, which was sometimes involuntary.

The experience of being tied down among the kin care providers is partly related to the the close relationship between the care provider and the receiver and to the continuity in this relationship. Not all providers had the experience of being tied down and not all of them were in a situation in which the question was relevant. It is, however, relatively easy to end up in a situation where the experience of being tied down increases. The results indicate that this process does not have to assume a negative form, nor must it become permanent if the assistance is of good quality and is administered at an early stage. Having insufficient assistance in the care work is, however, a health hazard for both the kin care provider and the care recipient.

Advantages of Employment

As has been discussed above the kin care providers do not have the same conditions as other health care assistants. Nor do they seem to have a salary corresponding to the work they do. In spite of this it was obvious that they were very pleased to be employed and to be paid. How can this contradiction be explained? One way is to see how the care providers' personal financial situation has been affected by employment. The third study included several questions about work and economy. Employment can be a positive alternative even if one's economy has been negatively affected, which means that other factors can be seen as more important. Some people may value the possibility to be a care provider, and see a low income as better than no income at all.

An important point of reference is which work tasks and which salary one had in one's previous job and whether one was employed part or full time before becoming employed as kin care provider. In this section two tables are shown where the first shows if one has experienced financial change after employment as kin care provider, and if so how. The next table shows changes in economic situation in the case of previous part or full time employment. (Table 4 shows only those who were previously employed).

The importance of employment as a kin care provider and the influence of this on economic situation will then be connected to changes in other employment in order to handle the situation as care provider, if such exist. More specifically, the question is whether the care provider can shorten other working hours in order to handle the care, and without loosing out economically.

Table 3. Experienced change in economy after becoming employed as a relative care provider. (Percent)

	Women	Men	Total
Better	45	28	42
Same	33	38	34
Worse	22	34	24
Total	100	100	100
N	963	167	1130

Thanks to the wages, the majority of the kin care providers did not suffer any economic losses due to becoming an employed kin care giver. The women's economy was on the whole the same as or better than it had been prior to employment, in part due to having made adjustments in working life before employment as a kin care provider, and/or in part because of having several years of unpaid work behind them. Naturally, receiving wages, even low ones, would be considered an improvement in comparison to not having an income at all. Spouses and parents were primarily the ones who did unpaid work to a large degree before employment and who also did so for a considerable period of time.

One-fifth of the women and one-third of the men, however, experienced a worsened financial situation. If the responses are divided according to whether respondents worked part or full time in an ordinary job, a clearer picture of who benefited or lost out economically respectively emerges.

Table 4. Changes in economy after employment as relative care provider related to ordinary work. (Percent)

	Full time		Part time	
	Women	Men	Women	Men
Better	23	22	50	19
Same	36	44	32	31
Worse	41	34	18	50
Total	100	100	100	100
N	257	121	444	16

It is above all the part time working women who have benefited from kin care employment and half have even experienced an improved economic situation. It is here necessary to take a closer look at the social class variable, as type of work and level of income can be of importance. The occupational status of the care providers is principally that of blue-collar workers and lower civil servants. Several studies have shown that working class women feel stronger obligations to care for a relative than do women from other socio-economic groups (e.g.Wærness 1987). One explanation for why those with non-professional work backgrounds are more likely to become an employed kin care provider is partly because the wages are similar. Another explanation is that the working conditions are similar.

Working class women more often have part time jobs and insecure working conditions, which resembles employment as kin care provider. Employment as a relative care provider can therefore be more acceptable to them.

Most of the men were in full time employment and had difficulty combining this with the needs of the care recipient. As changes in working life took place, their economic situation deteriorated, as was also the case for some of the women. The reason for kin care providers making changes in their working life, despite a less favorable economy, is that it was not possible to continue other employment to the same extent as earlier. The wages as paid kin care provider were not enough to compensate lower or no wages from a previous job.

Several views were expressed in the comment section of the questionnaire regarding economic matters. A common comment from those who had responded that their finances had become "worse" was that they earlier had had a better paid job. It could also however, be the case that both spouses had been working up to the day that one of them was disabled. This meant a loss of income for the one and a decrease in working hours and income for the spouse providing the care. This had a negative effect on the couple's economy. Another comment concerned the costs associated with having an ill or disabled relative; it might entail costs for traveling, doctors, facilitating equipment, medicine etc. These extra costs in combination with a decrease in income are two aspects that contribute to a considerably poorer financial situation.

Generally, women to a larger extent than men feel that their finances improved after becoming employed as kin care provider. Irrespective of sex, the majority of kin care providers have an economic situation that is as good or better than earlier. Even if several of the respondents changed their working hours or stopped working for wages on account of the informal care, they seem to have been able to do so without experiencing a financial loss. One interpretation of this is that the employment situation and the wages are positive alternatives in a care situation.

The Symbolic Value of the Wage

No consistent picture of the experienced situation of the kin care providers regarding their economic situation emerged. Responses show that some are relatively content while others are clearly discontent. The discontentment is due to the insecure conditions of employment and the poorer working conditions compared to other health care workers, which the kin care providers are well aware of. In spite of this discontentment they are also glad that they are employed and have a wage. Could it be that the positive responses express something else? One likely possibility is that a wage has a symbolic value. Apart from the bread-winning aspect, a salary is also seen as recognition of accomplishment. This recognition serves as a possible counterweight to the confinement and the heavy work often experienced by kin care givers (Furåker and Mossberg 1997b).

Care work has dimensions that many other occupations lack. It means working with human beings, being important to somebody, and it is seen as morally right. There are thus many positive aspects in health care work and in being able to assist a relative may be regarded as especially meaningful. The data were analyzed to see whether an experience of joy in one's work could function as a buffer in an otherwise heavy work situation. The most important dimension for experiences of joy seemed to be the appreciation of one's performance as a kin care provider. Those who gave such responses emphasized the positive aspects of the work to a great extent. Appreciation is thus a key factor and this type of social support may stem from different sources – from the care recipient, from other relatives, from neighbors and friends and from society. Society is an abstract concept but the kin care provider sees society's appreciation as very concrete; it is expressed in the form of wages and employment. Those with improved finances to a large extent claimed that they felt valued by society. Wages are viewed as a symbol for society's appreciation and it can be described as the municipality's special way of recognizing the work being done.

SUMMARY AND DISCUSSION

Sweden is a society in which women as well as men are expected to perform paid work in order to be eligible for the benefits provided by the national social insurance system. Care support allowance and other forms of economic support do not provide the privileges employment does, and are thus less advantageous to the care provider. Employment may therefore be regarded as society's chance to provide relatives with conditions comparable to other paid work. Kin care provider employment is a solution that works in several different situations, and it can in most cases be regarded as a good solution. One conclusion from this investigation is that employment and salary are much appreciated forms of support. Wages are compensation for work effort, and provide the possibility to quit or reduce other work in order to handle the care. The majority of the kin care providers are satisfied, although many desire better employment conditions and higher wages – or rather conditions which correspond to other health care work and wages corresponding to the effort.

The difficulties expressed in the study do not concern employment per se but rather the fact that formal rules of employment do not seem to be applicable to kin care providers. The insecure conditions of employment are a problem, as are the low wages and unsatisfactory division of duties between the kin care providers and the municipality. There is a conflict between recommendations given via governmental policy and the reality that the care providers meet in their everyday lives. The majority of managers or middle managers still seem to be unaware of recommendations for how to handle the employment of kin care providers, which also seems to be true for the relative care providers themselves.

The question is then how the kin care providers' work is valued and if wages are seen as compensation for other kinds of lost income, payment for duties performed, or as some kind of allowance. In spite of the fact that most of the respondents have been employed care providers for many years their work seems to be viewed as temporary by middle managers. It is apparent that wages do not correspond to work done or to what professional care providers earn. In one way the wages have made it possible for relatives of those needing care to decrease working hours in other areas in order to be a kin care provider without too great a financial loss. This was however true primarily for those who had previously held part time jobs in a working class, female occupation. Compared to full time work and/or better paid work the result was financially less beneficial. For some the lowering of other working hours was voluntary, while in other cases was more or less compulsory. A great risk of losing other career prospects exists if working hours are decreased. Leaving the labor market completely could be detrimental to career and salary development. The risk of losing income both in the present and in the form of future pension benefits is great. But informal care is not just a question for those of working age. For most, employment and wages as a kin care provider end when they turn 65. The need for care, and the work load, however, persist. Refusal to extend employment for those who turn 65 but who go on caring for a relative can be regarded as a form of age discrimation.

As far as the division between society and kin care providers is concerned, it may be said that a considerable proportion of the responsibility and work lies with the relatives. Some relatives do not want much societal interference, and are happy with monetary compensation. Others have an apparent need for assistance. The question of responsibility is not simple, and no general line can be drawn for what the municipality and relatives respectively should contribute with. A point of reference should, however, be that relatives are given choices in terms of their care commitment and that there are possibilities for a reasonable division of duties. This is difficult however when work tasks contain so many traditions and duties. It is difficult for kin care providers to make demands and avoid being subject to exploitation.

There are many implications concerning family care and money. Love and moral obligations are not always reconcilable with money and are often used as arguments against payment. A secure income and reasonable working conditions could, however, be seen as conditions that could facilitate good care and provide a possibility for love to survive.

Conclusion

Being an informal care provider on a long-term basis may effect life in many ways. The predicaments of informal care often include a problem of financial support. It may, for instance, prove difficult to combine care of a relative with work in the labor market. In this chapter I have discussed some results from an investigation concerning employment for family care. Employment means that the relative is seen as a member of the municipality's Home Help staff and is to have the same conditions as other employed personnel. The main focus in the chapter has been how informal care work was assessed and evaluated compared to professional care work. Another main question was the family care provider's own experiences of employment as a kin care giver, regarding both financial aspects as well as working conditions.

Compared to professional care work it is apparent that the family care providers did not have the same conditions. The wages did not correspond to the work done or to what professional care providers earn for comparable work. Still, when it comes to the family care provider's own experiences, employment and salary are appreciated forms of support. Employment provides social security and pension credits for the care provider. A salary is compensation for work effort, and also provides the possibility to quit or reduce time spent in other work in order to handle the care. Apart from the bread-winning aspect, a salary has another important significance; it is regarded as recognition of work done. The majority of the kin care providers are satisfied, although many of them would like better employment terms and higher wages. More specifically, they want conditions that correspond to other care work, and a salary that correspond to the effort.

RECOMMENDATIONS

- Make the cost of informal care visible.
- Ensure that the care providers are given the information they need about practical and economical help that may be available to them.
- Make advantages of employment instead of care support allowance visible.
- Adjust employment to the family care provider's specific situation.
- Provide reasonable payment.
- Encourage the possibility for family care providers to keep up with other work and activities.
- Ensure that the care providers' own health is considered by social services.

REFERENCES

Abel, Emily and Nelson, Margaret (eds.). (1990). *Circles of care – Work and Identity in Women's Lives*. Albany, N Y: State university of New York Press.

Age and Attitudes. (1993). Main results from a Eurobarometer survey. Commission of the European Communities.

Andersson, Lars (1993). *Äldre i Sverige och Europa.* (Elderly in Sweden and in Europe). Ädelutvärderingen 93:4. Socialstyrelsen. Report from the National Board of Health and Welfare.

Axelsson, Christina (1992). *Hemmafrun som försvann. Övergången till lönearbete bland gifta kvinnor i Sverige 1968-1981.* (The House wife who disappeared. The transition to employment among married women in Sweden 1968-1981). Stockholms universitet. Institutet för social forskning. (Dissertation).

Björnberg, Ulla (1992). Tvåförsörjarfamiljen i teori och verklighet. (Two-earner Family in Theory and Reality. In Acker, Joan et al. (eds.). *Kvinnors och mäns liv och arbete* (pp. 153-218). Stockholm: SNS Förlag.

Ds 1981:15 *Vårdbidrag för handikappade barn under 16 år.* (Care allowance for handicapped children below the age of 16). Betänkande från Anhörigvårdskommittén. Governmental report.

Eliasson-Lappalainen, Rosmari and Nilsson Motevasel, Ingrid (1997) Ethics of care and social policy. *Scandinavian journal of social welfare,* 3 (6) 189-196.

Evers, Adalbert, Pijl, Marja and Ungerson, Clare, (eds.). (1994). *Payment for care. A comparative overview.* Vienna. Avebury European Centre.

Finch, Janet and Mason, Jennifer (1993). *Negotiating family responsibilities.* London and New York: Tvistock/Routledge.

Furåker, Bengt and Mossberg, Ann-Britt (1997a). Vårdansvar och bundenhet. (Care responsibility and some of its consequences). *Socialvetenskaplig Tidskrift*, 1, 3-20.

Furåker, Bengt and Mossberg, Ann-Britt (1997b). Arbetsglädje bland anställda anhörigvårdare. (Work satisfaction among People Employed to care for Their Relatives). *Socialvetenskaplig Tidskrift*, 4, 305-318.

Glaser, Barner and Strauss, Anselm (1997). *The discovery of grounded theory: Strategies for qualitative research.* Chicago. New York: Aldine Publishing Company.

Graham, Hilary (1993). "Social Division in Caring". *Women's Studies International Forum*, 16 (6) 461-470.

Johansson, Lennarth (1991). *Caring for the Next of Kin. On Informal Care of the Elderly in Sweden*. Uppsala universitet. Department of Social Medicine. (Dissertation).

Johansson, Lennarth (1997). Anhöriga och frivilliga - lösningen på äldreomsorgens problem? (Relatives and voluntary work – the solution for Elderly care problems?) In Jennerbert, K. and Lagerkrantz, R. (eds.). *Äldrepolitik i förändring.* Välfärdsprojektets skriftserie nr 9. pp. 57-70. Socialdepartementet. Report from the Ministry of Social Welfare.

Mossberg, Ann-Britt (1996). "Jag tar en dag i sänder" - om ålderspensionerade anhörigvårdare. (I take one day at a time" – on retired Relative Care-providers). In Eliasson R. (ed.). *Omsorgens skiftningar - Begreppet, vardagen, politiken, forskningen.* (pp. 114-130). Lund: Studentlitteratur.

Mossberg Sand, Ann-Britt (2000). *Ansvar, kärlek och försörjning. Om anställda anhörigvårdare i Sverige.* (Responsibility, Love and Maintenance. On Employed Relative Care-providers in Sweden). Göteborg University. Department of Sociology. (Dissertation).

Regeringens proposition 1990/91:14. *Ansvaret för service och vård till äldre och handikappade m m.* (The responsibility for Service and Care for Elderly, Handicapped etc.). Governmental report.

Regeringens proposition 1997/98:113. Nationell handlingsplan för äldrepolitiken. (National plan for Elderly Care). Governmental report.

Sand, M. Ann-Britt (2002). Anhörigvård. (Family Care). Lund:Studentlitteratur.

Sand, M. Ann-Britt (2003). Var finns de gamla I den svenska familjen? (Where are the old in the Swedish Family?) In Kollind, A-K. and Peterson, A. (eds.). *Thoughts on Family, Gender, Generation and Class* (pp. 205-220). Research Report No. 133 from the Department of Sociology, Göteborg University.

SCB (2000). *Äldres levnadsförhållanden 1980-1998.* (Living conditions of the Elderly 1980-1998). Rapport 93. Statistics Sweden.

Sipilä, Jorma and Simon, B. L. (1993). Home care allowances – for and against. *Journal of Sociology and Social Welfare*, 20 (3), 119-34.

Sipilä, Jorma (1994). Why do the Scandinavian governments compensate family members who care for Elderly kin? *Care in Place,* Volume 1, Nr 3, Dec 1994. 261-271.

Sipilä, Jorma (1997). *Social care services: The key to the Scandinavian welfare model.* Aldershot:Avebury.

Sjöberg, Malena (1997). *I första hand kvinna.* (First of all woman). Välfärdsprojektets skriftserie. Nr 8. Socialdepartementet. Report from the Ministry of Social Welfare.

Socialstyrelsen 1993:4. *Äldre i Sverige och Europa.* (Elderly in Sweden and Europe). Ädelutvärderingen. Report from the National Board of Health and Welfare.

Sodei, Takako (1995). Care of the Elderly: A Woman's Issue. In Fujimura-Fanselow, K. and Kameda, A. (eds.). *Japanese Women. New Feminist Perspectives on the Past, Present and Future* (pp. 213-228). New York: The feminist Press at The City University of New York.

SoS-rapport 1994:22. *Familjen som vårdgivare för äldre och handikappade.* (The Family as Care providers for The Elderly and the Handicapped). Socialstyrelsen. Report from the National Board of Health and Welfare.

SOU 1983:64. *Ledighet för anhörigvård.* (Care leave). Betänkande från Anhörigvårdskommittén. Governmental report.

SOU 1994:139. Ny socialtjänstlag: Huvudbetänkande av Socialtjänstkommittén. (New Social Service Act). Stockholm: Fritzes Förlag. Governmental report.

SOU 1998:6. *Ty makten är din ... Myten om det rationella arbetslivet och det jämställda Sverige.* (For thine be the power... The Myth about the rational working life and the equal Sweden). Betänkande från Kvinnomaktutredningen. Governmental report.

Stark, Agneta and Regnér, Åsa (2001). *I vems händer? Om arbete, genus, åldrande och omsorg i tre EU-länder.* (In who's hands? About Work, Gender, Ageing and Care in three EU-countries). Linköping: Tema Genus. Rapport Nr 1:2001.

Sundström, Gerdt (1994). *Hemma på äldre da'r.* (Living at home in old age). Ädelutvärderingen 94:17. Socialstyrelsen. Report from the National Board of Health and Welfare.

Svallfors, Stefan (1996). Klass, kön och välfärdsstatlig integration: om attityder till välfärdspolitiken. (Class, Sex and Welfare State Integration: about attitudes toward the welfare policy). In Palme, J. and Wennemo, I. (eds.). *Generell välfärd Hot och möjligheter?* Välfärdsprojektet. Skriftserien Fakta/kunskap 3, pp. 65-86. Socialdepartementet. Report from the Ministry of Social Welfare.

Thorslund, Mats and Larsson, Kristina (2002). *Äldres behov. En kunskapsöversikt och diskussion om framtiden.* (The needs of the Elderly). Stockholm: Stiftelsen Stockholms läns äldrecentrum.

Ungerson, Clare (1996). *Gender, Cash and Informal Care: European Perspectives and Dilemmas.* EPS Fifth International Conference, August 5-9, Brisbane Australia. Unpublished paper.

Wærness, Kari (1987). Tvinga inte kvinnor att vårda! In Lundborg, Bitte. *De anhöriga är vi. Om anhöriga och hemtjänsten.* (Do not force women to become care-providers). (pp. 49-57). Socialdepartementet. Report from the Ministry of Social Welfare.

Walker, Alan (1995). Integrating the family into a mixed economy of care. In Allen, I. and Perkins, E. (eds.) *The Future of Family Care for Older people.* (pp. 201-220). London: HSMO.

In: Family Caregiving for Older Disabled People
Editor: Isabella Paoletti, pp. 319-332
ISBN 1-59454-808-0

Chapter 15

INTERPROFESSIONAL DECISION MAKING IN ELDERLY CARE: MORALITY, CRITERIA AND HELP ALLOCATION

Pirjo Nikander
Department of Sociology and Social Psychology,
33014 University of Tampere, Finland

INTRODUCTION

Talk and interaction between health and social care professionals form one central arena where statutory decisions concerning the care of elderly people are made. Cooperative work between members of different professional groups in meetings, or in teams is also a practical arena where various agreed upon policies and principles of elderly care are turned into practice through talk. In this chapter, I analyze interprofessional meetings as a practical site for decision making over service and help allocation to elderly people and their carers. I attempt to lay out for view some characteristics of professional deliberation and decision making. Discursive analysis of professional-professional interaction and talk is seen here as a powerful means of studying help allocation, and the unfolding of institutional criteria and morality.

The interdisciplinary field of discourse studies has in recent years produced an ample supply of work on institutional and lay caring relations. The existing literature already provides information on the construction of elderly identities (Paoletti 1998; see also Nikander 2002), on the discursive construction of frailty (Taylor 1992), of caring relations and the professionals' role as part of the care arrangements (e.g. Grainger 1993), on intergenerational relations (e.g. Cicirelli 1993), and on professional construction of client or patient cases (e.g. Nikander 2003, 2005).

Empirical research on professional or institutional discourses in elderly care falls roughly into three distinctive areas of interest (c.f. Linell 1998). Perhaps most prominently, research has focused on professional – lay discourse i.e., on encounters involving the co-presence of doctors and elderly patients (e.g. Coupland and Coupland 1998, 1999), elderly mental patients and attorneys (Holstein 1990), or for instance district nurses and patients (Leppänen 1998). A second area of research gives discourse *within* specific professional groups centre focus. Analysis of nurses' actions within a medical unit may for instance tease out specifics of how this professional group constitutes patient classes or patient types as part of their own everyday ordering work (Latimer 1997). Third, discursive analysis on care and caring relations has also been concerned with interprofessional discourse, i.e., encounters, cooperation and joint decision-making *between* individuals from different professional groups. Research in this area varies from managerial interests (e.g. Dockrell and Wilson 1995) to a focus on professional roles and narratives (Housley 2003), and joint professional categorization work (e.g. Nikander 2003, 2005). It is this area of research that this chapter also hopes to contribute to.

In terms of its methodological stance, the current chapter draws on prior work on discourse analysis, categorization in institutional settings as well as work that analyses categorization in talk more broadly (e.g. Antaki and Widdicombe 1998; Baker 1997; Boden 1994; Hester and Eglin 1993; Housley 2003; Nikander 2000, 2002). It provides numerous illustrations and detailed analyses of professional care allocation. Doing this, the chapter hopefully shows how the criteria and morality of decision making are jointly constructed in interaction, and how the responsibilities of professionals as well as the rights and responsibilities of elderly clients and of their carers are discursively carved and talked into being in institutional meeting talk. Special focus in the chapter will be given to the ways in which professionals use *imageries and ideals concerning the caring relationship and the life course* as part of their descriptive work.

In the remaining sections of this chapter I will first introduce the data and the institutional setting in which they were collected. Following this, I will then move to the analysis of two elderly client cases and provide several data excerpts on both. To conclude, I will briefly discuss possible benefits and practical implications of discursive analyses of professional argumentation.

THE MEETINGS DATA: INFORMAL HOME CARE ALLOWANCE

In the Finnish care system, the state and municipalities are to a large degree responsible for arranging social and health services for the elderly. To date, public funds have secured the services provided, and citizens have received them either against a moderate fee or for free (Anttonen and Sipilä 2000). More recently a variety of market-based service systems are also available and there is an increasing tendency towards supporting informal care at home (Vaarama and Kautto 1999).

The data and analysis in this chapter elucidate the practical institutional work whereby decisions about care allocation are reached. The data originate from a wider research project titled *Constructing Age, Health and Competence: Argumentation and Rhetoric in Institutional and Personal Discourse*. In the course of this project, 42 hours of video taped materials were collected from two types of interprofessional meetings in the Finnish social and health care.

1. Meetings making decisions over informal home care allowances for the elderly (15 meetings)

2. Meetings making decisions over long-term nursing home placements (15 meetings) [1]

Given the shared interest in family care giving in the chapters of this book, I focus here only on the first of the meeting types mentioned above. In the course of this chapter, I attempt to provide one concrete example of how formal – in this case financial support – is allocated to people who take care of elderly relatives living at home, and how members of interprofessional teams argue for, and advocate specific decisions to be taken.

The meetings making decisions on informal home care allowance are attended by (community) nurses, members of home help teams (home helpers, home helpers in charge, and head of home help), a medical doctor and a secretary. The participants not only represent a mix of professionals from both the social and the health sector, they are also somewhat differently positioned in the professional power hierarchy. Consequently interprofessional encounters like these are often also about displaying professional knowledge, power and competence and, at least potentially, saturated with boundary marking between professional tribes (see Housley 2003; Nikander 2005).

The meetings in focus are task-oriented. The practical business for the participants is to go through applications sent in by elderly people who currently still live at home and are cared for by a family member or an outside lay carer. According to the Finnish elderly care system, carers are eligible to apply for financial support when taking care of elderly relatives in their homes. Finland has a long tradition of supporting informal care which is also seen as an effective means of saving in the costs of long-term institutional care. This form of financial support becomes available once a year, and carers who have received it previously need to re-apply yearly. Carers are normally family members or relatives of the elderly client, but also so called outside carers with no relative status are eligible. The amount given to caregivers varies from two hundred to a thousand Euros, and the benefit is considered taxable income. This means that in addition to its financial importance, the benefit also carries symbolic meanings to caregivers: it says that that their caring work is officially acknowledged and appreciated as paid work. The funds available, and the monthly sums allocated to support informal elderly home care vary regionally within Finland. As a rule, however, funds are insufficient, and typically run out midway to the year. This means that despite the cost-effectiveness of this form of allowance, in practice the majority of informal care by relatives happens without such outside recognition and direct financial support.

The elderly client or the carer is not present in the meetings. Instead the absent client's case is presented to the meeting via textual documentation and through the detail that members of the interprofessional team take up and describe as relevant (see also Nikander 2003). Participants in the meetings have a pile of applications in front of them and they present client cases and follow the flow of the meeting using these textual materials. Each application also includes a doctor's certificate detailing the elderly person's medical status. Documentary realities and paper work (Atkinson and Coffey 1997) on client cases as well as discussion and development on the basis of these documents thus form the basis on which the meeting interaction in question unfolds.

[1] The project was funded by the Academy of Finland. The meetings were video taped and the researcher was not present in the meetings. The data were then transcribed into text. Both meeting types were video taped routinely in the course of one year.

Additional information on the elderly persons and their carers is available to the meeting as one member of the team always makes a home visit before a decision for or against financial support can be made. As the data excerpts in this chapter show in detail, home visits provide first-hand detailed information on the housing, caring and family circumstances of the elderly person, on how well both the carer and the cared for are coping, and on whether any significant change has happened that favours the possible earlier care benefit to go up this year.

One further detail is perhaps worth mentioning here. Despite being task-oriented, the informal home care allowance meetings discuss issues to do with the well-being and coping of their elderly clientele more generally. The discussion is rife with longer and detailed narratives about carers and the elderly clients themselves. The interprofessional team also discusses issues that have to do with the wider mix of formal and informal eldercare: the number of home help visits and short term admissions, meal services, housing and family arrangements and special aids. They also discuss forms of support to the carer: trips to day centres that allow time off, and care vouchers that allow for holidays from the caring relationship. Discussions also cover wider moral and ethical issues concerning the whole decision making process. During all this, speakers often move between their own professional perspective and financial imperatives and the concrete life situation, worries and perspectives of their clients. In the previous chapter, Sand pointed out that decision about terms of employment of kin care providers can often completely differ, depending on the municipality, since they depend on individual civil servants' assessment. In this chapter we can observe this type of decision making process in its making. That is, institutions are seen at work, through the analysis of actual instances of institutional interaction.

In sum then, the meeting data in this chapter illuminate some of the core elements and key questions topical to all ageing societies (e.g. Walker 1995; Gilleard and Higgs 1998). What constitutes a proper mix between professional care and informal care given by family members and relatives? How should we define and demarcate the rights, obligations and responsibilities of elderly citizens and their relatives on the one hand, and of the official system of health and social care on the other? Can ageing societies find better means of supporting good quality home care in ways that secure the well-being and coping of all involved? As I am about to show in more detail, these are questions that professionals in the meetings data in focus also tackle and seek to resolve.

PRACTICES OF INSTITUTIONAL DECISION MAKING: DATA ANALYSES

The excerpts chosen for analysis in this chapter, deal with two client cases discussed in the same three-hour long meeting. The meeting was attended by nine professionals: four community nurses, two home care workers, the head of home help, a medical doctor and a secretary. The number of client cases in the whole meeting was 31. The interaction during the decision making phase of informal home care allowance meetings routinely consists of case or client presentations. The professional most familiar with the elderly client's history and current situation normally takes these longer turns of talk. The same professional has often also made the home visit required before a decision on a potential allowance can be made.

The first excerpt is an example of a case presentation that was made 31 minutes into the meeting in question. In it, one of the home-helpers describes a female elderly client who lives at home cared for by her daughter who visits daily. The case description below includes many elements typical to client description in this meeting type. The transcription symbols used in the excerpts can be found at the end of this chapter.

Excerpt One: Mother and daughter I (HCA4, 31:35-36.32)
Speakers: HH = home helper, HHH = head of home help, S = Secretary,
? = unidentified speaker

01 HH: Then the next one is this (0.8) ((*last name-middle name-first name*))
02 (3.8) *((hands the doctor's certificate over to the doctor sitting next to her))*
03 HH: I went there *yes*terday (8.0)
04 HH: Lives there in ((*name of town district*)) (0.5)
05 in a flat with all modern conveniences and the house has
06 a lift fortunately so (.) this lady m*o*ves about (1.5.) poorly (1.5)
07 Here the (.) carer is the daughter ((*first name + last name*))
08 and she was present there yesterday (1.0) also and-a
09 (2.8.)
10 HH: Here the (.) situation has remained er approximately the same
((meeting jointly discuses the client's medical condition and physical aids in use))
11 HH: ((the daughter)) terribly actively wants to keep her mother
12 (0.2) [keep her in good shape and the mother
13 HHH: [mmm
14 HH: wants to [keep herself in [shape
15 S: [mm: [yes sure she herself wants that [too
16 HH: [ye:s
17 HH: heh but this lady still needs help in getting dressed like she
18 no longer (.) is able to deal with poppers or zippers and all these so
19 and needs help showering and meals the daughter takes care of
20 and then she (.) eats unassisted (0.8) with the other hand
21 and ((the daughter)) takes care of clothes maintenance
22 and shopping and (1.0) the length of care is roughly
23 two to f*ou*r hours a d*a*y and (1.5.)
24 w*ant*s to live at h*o*me (0.8) and at this stage they don't want any
25 short term admissions or anything (.) nor care vouchers, nor anything
26 else like this cause the lady said that she is so h*a*ppy h*e*re at h*o(h)*me
27 ?: mmm
28 HH: and-a (.) and she still has a s*o*cial network so a group of friends
29 that visit her there (.) and-a
30 So they've had this lowest rate and they said that for them it is
31 quite (1.5) all right and then if there's some quite radical [change
32 S: [mm
33 HH: then they'll get in touch and we can have another look at the situation

The home helper moves the meeting forward by mentioning the next client and by identifying her by her last, middle, and first name. The mentioning of the name in this order (usually in the form last name – first name) follows the documentary format on the application forms everyone in the meeting has in front of them. Having identified the client, the home-helper then opens the file, and hands the medical documentation on the client to the doctor sitting next to her. By this simple move that often follows the introduction of a new case, the home-helper simultaneously demarcates medical knowledge and the physical status of the client as something belonging to the doctor's professional area of expertise.

In what follows, the home-helper then moves to list specifics of the client in question. In the beginning of the client description that lasts five minutes in all, the home helper delivers detail about the client's living arrangements (lines 4-6), her physical state (*moves about (1.5) poorly*, line 6) She also makes reference to the fact that she has made the home visit the day before (line 3), and that the daughter of the elderly client, who is also the carer, has been present during the visit. On line ten we learn that the situation within the past year has not changed significantly. This indicates implicitly that the elderly client is already within this particular form of support, i.e., she has previously already received the informal home care allowance. In case of such 'old cases', the task for the meeting is to check whether any significant change has occurred in the medical status of the cared for, and whether the amount of care needed per day has risen to a degree that favors the amount to be raised.

Despite the no change –status of the elderly lady in question (line 10), the home-helper nonetheless continues to describe the caring relationship between her and her daughter in some considerable detail. This is in line with the how such seemingly 'routine' cases are treated in the data more generally. After jointly discussing the medical status of the client and the level of physical aids provided by the home help team (discussion omitted from excerpt), the home helper and the secretary of the meeting in co-operation make reference to the committed nature of both mother and daughter alike: they both do their best to keep the elderly lady in good shape (lines 11-16). The home-helper also points out that despite these active efforts and the ideal initiative shown by both, the elderly lady still needs help with daily chores. She also outlines the detail of acts that go into the caring relationship (lines 17-23: dressing, showering, clothes, shopping). On line 23, the home-helper then summarizes the care with quantification: two to four hours of care work per day. This type of quantification is crucial information for the meeting to reach a decision on the exact level of support and the sum of money to be allocated.

From line 24 the home-helper then moves to summarize the opinions and viewpoints of the elderly client herself. Stating that the daughter and her mother do not want short-term hospital admissions nor care vouchers[2], she simultaneously makes clear that she, as the professional has made clear all the options open to her clients. Note, how she also resorts to active voicing (Wooffitt 1992) when describing the elderly lady's own wishes. On line 27 she reports the words of the elderly client herself, and does it in a way that repeats her own exact words "h*app*y h*ere* at ho(h)me" (here instead of there). This direct active voicing that repeats the words as they were uttered the day before adds to the factuality and authenticity of the report delivered. The wishes to continue living at home are then further fleshed out and supported with detail about the client's wide network of friends that still visit her there. The excerpt then closes with the statement of both the mother's and the daughter's wishes of maintaining the home care allowance at its current level.

What we have here then is an account of a fairly well-functioning caring relationship. The elderly person's home is depicted as the ideal place that allows the maintenance of

[2] Care vouchers are part of the municipal means of supporting informal home care. Using service vouchers granted to them, family carers can buy necessary services from private service providers and take some time off.

ongoing friendships in familiar surroundings. What I find particularly noteworthy in excerpt one is the agency attached to both the carer and the cared for. They are both depicted as responsible, as good and devoted people who do their own share. Both mother and daughter want to do their utmost to keep the mother in good shape, *but* (line 17) help from the daughter is still crucial. This raises two further analytic points. First, describing the current devoted activity of the carer and the cared for, the home-helper also evokes moral notions concerning the responsibilities of elders and of their formal and informal carers. The home-helper's account also makes available the possible trajectory that, should the best efforts of the mother and daughter fail (*radical change* line 32), potential next steps then need to be taken by us, the professionals.

In excerpt two, moral and ideal notions of devoted care by the daughter become even more pronounced as the case description unfolds further.

Excerpt Two: Mother and devoted daughter (HCA4, 32:15-36.32)

HH: ((talking about the mother)) [She] copes on her own while the daughter
goes to work at this moment (.) she's she works at the town library
(0.8) in some library she's at work sort of 50 percent
(1.8.)
HH: But the daughter said that a realistic time for the mother to stay on her own
is (0.8) something like eight hours but she still needs to phone up several
times in between (1.0) what with the recent tendency to fall she's now
taken up work half time
(1.5)
S: yes
HH: so
(0.5)
HH: they do want to do a great deal for the (0.8) mother (0.2) I mean
with the daughter also like sacrificing for her mother
All: mm, yes
HH: a part of her *work* too but I mean they said that they understand
that there are lots of applicants and they'd like this (.) lowest level

In excerpt two, the daughter is depicted as someone who is willing to sacrifice a part of her life in order to take care of the mother (line 14), while not demanding full financial compensation for the caring. Both daughter and mother are described as people who understand the institutional scarcity involved and as people who therefore are ready to settle for less.

Of all excerpts, one and two seem to construct something of a moral balance between the actions of the client and her daughter on the one hand and the public professional eldercare on the other. This public–private divide is also placed on a continuum where the situation and the efforts of all involved today are depicted, while potential changes along the caring trajectory are suspended to the background. Therefore, should changes despite all the moral and ideal devotion depicted occur, we, as the professional providers of care should be prepared to act accordingly.

LIFE COURSE IDEALS AND CULTURAL IMAGERY AS PART OF DECISION MAKING TALK

In the two excerpts shown so far, we already saw how professionals evoked notions of good and devoted family care. In what follows, I would like to provide further examples of how notions of ideal circumstances and surroundings for ageing well, as well as moral notions of devoted care by family members are brought to bear and used in support of decision making.

The interaction I chose to present concerns a case marked as exceptional by the meeting participants. This time the caring relationship consists of two brothers living together. This is a case where an elderly male carer is actively involved in the daily care of his own brother. In addition, as the excerpts below show, he is also partly responsible for another brother of his who is in long-term institutional care.

Male caregivers are not a rarity in the data as a whole. However, care provided by one brother to another is fairly rare, and also discursively marked as such in the excerpts below. Excerpt 3 begins 40 minutes into the meeting. The professional describing the case is the same speaker as in excerpts one and two. She again starts by identifying by name both the carer and the cared for, and by stating that a home visit has been done the day before. After this, however, she immediately moves to what can be analyzed as moral talk about the caring relationship in question. This time, the description also builds on some interesting discursive detail that evokes cultural ideals of good ageing as well as positive life course imagery.

Excerpt Three: The brothers (HCA4, 0:40-0:53)
Speakers: HH = home helper, S = secretary
Pseudonyms: Roundhill = a hospital

01 HH: <Then there's> er ((*last name* + *first name*)) I went there *yes*terday and-a
02 (3.5)
03 HH: hh and here the carer is the brother ((*last name* + *first name*))
04 (1.8)
05 HH: It was a such a (1.8.) an ext*re*mely g*oo*d feeling to
06 to make the (0.2) home visit because just how ((*name of the carer*))
07 had taken it to his heart to care after these brothers
08 He's had £several brothers in his care£ and now
09 one of them has gotten a place in Roundhill
10 (0.2)
11 S: yes
12 HH: a permanent [placement and
13 S: [he has
14 (1.0)
15 HH: and (0.8) it's with such joy and with a sincere heart
16 he does this
17 (1.5)
18 HH: So this ((*name of the cared for*)) has er (1.8) turned eighty hh
19 said he just (0.2) er (1.0) in September turned eighty and
20 (.) has lived *all* his l*i*fe in the same house and was *born* in it
21 and lived in it *all his* l*if*e this house that's not quite well-equipped

22 so there's no .hh (0.4) no Sauna or any other proper bath facilities
23 a sort of olden times house in ((*name of town region*))
24 (1.5)
25 and er so (2.2) this ((*name of carer*)) takes care of all shopping
26 handles all (.) all money matters and shopping and (0.4) takes
27 care of meals. He is (2.2) a g*oo*d c*oo*k has become a good cook
28 in the course of all these years, takes care of the dishes and
29 cares for the clothes of this ((*name of the cared for*)) a:nd (0.8)
30 the cleaning and (0.8) helps him get dressed and (1.0)
31 washed up. Cares for him during the *night* if needed but he
32 says that l*u*ckily t-this ((*cared for*)) sleeps well at night

In the excerpt the home-helper clearly sets out to depict the carer as someone fully and admirably devoted to the caring of his brothers. The attributes attached to him evoke notions of genuineness and of honesty: he has taken it to his heart to care for his brothers (line 7) and does this with joy and sincerity (line 15). The home-helper also describes her own feelings when coming face-to-face with such an ideal caring relationship (line 5)[3].

As the case description continues, we learn that the existence of such a devoted carer also ensures ideal surroundings for the ageing 80-year-old brother. Secured by the care by his (presumably somewhat younger) brother, he is able to continue living in the house of his childhood where he has lived all his life. In the home-helper's narration, the notion of continuity and the romantic, and in many ways old fashioned idea of living in the same house throughout one's entire life course also clearly surmount small deficiencies in the housing arrangements of the brothers (line 21-23). In all, the case is constructed as something of a nostalgic and rare glimpse into a way of living and to a form of devoted care that is about to become extinct. Moral, emotional and nostalgic overtones, in other words, clearly mark the case description.

The meeting still needs to deal with the practical question of whether and how much economic support is to be given to these brothers. In the next excerpt, the home-helper starts by pointing out that the applicants have received a modest amount so far, and that the brother in charge of the care giving has implied that the benefit should perhaps be revised.

Excerpt Four: The brothers II (HCA4, 0:43:08-0:53)
Speakers: HH = home helper, S = secretary, HHH = head of home help

01 HH: they've had this lowest er this (.) I mean this (0.2) .thh
02 ((*the carer*)) suggested that couldn't he like get a little bit more
03 than the lowest rate cause (0.2) everything (0.2)
04 he never sees any of that money himself
05 like he's done a lot of wo(h)rk for the society
06 £having taken [care of all
07 S: [he has
08 HH: his brothe(h)rs£
09 ?: that's right
10 HHH: >What< about the leg sore on ((*the cared for*)) at the moment
11 like how many medical home visits do they get nowadays?

[3] For a detailed analysis of emotion evocation and emotion categories in meeting talk, see Nikander forth.

The home-helper (on line 2) makes reference to the wishes of the carer and describes how, probably due to taxation, he hardly sees any of the money currently granted to them. She then goes on to argue for a raise in the allowance due to the long-term nature and the cost-effectiveness of the care given. In this context it is not quite clear whether the home-helper is quoting the words of the carer himself, or whether "the work for society" argument is something she herself is advocating. The laughter tokens and the smiley voice might suggest that she is in fact quoting the carer's words and marking them as delicate or as a fitting argument made by the carer. Despite the agreement by the meeting secretary, other members of the meeting do not join in or express their opinion on the home-helpers indirect suggestion. Instead, the head of home help changes the course of the discussion by asking a specific question on the elderly brother's health (>*what*< *about the leg sore*, line 10). Note how the temporal marking in the question (*nowadays*, line 11) infers that she too has access to specific information on these two brothers and their care history. The head of home help, in other words, also has a platform from which to participate in the discussion. By asking a direct question she also marks the case description as lacking in some crucial detail, and as incomplete.

It is only later in the discussion over the two brothers' case that the team comes back to the question of whether the allowance should remain on its current level or whether it should be raised. In excerpt five, the question is raised by the home-helper in charge who asks the team's and the case presenter's views on the matter. Instead of providing an answer the home helper continues by providing additional information on the case.

Excerpt five: The brothers III (HCA4, 45.00-)
Speakers: HHC = Home helper in charge, HH = home-helper, S = secretary

01 HHC: So what are we going to thin- (0.2) decide what do all you think
02 (.)
03 or what do you yourself (0.5) think about this
((*addressing the home-helper who is the case presenter*))
04 HH: then this ((*carer*)) also asked me to say (.) inform the meeting that he also .hh
05 (.) continuing (.) like this brotherhood and brotherly love (.) in a way
06 er so (.) he like (.) now that the othe- this other brother is there in Roundhill
07 S: mm
08 (0.8)
09 HH: then every other weekend cause he misses home so much
10 HHC: but the task [here is to
11 HH: [and he then every other weekend brings him home and-a
12 takes care of them both he heh he
13 ((*general laughter, talk and nodding*))
14 S: That's lovely
15 ((*general laughter and talk*))
16 HH: £so I mean brotherly love like that I haven't come across£
17 for a few years (.) not like what you can see in that house
18 S: (( )) but then surely the carer too (0.2) is tired
19 HH: that's right
20 ??: mm[m
21 HH: [yes that is what I told him too that he should think about that other
22 day in the day centre in Roundhill that they've been offered

((a few lines omitted))
HH: They've received the lowest rate before (0.2) but this ((*carer*))
just said that couldn't it be raised somewhat and I said that
I can always take the message but like I cannot ((*talk cut off*))

The home helper in charge directs the question concerning the amount of the allowance first to the whole meeting but then addresses the case presented directly (*what do you (0.5) yourself think about this*, line 3). The case presenter is reluctant to move to the decision phase, and instead, quoting the caring brother, proceeds to present further information to the meeting. What follows is further evidence on the devoted nature of the carer who, out of brotherly love, also takes his other brother out of the hospital and thus takes care of two of his brothers for shorter periods of time.

The home-helper's turns here clearly advocate a specific outcome. She continues her narrative despite the interruption on line 10 and manages to get a general, understanding and sympathetic reaction from the meeting participants (*that's lovely*, line 14). On lines 16-17 she sums up the case in a way that marks the caring relationship between the three brothers as one of a kind and exceptional. In her case description the "house of brotherly love" seems to encapsulate or turn into something of a metaphor of rare and devoted care. Discursively constructing the case as special, as something that she, as a professional, has not come across for years (lines 16-17), the speaker simultaneously advocates a specific favourable decision to be taken. Note also that towards the end of the excerpt the case presenter pronouncedly distances herself from any direct advocate work. She positions herself as simply an even-handed messenger who passes on the wishes of the client to the meeting and leaves it at that (lines 23-25).

In sum, the two cases presented above bring forth three interesting discursive phenomena. First, I have been focusing on how notions of ideal circumstances for ageing as well as positive (romantic) life course imagery are evoked when describing elderly clients and their carers. Second, I have attempted to show how such imagery trades in and calls into being moral and emotional notions of both formal and informal care and responsibility. Third, the excerpts also showed how professionals when presenting and describing their clients, walk a discursive tight rope between advocacy and notions of neutral descriptive institutional work. In both of the cases shown here, and despite the advocacy work done by one of the members, the team decided to keep the informal home care allowance at its current level.

CONCLUSION

In this chapter, the analytic focus has been on the local decision making level and on the logic and argumentation via which practical decisions about elderly care are made. This type of decision making takes place in the delicate area where the strengths, coping and abilities of individual elderly people and their carers must be appreciated and supported to the full. Simultaneously, a crucial part of any professional deliberation includes the capability of making well-informed and ethical decisions about the timing, form and level of outside support. As we have seen, interprofessional deliberation and joint decision making evoke notions of justice and morality and make use of imagery concerning the life course and "good ageing" as part of the argumentation. It seems then that professional decision-making hardly ever escapes more general ideals, and moral notions about the responsibilities of 'us' as professionals vis-à-vis those of the relatives or the elderly clients themselves. Decision making practice also trades in and discursively establishes distinct characteristics for what constitutes good and devoted care, and what the life circumstances of individual elders should ideally look like.

In sum, the key message in this chapter has been that institutional decision making over home care services consists of more than mere rational people-processing. Close discursive analyses of professional argumentation, categorization and decision making reveal the reflexive, sensitive practices whereby the morality, criteria and ethical basis of care and support allocation are negotiated. The complexity and conflicting demands under which professionals work within elderly care is hardly going to become easier in ageing societies. Therefore, close discursive analyses of professional everyday practices today, be it in meetings, by the bed side or in the cabinets of policy making may, in part, help us better understand the dynamics, ethics and challenges of elderly care tomorrow.

Practical Considerations and Recommendations:

1. Close analysis of institutional interaction lays out for view the day-to-day logic and argumentation of professional deliberation and decision making.
2. The training and schooling of elderly care professionals could make better use of discursive studies and analysis on professional practice.
3. Work arrangements and time budgeting within elderly care should enable and support professionals' joint reflection and analysis of their work and decision making practices.
4. Forming and maintaining an outspoken set of criteria on the local level helps professionals work and makes the processes of decision making accessible and transparent to all involved.
5. Analysis and awareness of shared ideals, morality and criteria helps prepare for the ongoing changes and challenges within elderly care.

References

Antaki, C. and Widdicombe, S. (eds) (1998): *Identities in Talk*. London: Sage.

Anttonen, A. and Sipilä, J. (2000): Suomalaista sosiaalipolitiikkaa [Social Policy in Finland]. Tampere, Vastapaino.

Atkinson, P. and Coffey, A. (1997): Analysing Documentary Realities. In D. Silverman (Ed.): *Qualitative Research. Theory, Method and Practice*. pp. 45-62 London, Sage.

Baker, C.D. (1997) 'Ticketing rules: Categorization and moral ordering in a school staff meeting.' In S. Hester and P. Eglin (eds) *Culture in Action: Studies in Membership Categorisation Analysis.* pp. 77-98. Lanham, Maryland: International Institute for Ethnomethodology and Conversation Analysis and University Press of America.

Boden, D. (1994): *The Business of Talk: Organizations in Action*. Cambridge, Polity Press.

Cicirelli, V.G. (1993): Intergenerational communication in the mother-daughter dyad regarding caregiving decisions. In Coupland, N. and Nussbaum, J.F. (Eds.): *Discourse and Lifespan Identity*. (pp. 215-236) Newbury Park, CA: Sage.

Coupland, N. and Coupland, J. (1998): Reshaping lives: Constitutive identity work in geriatric medical consultations. *Text*, 18(2): 159-189.

Coupland, N. and Coupland, J. (1999): Ageing, ageism and anti-ageism. Moral stance in geriatric medical discourse. In Hamilton, H.E. (Ed.): *Language and Communication in Old Age. Multidisciplinary Perspectives.* (pp. 177-208.) New York: Garland.

Dockrell, J. and Wilson, G. (1995) 'Management issues in interprofessional work with older people.' In K. Soothill, L. Mackay and C. Webb (eds) *Interprofessional Relations in Health Care*. pp. 281-296 London: Edward Arnold.

Gilleard, C. and Higgs, P. (1998): Old People as Users and Consumers of Healthcare: A third age rhetoric for a fourth age reality? *Ageing and Society* 18, 233-248.

Grainger, K. (1993): That's a lovely bath dear: Reality construction in the discourse of elderly care. *Journal of Aging Studies*, 7(3): 247-262.

Hester, S. and Eglin, P. (eds) (1997): *Culture in Action: Studies in Membership Categorisation Analysis*. Lanham, Maryland: International Institute for Ethnomethodology and Conversation Analysis and University Press of America.

Holstein, J.A. (1990): The discourse of age in involuntary commitment proceedings. *Journal of Aging Studies*, 4(2): 111-130.

Housley, W. (2003): *Interaction in Multidisciplinary Teams*. Cardiff Papers in Qualitative Research, Hants, Ashgate.

Latimer, J. (1997): Giving patients a Future: The constituting of classes in an acute medical unit. *Sociology of Health and Illness* 9(2), 160-185.

Leppänen, V. (1998): *Structures of District Nurse – Patient Interaction*. Lund Dissertations in Sociology, University of Lund.

Linell, P. (1998): Discourse Across Boundaries: On recontextualizations and the blending of voices in professional discourse. *Text* 18(2), 143-157.

Nikander, P. (2000): 'Old' vs. 'Little Girl': A discursive approach to age categorisation and morality. *Journal of Aging Studies*, 14(4): 335-358.

Nikander, P. (2002). *Age in Action: Membership work and stage of life categories in talk.* Helsinki, Finnish Academy of Science and Letters.

Nikander, P. (2003). The Absent Client: Case description and decision-making in multi-professional meetings. Interactions, identities and practices. In Hall, C., Juhila, K., Parton, N. and Pösö T. (Eds.) *Constructing clienthood in social work and human services*. (pp. 112-128) London: Jessica Kingsley.

Nikander, P (2005): *Managing Scarcity: Joint decision making in interprofessional meetings.* In Heinonen, T. and Metteri, A. (Eds.): Social Work in Health and Mental Health: issues, Developments and Actions. pp.273-299. Toronto, Canadian Scholar's Press.

Nikander, P. (forth): Emotion Categories in Meeting Talk. In A. Hepburn. and S. Wiggins (Eds.): *Discursive Research in Practise. New Approaches to Psychology and Interaction.* Cambridge University Press, Cambridge.

Paoletti, I. (1998): *Being an Older Woman: A Study in the Social Production of Identity.* Everyday Communication: Case Studies of Behavior in Context Series. Mahwah, NJ: Lawrence Erlbaum Associates.

Taylor, B.C. (1992): Elderly identity in conversation: Producing frailty. *Communication Research*, 19(4): 493-515.

Vaarama, M. and Kautto, M. (1999): Social Protection for the Elderly in Finland. Saarijärvi, Gummerus.

Walker, A. (1995): The family and the mixed economy of care. In I. Allen and E. Perkins, *The future of family care for older people*. pp. 22-35. London: HMSO.

Wooffitt, R. (1992): *Telling Tales of the Unexpected: The Organization of Factual Discourse.* London: Harvester Wheatsheaf.

In: Family Caregiving for Older Disabled People
Editor: Isabella Paoletti, pp. 333-357
ISBN 1-59454-808-0

Chapter 16

EXPLORING THE CULTURAL BORDERLINES OF FAMILY CAREGIVING IN FINLAND

Marja Saarenheimo, Suvi Nikula and Päivi Eskola
The Central Union for the Welfare of the Aged,
Malmin kauppatie 26, 00700 Helsinki, Finland

INTRODUCTION

Family care is currently carried out as the joint work of families and professional carers. It is a mixture of everyday practices and administrative activities, such as the actual care work performed by the family members and the decisions made by the authorities to allocate services to the families. Consequently, family care consists of several different and even possibly incommensurable "microcultures" and discourses, This complicates the cooperation between the families, service providers and decision-makers. Our aim is to explore how everyday care is conceptualized and how service needs and solutions are defined within these microcultures. Specifically, we focus on the critical points where controversies and misunderstandings between different actors within the field of family care are manifested. These puzzling occasions are called here 'cultural borderlines'.

DIFFERENT WAYS OF CONCEPTUALIZING FAMILY CAREGIVING

Family care is typically conceptualized in two alternative ways. The first of these focuses on the reactions, actions and experiences of the persons or other stakeholders involved. The second concentrates on the formal structure of family care and its role as a vehicle of social and health policy. Both conceptualizations are, however, closely tied to the paradigms of disability and dependency, as is the case with research on fourth age phenomena in general. (Gilleard and Higgs 2000, preface; Blaikie 2002). Research on family care can be divided into practically oriented research, such as intervention studies, and more theoretically oriented research, where the focus is on the process and act of caregiving itself. Next, some of the previous research is presented and we argue that despite voluminousvery little evidence for the effectiveness of current methods of supporting families.Tthere is also a need for theoretically oriented research to support creative planning in indicating the conflicts in the current experiences of the caregiving families.

From the caregiver's perspective, family care has been conceptualized as a burden, a moral duty or a mutually dependent complex relationship. Empirical research has widely demonstrated the burdensome nature of the care work carried out by family members of the elderly and frail (Knight, Lutzky, and Macofsky-Urban 1993; Toseland, Smith and McCallion 2001). The most plausible evidence links family care to psychological stress, and especially the spousal caregivers to the demented elderly are found to suffer from depression, anxiety and other psychological symptoms (Neundorfer 1991; Jutras and Lavoie 1995; Schulz et al., 1995). There is no similar consensus concerning threats to physical health during the care work, although the family carers frequently report physical complaints such as sleep disturbances, chronic fatigue and muscle aches (Toseland et al., 2001). However, a recent meta-analysis (Vitaliano, Scanlan, and Zhang 2003) verifies the greater risk of physical health problems and higher levels of stress hormones in caregivers compared to demographically similar non-caregivers.

The Support Services

As family care is currently being established as a promising component of the public service system in many societies, it has become necessary to consider the nature of support systems needed to sustain it, as well as to figure out what type of support is most beneficial to families and society. A large number of intervention programs have been conducted in order to pursue these questions. Here, as Toseland et al. have pointed out that the policy-makers and researchers are faced with two contradictory imperatives, with the first focusing on the alleviation and/or prevention of the caregiver burden and the second emphasizing the maximization of the amount and duration of family care and, accordingly, the minimization of the need for institutional placements (Toseland et al., 2001). Intervention studies apply a variety of different aims and objectives and consequently, the findings strike one as heterogeneous and even contradictory (Knight et al., 1993; Flint 1995; Bourgeois et al. 1996; Thompson and Spilsbury 2000; Green and Brodaty 2002). Overall, the benefits of intervention programs have at best been only moderate (Zarit and Leitsch 2001). Some well-designed and well-targeted programs have managed to increase caregiver satisfaction and alleviate the caregiver burden, but when the primary aim is to delay the institutional placement of the care recipients, the effects have usually been minor (Hyvärinen et al., 2003).

The diversity of intervention programs is enormous. A program may involve many types of care recipients and caregivers or be targeted only on a specific group, for example spousal caregivers of demented patients or adult children caring for their physically disabled parents. The problems and challenges vary from one family to another and although a program may benefit some participants, the overall effects can still be modest. Also, the type of support given to the families varies across the programs. Some consist mainly of treatments and services given to the care recipients, like respite care and day-care services. In others, the services are designed more directly to meet the needs of the caregivers, for example through peer groups or educational groups. Individual or group counseling and even psychotherapy may also be involved. The best outcomes so far have been attained in comprehensive counseling programs that are able to address the specific needs of each family and involve services to all family members (Mittelman et al., 1993, 1995; Eloniemi-Sulkava et al., 2001).

In most intervention programs, the support services are standardized to fit all families irrespective of their unique life situations. The caregivers, not to mention the care recipients, do not generally participate in planning, implementing or evaluating the services and thus the services may not meet the expectations of all families. In Finland, family caregivers are entitled to a caregiver's monthly allowance, including care arrangements for two days a month to allow time off for the caregiver. The system is sustained and administered by the municipalities. In spite of the obvious benefits, there remains considerable discontent with the organization of Finnish family care, both on the part of families and practitioners. On the one hand, the families commonly experience difficulties in finding appropriate and good-quality services, especially during the caregiver's holidays. On the other hand, the service providers often regret that families are reluctant to use the services offered to them. According to Zarit et al., the issue of why families do not use respite services more is one of the major, unanswered questions in the caregiving field in general (Zarit and Leitsch 2001).

The Reasons for Caring

What makes the families continue care despite the experienced stress and without sufficient societal support? Betty Kramer, among others, suggests that instead of focusing solely on the negative consequences of caregiving, the researchers should pay more attention to the motives, incentives and resources that make families accept the caring duty in the first place (Kramer 1997; see also Lawton, Kleban, and Moss 1989; Farran 1997). Understanding such positive aspects of caring may, according to Kramer, help practitioners work more effectively with the families. Recognizing the strengths and resources of the families is consistent with the idea of empowerment in the sense of helping the families to make decisions and to prepare and/or access support systems needed to help them face future challenges (Clark 1989, 270-271).

One way of studying the caregivers' strengths is to observe "successful caregivers" or successful strategies in family caregiving (Noelker and Wallace 1985; Silverman and Huelsman 1990; Farran 1997). In qualitative research interviews, the family caregivers frequently bring up positive meanings of caring (Farran 1997; Kramer 1997). As burdensome as the care work may be, the carers report feelings of satisfaction and pride in their ability and endurance in taking on the caregiving duty. Meeting the challenges of caring may also increase the carers' sense of being useful and the sense of being recognized by others for their work. (Gatz et al., 1990; Pearlin et al., 1996.) For some, the mutual inter-dependency between carer and care-recipient acts as a source of increased emotional intimacy.

A slightly different perspective on caregiver strengths is offered by ethnographic research on family care. In his insightful study, Steven Albert has explored the adaptation to caregiving demands in different families. His interpretations highlight the importance of specific adaptation strategies that emerge in response to concrete caregiving demands and allow families to render care more effectively (Albert, 1990). The participants in this study were middle-aged daughters and sons caring for their disabled parents at home. The crucial issue for the interviewees was how to draw lines between caregiving tasks and other components of family life. According to Albert, the families used two broad sets of strategies, establishing routines for caregiving tasks and redefining the roles of the carers and care recipients. Albert's study highlights the relevance of considering the embeddedness of the caregiving dyad within the microcultural context of family life.

A Cultural Perspective

In this chapter, our aim is to explore the field of the family care of the elderly from a cultural perspective. Here, the cultural perspective means that family care is not studied as an established phenomenon with universal or stable meanings in relation to social policy, responsibility and experience. Rather, our purpose is to look at family care as a "phenomenon under construction" and pave the way for alternative conceptualizations of care and related subjects. After a brief discussion of the methods and the source of the data, we present interpretations concerning how the different microcultures are manifested in everyday care. Specifically we will highlight the meanings given to the changes taking place within and controversies between these microcultures. The analysis is presented in three parts. The first part addresses changes within the domestic culture of caregiving families during the care process. Here, we focus on two interrelated issues: the changes in the spousal relationship and the cultural meanings of home as components of home care. In the second part of the analysis we turn to changes taking place in the social networks of caregiving families. The third part takes us to the encounters between families and service providers, where cultural controversies are most obvious. Our interpretations are based on a social-constructionist perspective dealing with how the phenomena of everyday life are construed in the dialogues between different actors. In the next section the method of data collection and data analysis are presented.

Data and Methods

The Participants

This study is a part of a larger research project focusing on the situation of elderly family caregivers in Finland.[1] Our research material is drawn from a corpus of thirty encounters with elderly caregiving families in different parts of Finland. The encounters took place mostly in the homes of the families. The families were contacted through care professionals working in five Veteran Rehabilitation Centres. For this particular chapter, we selected twelve families to represent varied care situations and diverse living environments. Three of the caregivers were men and the remaining nine were women. Family care had been of varying duration and the

[1] The study was carried out in the Central Union for the Welfare of the Aged in Finland. It was funded by the Finland's Slot Machine Association, which supports most third sector health and welfare organizations in Finland.

condition as well as the primary illness of the care recipient varied across the families. For this generation, 70-80 year olds, it is common that the wife takes responsibility for household tasks and especially with the wife as the caregiver, it is sometimes difficult to indicate the precise moment when the actual care has begun. The change of roles may take place over months or years, as the caregiver has to take increasing responsibility for the household and finally is responsible for the personal care of the spouse, too. Also the burden of care varies considerably. In some families carers have been trained by community nurses to perform some nursing tasks as well, and in some families, care mostly consists of taking increasing responsibility for running the everyday life of the household.

The core of the home care in our study is invariably an elderly couple. All the twelve couples had been married for more than 40 years and some almost 60 years. The length of the shared lives had taken some of the caregivers by surprise, as around the time they got married (mostly in the 1940s) life expectancies were shorter in general and becoming a widow(er) at middle-age was quite common. Therefore, the remarkable length of the shared lives was highly valued and it created a strong base for the mutual care. Currently, it is well known, that when available, the spouse is the primary option for giving care (e.g. Montgomery 1999). Women become caregivers more often than men. Furthermore, caregiving tasks are often taken for granted as responsibilities related to the person's role in the family, e.g. the role of the wife, and caregiving tasks may be assumed without conscious recognition of the role of a family caregiver (e.g. Levine 1999). Three of the twelve caregivers here were men. Research on husbands caring for their wives shows that they are not common in western cultures (Brewer 2001), but some can be found (e.g. Kirsi, Hervonen, and Jylhä 2000).

An Ethnographic Approach

As the focus of our study was on the meanings given to care and related issues, a sensible choice for the method of data collection was that of ethnography. We have applied ethnography here to study the social setting where the family care takes place and to observe the care situation at home. The central task of an ethnographer in culturally remote settings has been described as making the strange familiar. Paradoxically, in ethnographies carried out in familiar settings, the task of the researcher could be defined as making the familiar strange. (Spindler and Spindler 1982; Delamont and Atkinson 1995; Gordon, Holland and Lahelma 2001.) The family care setting is a peculiar mixture of the familiar and the strange. The familiarity arises from the implicit meanings of home and family that are rarely either explicated or (less still) questioned in everyday conversations. The strangeness, on the other hand, arises from the Western cultural tendency to understand illness and care as private matters to be protected from public view. More than a decade ago, Gubrium and Shankar (1990) encouraged researchers to use ethnographic methods and analytical techniques to understand the home care experience, but apart from a few exceptions (e.g. Albert 1990), researchers have not tried to observe how the caregiving families actually get through the day.

Some of the principal functions of participant observation are to understand the context of the phenomenon under investigation and to work out what the important questions to be asked are (Darlington and Scott 2002). The level of participation can vary from non-participation to complete participation in the sense of sharing most of the everyday routines and practices with the people to be observed (Spradley 1980). In this study, the actual observation took part in two lengthy (3 – 7 hours) visits per family. Before getting to the field, however, it was essential to figure out what in the first place constituted the field to be observed. If family care is defined as the joint work of families and professional carers, then the observation should not be restricted to the inside of the home but embrace the varied occasions where care arrangements and decisions are made. Besides, observation alone cannot tell us why people do the things they do and what a particular activity means to them (Darlington and Scott 2002). Other research tools are needed to capture the cultural and personal meanings attached to care and other everyday practices. For this purpose, ethnographic interviews were conducted with caregivers. Barbara Sherman Heyl has defined the ethnographic interview as one in which the researcher has established respectful, on-going relationships with the interviewees, including enough rapport for there to be a genuine exchange of views and enough time and openness for the interviewees to explore purposefully with the researcher the meanings they place on events in their worlds (Sherman Heyl 2001).

In order to understand the unique context of family care in each family and the nature of family care as practical, day-to-day activity, it was necessary to spend a sufficient amount of time with the families and to interact with the wife and husband together. This was also essential for creating a good rapport. The initial visits consisted mainly of casual conversations with the family and observations of the home and the relationship between the husband and wife. The researchers also offered their help with domestic duties. In the second visit, a qualitative interview was conducted with the caregiver. In most cases, there was a day-care arrangement for the care-recipient to enable the lengthy interview with the caregiver. All interviews were tape-recorded as well as parts of the conversations on the initial visits. To grasp the wider cultural context of family care in contemporary Finnish society, familiarity with public support systems and professional practices was also fundamental. For this purpose, encounters with the contact persons in Rehabilitation Centers, as well as with local care professionals were arranged. These encounters, together with public documents concerning family care, constitute a kind of background data for the study. The actual empirical data to be analyzed consists of transcripts of interviews with the caregivers and conversations with the families, as well as researchers' field notes.

The Analysis of the Data

At the core of our analysis are the family carer's and other stakeholders' meanings and conceptualizations of care and related issues. Our methodological tools are drawn from social constructionist and discourse-analytical research, as defined among others by Wetherell et al. (2001). The use of the term "microculture", instead of, for example, "discourse" is justified by our specific focus on meanings that become apparent not only in verbal accounts but also in everyday practices and actions. A microculture can be defined as a system of practices and patterns descriptive of a group of people, for example a family or service providers. Using the social constructionist perspective, the conversation and interview transcriptions, as well as the researchers' field notes were interpreted in relation to three domains where the different microcultures of family care became apparent and were recreated. These are the domestic sphere (specifically the relationship between the carer and care-recipient and the home as the context of everyday care), the wider social network of the caregiving family as a source of support, and the service system as the context for cooperation. Our specific interest lies in the changes and controversies taking place within and between the different microcultures of family care. The term "cultural borderline" was invented to exemplify these occasions. To elucidate the process of analysis, we use a number of citations from the interview transcripts. These provide insight into how the caregivers conceptualize the care process and what strategies they use in explaining and justifying their actions and experiences. In the next section, we present the result of the analysis starting with the examination of the changes within the family context.

Changes in the Domestic Culture of a Family During the Caring Situation

Family care affects the domestic culture of an elderly couple on at least two levels: the relationship between the spouses and the home as a social and psychological context of care. Caring at home is thought to have more benefits than disadvantages, but there is no doubt that considerable problems and compromises are also involved. Next, we focus on the changes in the domestic culture that take place in a caregiving situation. First, we explore how family roles and relationships were construed in the interviews and how the changes in the marital relationship were interpreted. After that, we consider the meanings given to the home and how the alterations of the home during the care situation became important constituents of caregivers' experiences and actions.

Changes of Roles within the Couple

The interviews revealed two critical changes in the mutual relationships of these elderly couples. First, as the one person becomes more and more unable to take responsibility for his/her share of the household tasks, the responsibilities of the carer expand beyond caregiving to include an increasing proportion of everyday chores. The burden of care is not therefore only related to the possible caregiving tasks, including e.g. personal care, but is also related to a growing amount of housework while the carer's own physical health and endurance are also deteriorating. This phenomenon is easier to demonstrate for husbands, as they fill in the daily chores when their wives become unable to perform their domestic tasks (e.g. Kirsi et al., 2000). For wives this transition of responsibility is more difficult to indicate, as the domestic sphere has mostly been dominated by them according to the traditional division of labour (e.g. Avlund, and Schultz-Larsen 1991). From a husband's perspective it may seem that the gender roles are exchanged but based on the wife's description of the process, it is not merely an exchange but an expansion of roles and responsibilities that takes place in a family where one becomes dependent on the other. As a fairly practical topic, this point was well described in many interviews. The next extract demonstrates a husband giving an explicit account of his 'new' daily chores after his wife has become unable to take responsibility for shopping and cooking.

Caregiver: (...) and after the last time at the country place it has been very, very difficult. Ehh (.) little by little, already since a fairly early stage, doing grocery shopping and planning meals. She really hasn't, about the time of the diagnosis or after it, prepared hardly any food.

Interviewer: Hmmm.

Caregiver: Although she was very, very much a kind of kitchen person. She was very, very, she had a good feel for it. A good cook.

Interviewer: Yes. But she then lost interest in it?

Caregiver: She lost interest and apparently also the ability to do it.

Interviewer: Hmmm.

Caregiver: I have then, for the last few years, taken care of these things.

Later, the husband explains, that despite some experience in cooking, the greatest change has been taking responsibility for the kitchen chores in general, including planning, shopping and seeing to cleaning as well. For wives, describing the daily chores was more difficult as most of them were self-evident. When the couple lived in a house of their own, the husband had usually been responsible for the outdoor tasks such as taking care of the firewood or snow shoveling. When the couple lived in an apartment building, the responsibilities of the husband were more difficult to indicate. However, it had often been the husband who had taken responsibility for financial decisions. Thus, along with the caregiving role, the wife had to learn to take care of financial matters as well. The next extract demonstrates how the wife indicates the beginning of increasing caring responsibilities through negotiation about moving. The wife had become aware of the fact that in their current residence she would not be able to continue caring for much longer and decided they should find a new apartment and sell the current one. This meant that the wife had to make considerable financial decisions that used to be taken care of by her husband.

Interviewer: When did it begin, what did it feel like? Eh (.) how has the change been in that way, who takes responsibility and ...?

Caregiver: Yes. I take the responsibility alone and I really feel it, because my husband was not very keen on moving [from this apartment] when he said that he wants to suffer his illnesses here and die here.

Interviewer: Yes.

Caregiver: But that's where I was [according to the others] brisk. I noticed, that I have to take the reins.

Interviewer: Hmmm.

Caregiver: I said, that now we will look at what is best for me and you are close to the end already. Well (he) can't do a thing anymore. Hardly can take care of himself and so on. But I told him I am the one taking responsibility, I will take care of you as long as I am able to.

The second critical issue is the change of the relationship from a spousal to a care relationship.

CHANGES IN THE MARITAL RELATIONSHIP

This is possibly the most difficult process to address in empirical caregiving research for at least two reasons. Firstly, family care is often studied from the perspective of the service provider and while the home is "cleaned of the family life" when the formal services enter the home (e.g. Tedre 1999; Ala-Nikkola 2003), maintaining the expressions of an intimate relationship may become impossible. Secondly, the illness itself may have caused a loss of intimacy because of physical care needs and sometimes because of changes in personality. Despite the changes, the carers found ways to see the relationship as precious and meaningful for them. The next extract presents a wife's conceptualization of the changes in the marital relationship with a demented husband.

> *Interviewer*: And how are the (.) how would you describe the relationship between you two?
>
> *Caregiver*: Now, with Antero? (.) Well we do have a stable relationship, that, that somehow one knows one another and that (.) that there is, there is old friendship and being mates remaining now and (…)
>
> *Interviewer*: Yes.
>
> *Caregiver*: And like that. And emotional values exist, although if one would be cross about something, the other will not care about it or be shaken by it.
>
> *Interviewer*: Okay, yes.
>
> *Caregiver*: Then in the beginning one was hurt a little and it felt that now he did, he did (…) But then as years go by the sharpest corners have worn out, and what has become of it, is a kind of friendship.
>
> *Interviewer*: Yes.
>
> *Caregiver*: And unity, like that, that. Don't know, it is the kind of thing you just know.
>
> *Interviewer*: Yes, well, after being together for 45 years.
>
> *Caregiver*: Well, yes, so we have.

Caregivers commonly described their current relationship as a "friendship or being mates" and the history of their marital life as "having never had many conflicts". In most families it is clear, however, that the disabled spouse has become easily irritable or that there is hardly any conversation between the spouses. Based on the interviewees' accounts communication between the spouses may be mostly based on mutual non-verbal interaction that has been learned during the long-lasting companionship. Therefore, one clear change in the family life that the carers describe is the requirement to know the care recipient's needs without them being explicitly spoken. In some ways, the couple acts as a solid unit and as one's condition deteriorates the other tries to fill in the parts that are deteriorating. When asked about what is most demanding in their current situation, it is more often the emotional than the physical stress that is mentioned. One of the most difficult things for many carers seemed to be the incessant need to be there for the disabled spouse. In the next quotation, a female caregiver gives an explanation for the couple's shared reluctance to use respite services or granny sitting based on an encompassing dependency between the spouses.

> *Interviewer*: Yes (…) have you already tried that someone would come here? To be with him or (.) It hasn't worked out, has it?

> *Caregiver:* I really don't know (...) I really don't know. It seems as if he only likes me better, that I know all his desires and thoughts you see and no, no one, no other will understand [laughs] him, the way (I do).

Some caregivers explained how they were able to better guide and support their spouses to do things that had become difficult for them with their illnesses, such as moving around for someone who had had a stroke. The long history together supported caregiving in numerous ways. It helped on a practical level to know the spouse's needs and difficulties but it was also essential in conflicts, which were easier to solve in ways familiar from earlier years. As the verbal communication often became less frequent between the wife and the husband, caregivers were able to maintain the friendship with their spouses based on their earlier knowledge about them.

Based on the accounts of the respondents in this study, it is clear that becoming a family caregiver is far more complex than just providing increasing care to the cared for. A large proportion of the responsibilities involve the expansion of housework and seeing to things that used to be taken care of by the spouse. Sometimes it is difficult, for even the caregiver himself or herself to indicate all the responsibilities that they now take care of. Secondly, the process of becoming carers and care-recipients is a remarkable change for most couples. Mostly the carers accepted it quietly, but some expressed sorrow related to the loss of the partner that the spouse used to be. Old friendship was much valued and sometimes the memory of earlier times helped to cherish the relationship. In both cases, the caregiving spouses show remarkable ability to adjust to and cope with changing family life. Therefore, the changes are constantly compensated so that the domestic culture of the home can be recreated according to the requirements of care.

The Home Arrangements

There is a widespread belief in the overall benefits of living at home even in a very old age. Home care has important emotional and economic grounds, but there appears to be even more at stake in the care decisions of elderly families. The home is one of those obvious concepts that are rarely problematized in everyday thinking and talk. Yet in a more detailed analysis a variety of diverse psychological, juridical, developmental and socio-cultural meanings become apparent. The home contains elements of control, security, family development, independence, comfort, protection, feelings, and the presence of people (Rubinstein 1991, 39). Fundamentally, the home represents safety and self (Csikszentmihalyi and Rochberg-Halton 1981), and being able to live at home contains a possibility of controlling one's own life and sustaining one's lifestyle even in frail old age. Based on our data, the personal and cultural meanings of the home are rarely portrayed in the interviews as direct reflections. Rather, they offer themselves for interpretation from between the lines, as small fragments of stories or through distinctions of home and "not home". The meanings of home are thus constantly recreated, reinforced or transformed through the cultural exchanges that take place during the process of family care.

THE MEANING OF HOME

For most of our interviewees, keeping their disabled spouse at home was a matter of course, something that did not require any special justification. In fact, many had not even considered other options. Not surprisingly, this matches well the dominant guideline of today's old age politics in Finland and also elsewhere. When asked about the decision to accept the responsibility for care, the answers covered a spectrum from expressions of constraint and necessity ("Well, I had to"/ "There were no other alternatives"/ "Who else would take care of him?") to expressions of unquestionable willingness ("I have never thought of any other alternative and I never think that it will end some day"/ "We always hoped that we could live here just the two of us"). Should the reasonableness of the home care be questioned, for example, by their children or the care professionals, the carers appealed to their marriage vows that obligated them to stand by their spouse "in sickness and in health, until death do us part".

Rubinstein has argued that to live at home represents a more active personhood and therefore, to keep a sick family member at home means that she or he is not fully sick (Rubinstein 1990, 39). Besides, it seems that in the context of the home, institutionalization can be interpreted as a violation of an important cultural imperative, according to which each person should have the right to live at home as long as possible. (An interesting question is whether the imperative will in fact be changing, as there is some evidence that the adult children in Finland encourage the elderly caregivers to place their disabled spouses in residential care). In the next transcription, a moral dilemma is constructed around the decision concerning respite care.

> *Caregiver*: We have been together so long and I always tell him that it is my duty to take care of him. And when I took him to [the rehabilitation hospital] for the first time, it was somehow difficult for me and I thought: what if he had understood where we were taking him (...) and I kind of thought it was needless to put him there. I could imagine the opinions of the relatives when I take him there. Like "why doesn't she take care of him at home?"
>
> *Interviewer*: Yes, what did the relatives actually say (.) because you were afraid of what they might think about it?
>
> *Caregiver*: Well, they have not asked me, why I don't take care of him myself (...) And his sister, who is a nurse herself and has worked with old people (.), she said that if only you get a place for him for two weeks, you should take it. Don't say "no", because there are not so many places like that available.

The reluctance to accept the respite care was based here on the caregiver's conviction that it is the moral duty of a wife to manage the care at least while her husband is still able to walk. Not being able to walk would, for this interviewee, create the justification for sharing or even giving up the care. In addition, her conviction that her demented husband was not aware of the destination, made her question whether she was acting in a morally defensible way. Confirmation was needed from others that she considered important.

What specific consequences does intensive home care have for a household? Corbin and Strauss (1990) talk about the "making of arrangements", when referring to the process of negotiating and agreeing about necessary changes in household tasks and practices because of the care situation. In our data, the caregivers brought up three kinds of changes in the household arrangements. First, the illness of the spouse sometimes necessitated the concrete reorganization of the room order or of the furniture. Secondly, most families had made or experienced radical changes in their social life. Thirdly, in most cases there were care professionals in the house more or less regularly. In this section, we consider the first two issues; the encounters with professionals are examined in a later section.

FAMILY RITUALS

In elderly families, the rituals and practices of everyday life have taken shape during decades of family life. Many of these practices are based on tacit understandings between the spouses rather than actual negotiation. For this generation, the women are more likely than men to control the domestic order of the home, as it is often the women who have created a home inside the house (see Csikszentmihalyi and Rochberg-Halton 1981). For women, being a caregiver often meant giving up, at least in part, on their standards of household management. A hospital bed might, for example, occupy the living room or the women had to give precedence to the caring duties over the housekeeping tasks. For the men, on the other hand, the caregiver's position could even open up new domains of family life, such as cooking or laundry. As a consequence, the control of the home shifted from the wife to the husband.

Even if home care enables a more active personhood for the disabled family member, it often means a simultaneous change in the home as a social and cultural arena, at least temporarily. Nearly all our respondents reported changes in socializing with friends and relatives. This might result partly from the caregiver's lack of time or simple exhaustion, but it may also be a consequence of rigid cultural rules of family life that do not allow for new forms of interplay inside the home. In most cultures there is a distinct set of rules regulating the visits of friends and relatives. In Finland, the "visiting schema" includes at least some kind of hospitality, usually including coffee and pastry. Having nothing to offer guests at all would violate the cultural rule. A safer alternative is, therefore, to refrain from inviting guests altogether. The field notes, together with some theoretical conceptions, offer one more potential explanation for the reluctance of the caregivers to invite guests to their home. If the home is psychologically best understood as "a shell of the self" (Csikszentmihalyi and Rochberg-Halton 1981), all radical changes in the domestic order can be interpreted as challenges to maintaining the continuity of the self. In this respect, the "signs of illness", such as the presence of special hospital furniture, care equipment or particular odours and noises, get easily interpreted as obstacles for social interaction at home.

In this section we have tried to identify some of the critical issues in the everyday life of elderly couples in family care. From a cultural point of view, some of the most important changes involve a new division of responsibilities, an increase in the complexity of roles and an ambiguity in applying the traditional meanings of home to the process of care. In the next section we will extend the analysis to the broader social networks of the caregiving family.

FAMILY CARE AND SOCIAL NETWORKS

The social networks of a family change during the family's life cycle. Contacts with people become more frequent in some areas of life and less in others. In elderly families, the reduction of contacts usually takes place in the sphere of informal networks (i.e., relatives and friends). An increase of contacts typically occurs in the formal network, with more or less involuntary relationships developing with home help and community nursing, for example (Marin 2003). Having friends, neighbours and relatives of the same age becomes less and less common in old age. These relationships are eventually at least partly replaced by people from younger age groups, such as children and grandchildren. However, not only the size or shape of the network changes with age; but also the contents and functions of the existing relationships may be transformed. The social networks of the caregiving families have mostly been examined with respect to the support they provide or fail to provide to the caregiver (Barker et.al., 1998; Clipp and George, 1990; Rimmerman and Muraver, 2001; Wallsten, 2000). It has been argued that the family caregiver's ability to cope with the demands of caring is influenced by the presence or absence of personal, social and spiritual support, as well as by the knowledge and use of outside resources (Phipps, et al., 2003). The function of such social networks is not, however, limited to direct support, but includes many other cultural, social and psychological aspects. Next, we examine how the functions of social networks were defined by the elderly caregivers themselves and what resources they made use of when striving to manage their networks.

THE HELP RECEIVED FROM CLOSE KIN

All the couples in our data had children. Most of them had grandchildren and even great grandchildren. The adult children were involved in the everyday life of the respondents in various ways and in various measures. In some interviews, the children were hardly mentioned while in others they occupied an important role in the social life and/or in the care arrangements of the interviewees. Typically, the caregivers emphasized that they did not want to bother their children too much, because "they have a life of their own with the work and the children". The ideal of a self-sufficient individual seems to dominate even in moments of utmost distress. At the same time, however, it was often underlined that if help were needed, the children would be there:

> *Caregiver:* Of course she [the daughter] shares the difficulties with us, and all that (...) you know that all these things with paperwork and forms are so difficult nowadays. She knows them better and also knows how to apply for the compensation for medication expenses, for example. (...) She sends them over to the [State Treasury] and we get the money back.

In this family, help was needed in applying for allowances and filling in forms, which required specific knowledge and was thought to be easier for the daughter, with her higher level of education. In addition, the sympathetic attitude of the daughter was emphasized. In other cases, especially in the rural areas, the caregivers often mentioned a son helping with heavy domestic duties; for instance, carrying the firewood in or clearing the snow off the driveway. If there was no son there could be a male neighbour who ploughed the farmyard or chopped wood. In these cases the caregiver often paid for the service, because, as one of our respondents said: "Otherwise they won't come next time". The help of daughters or other female relatives was mentioned in relation to the inside house chores, regardless of the living environment. Typically the child who lived nearby was considered the main support with regard to the practical tasks. The children were also mentioned as sources of emotional support. The next transcription presents a male caregiver whose wife was temporarily staying in an old age home:

> *Interviewer:* Talking about the present situation, you said earlier that [your wife] doesn't like it in the old age home. How did you come to the decision (.) for her to be staying there for a while?
>
> *Caregiver:* We made the decision together with [my son], and with my daughter, too, because the doctor had earlier prescribed this treatment (...) did I already mention that to you (...) a kind of short-term care (.) one week (...) It didn't take place at that time, though, because there was no room at the old age home.

When asked about the decision to give up his caring duties for the time being, the respondent explained that he called on his son and daughter, as well as the doctor to share the responsibility. Typically, the caregiving spouses found the decisions concerning institutionalization – be it temporary or permanent – too difficult to justify through their personal experience alone. "A second opinion" was usually needed to construct the institutionalization as a morally justifiable act.

Based on our data, elderly caregivers do not define themselves as mere receivers of support. They also reported providing support for others and contributing their own share of the reciprocity in their networks. One of our female caregivers said that when her daughter needs help with the grandchildren, she takes her husband to an old age home and drives 200 kilometres to help the daughter. The same caregiver defined her role in the social network of the small village where she and her husband live:

> *Caregiver*: We have good relations. Everyone here calls me [and asks] "Are you going somewhere", "when are you leaving" or "are you leaving". They feel free to call and ask (...) They consider me as a friend (...) Just recently a neighbour went to hospital and called me (...) "I just wanted you to know that I'm in the hospital in case someone wonders why there are no lights in our house. You may let them know that I am well and safe".
>
> *Interviewer:* Yes. That sounds a very nice way to handle that [situation].
>
> *Caregiver:* Well, yes. And the same [neighbour] reported, that she is staying four days in Lapland. We inform one another (...) where we are and where we are going.
>
> *Interviewer:* That sounds very good (...) in that way one doesn't have to worry in vain.
>
> *Caregiver:* Yes. The whole village community knows all about each other.

In the above interview excerpt the caregiver underlines the various good relations she had managed to create and preserve with the neighbours. The text highlights the significance to the interviewee of caring and being cared for. It is not exactly clear how close the relationships with the neighbours are, but at least they "consider" her as a friend. Being friends in this context seems to mean informing one another of one's comings and goings, and being aware of what happens in other people's lives.

Support Groups

Sometimes it is the illness of the spouse that stimulates positive social engagement via support groups. In particular, caregivers who participate in support groups talked about making new friends with whom to share their experiences. New friends can also be made through the care settings outside the home. This was the case with the caregiver in the next quote.

> *Caregiver:* I am friends with the residents [in the care home] and they always invite me to visit them there. It was just yesterday, when there was this Deaconess, who was there for an hour of prayer and I was asked to have a cup of coffee there.
>
> (…) Yes. They like to consider me as one of them and it was my idea to take them on a cruise on the lake the other day (…) and they were so pleased.

Active participation in social networks presupposes that the caregiver is able to manage and coordinate support resources. The care of the ill spouse requires certain routines, like giving medication, to be performed at specific times of the day or the week. The timing of the care duties is only possible through careful planning. The daily routine as a whole may be strictly planned but even single care practices, such as giving medication at a certain time, may require the regular presence of the caregiver throughout the day. With demented spouses there are often problems in taking care of daily routines, not to mention engaging in one's own hobbies. Caregivers may give up their own interests because they are reluctant to have, or it is too difficult to arrange "granny sitting" at home. One of our male respondents told of his difficulties in participating in gymnastic exercises because the group starts exactly at the same time his demented wife is being collected for day care. The wife cannot be left alone even for a short while and there are no friends or relatives available at that time.

The commitment to care has been found to isolate the caregivers and increase feelings of loneliness (Toseland et al., 2001). Old friends may draw away for a variety of reasons. There may be good intentions on the part of friends not to cause extra inconvenience to the caregiver, or uncertainty over how to converse with the sick person and the caregiver in a new situation. The caregiver, on his or her part, may interpret the distancing as rejection or even as a "fear of contagion". (see Blieszner and Adams, 1998.) One way of protecting the continuity of one's social network, though, is by "hiding" the truth of the family situation. One of our male caregivers described this kind of strategy in relation to his friends, whom he had noticed were embarrassed if he told them about his demented wife. Recently he had adopted the habit of saying "She's okay" whenever a friend would inquire about his wife's present condition.

The management of the social networks requires varied psychological, social and cultural resources. Having access to the resources varies between caregivers and may be dependent on contextual issues and the life history of the family. It seems that if the social network is thin to begin with, the care situation is likely to isolate the family even more. The caregivers with strong and dense networks, on the other hand, are able to employ several sources of support and they do not have to rely on a single relationship. From the cultural perspective, our data shows that managing the networks is a process where relationships are negotiated and renegotiated as the situation of the family changes. The illness of the spouse may, at least temporarily, limit the amount of cultural discourses that appear meaningful to the family members and thus favour certain relationships against others. Borderlines are sometimes created between old friends and even relatives who live in a completely different social and cultural world. Moreover, borderlines are created in the encounters between the family and the support services, an issue that we are going to discuss in the next section.

Encounters Between the Family and the Service System

Finnish elderly services are organized by local authorities (municipalities) and include both primary health care and social services such as home help. The caregiving families usuallyhave at least some need for support services, such as home help or home nursing, transportation or temporary institutional care. Merja Ala-Nikkola's (2003) research deals with the decision-making at the grassroots level concerning services for the elderly. Ala-Nikkola approaches decision-making from the professionals' perspective. Based on her data, it is clear that there are several sources of tension between service providers and family caregivers, as well as other close relatives of the service user. In chapter 18, Jeary and Stevenson discuss in detail the issue of conflicts between support services and families, reporting a case study in the UK. A focal point for the tensions seems to be the differences in defining the needs of the service users. The needs of the service users do not necessarily coincide with the categories of the service providers. Another source of tension seems to be identifying the client in a family care situation. Within the logic of the service provider, there are mostly individual clients with their individual needs. However, in caregiving families, especially with elderly couples, the needs for a particular service are typically shared needs. To benefit the whole family, the services should be provided while paying attention to the whole family and the unique microculture of each family. In this study, we tried to find out the logic of the need for services from the point of view of the caregiving family.

Different Orders of Priority

The differences in definitions of need and logic of actions between the service providers and the elderly clients are best manifested in the interpretations given to conflict situations. Refusing a given service, for example short-term care or "granny-sitting", is often interpreted by the professionals in psychological terms as a sign of excessive dependency between the carer and the care recipient. From the caregiver's point of view, there may be realistic doubts about the quality of care in the institution. Based on their past experiences, the families might also have doubts about the benefits of short-term care in general. Our interviewees' accounts include stories about bedsores or other signs of deterioration during the respite care. Also, what, from an outsider's perspective looks like dependency or rigidity, might, from the caregiver's point of view, be experienced as genuine worry and attachment.

The controversies between families and professionals were even more pronounced when it came to the services delivered at the client's home. On the one hand, the interviewees expressed gratitude for the services they had been provided by the municipal authorities, because they knew of the present scarcity of services in most of the municipalities. On the other hand, the professionals were seen as strangers with respect to the caregiver's desire to feel at home in her/his own house. To feel at home, for many people, means being fully in control and feeling no need to justify one's behaviour to anyone else. One of our interviewees described the freedom of home as being able *"to do whatever I want to do, even stand on my head"*. In her ethnographic study of Finnish home help workers, Silva Tedre concluded that in spite of its client-centred guidelines, the home help with its rationalizing tendencies tends to "clean" the clients' homes of their non-rational cultural meanings (Tedre, 1999). Thus, home help professionals act as a potential threat to the private order of the home and consequently to the identity of the family. The anticipation of a future visit alone can disrupt the daily routine of the family, especially if the caregiver does not know the exact time of the visit. On the other hand, the family's determination to defend the domestic order and continuity of the home might be interpreted by the professionals as a refusal to face the realities of life.

The following citation comes from a female respondent who has been caring for her paralyzed husband at home for ten years. About a year ago, she was offered home help up to five times a week:

> *Caregiver:* (.) and when the rehab [of my husband] was terminated at the health centre, they offered me home help for up to five days a week. But I thought that it (deprived me) totally of my independence [laughs] (…) because there was always someone here. (…) And it is kind of hard if there is always someone on her way in or out and you always have to follow a strict schedule.

The moments when there is a stranger in the house – and even the moments when she anticipates the visit of the home help worker – were interpreted by this caregiver as violations of her feeling at home. Another reason for the refusal was that she preferred to use her money to hire a physiotherapist twice a week for a rehab session. In this case, the caregiver presented herself as a competent actor with respect to the professionals. This was not the case with all caregivers in our data. For some, the relationship with professionals was described as a mixture of respect and fear and according to their accounts, they found it very difficult to act against the professionals' recommendations. Sometimes, the recommendations were seen as commands to obey even when one did not feel comfortable with the consequences:

> *Interviewer:* Do you get any state subsidy for being a caregiver?
>
> *Caregiver:* Well, not really.
>
> *Interviewer:* Was it a matter of course for you to start taking care of [your husband]? Was it a shared decision?
>
> *Caregiver:* Well, it just went that way.
>
> *Interviewer*: Did someone ask you how you manage at home (…) whether you have the strength to do that?
>
> *Caregiver:* No-one asked. No (.) the first time when he returned home [from the hospital] (…) I just took care of him and that's that. Probably I could have had help if I had known how to ask. But you don't think to, do you?
>
> *Interviewer:* What kind of help would you need just now?
>
> *Caregiver:* Well, no special help. The home help comes (…)

Interviewer: Do you think it's enough that they come once a day?

Caregiver: They would come twice but *think of the distance*! The municipality will not pay their travel expenses.

Interviewer: Otherwise, would they come back in the evening?

Caregiver: Yes, that's right. In the evening, when they start the evening shift. But no, it doesn't happen.

Interviewer: How do you feel (.) that it depends on the money?

Caregiver: It's always the money that counts (...) it's all about money.

This caregiver had a very difficult situation with the husband bed-ridden and the house practically without modern facilities. She was not receiving the official family carer's allowance, which is nowadays an important part of the Finnish social policy. According to the caregiver's account, the authorities did not show any interest at all in how she gets through the day with her caring responsibilities. However, she mainly blames herself for not understanding how to apply for support services. Later, the home help started to visit the family once a day, with an option for an additional evening call if necessary. This, however, did not work out because of the shortage of money allocated to the travel expenses of home helpers by the municipality. The caregiver sympathizes with the home help workers and asks the interviewer to consider the long distance between their home and the village centre. Her criticism focuses on the anonymous municipality or still more anonymous "money".

THE MEANINGS ATTACHED TO DIFFERENT SUPPORT SERVICES

The couples in this study all had a history of being clients of the Finnish Veteran Administration because of their status as war veterans. In most cases, the husbands had a varying level of physical disability caused by a war injury and therefore they had easier access to certain services than non-veterans. Also, the Veteran Administration provides the wives certain services based on their long-lasting role as support for Veteran spouses. However, in relation to the family caregiver role and increasing need for services, the couples will eventually become users of public services. It was here that the conflicts and disappointments appeared. This may be due to many overlapping issues. From the interviews, it became obvious that the Veteran services were understood as a reward for the veterans' war service. The municipal support, on the other hand, has been traditionally seen as social assistance for the poor. Some of the interviewees described their experiences with local authorities as humiliating. The next example is from the interview of an 82-year-old male caregiver whose wife is severely demented:

Caregiver: In September I felt that I did not have the strength any more to do everything by myself (.) I needed help (.) especially in bathing her (.) and our doctor (.) she said that I should get some help (.) that it could even be dangerous to try to manage all by myself. So I finally called them at the benefits office (...) if somebody could come twice a week or so (...) for an hour or two.

Interviewer: Yes and what happened?

Caregiver: Oh yes, two weeks ago this young man came with his papers and forms and we sat here as we sit now and he talked and talked (...) half of it went in one ear and out the other but the end result was that I was to report our financial situation (...) the savings and the

> value of the apartment and what we earn (.) and the pensions (…) I told him to take his papers with him and I would try to manage by myself rather than start reporting (…) I mean I only asked somebody to come and help her with bathing twice a week.

For a caregiver who has struggled to manage without help from outside the family, the threshold in turning to the public services can be very high. In this case, the decision to finally call the benefits office originates on the one hand from the caregiver's own worsening condition and on the other, from the "doctor's order" to get some help. Yet the disparity between his modest request and the demands of bureaucracy struck him as humiliating. In addition, he interpreted the request to "report" their finances as violating their privacy.

In this section of the chapter, we have tried to give voice to the caregivers as clients and partners to the service providers. In many cases, the caregivers seem to feel obliged to accept the care decisions recommended to them. On these occasions, we identified a strategy of "giving in" and trying to cope with the inevitable. On other occasions, acts of resistance were recognized with caregivers actively trying to sustain their autonomy in relation to the services.

Discussion

As a concept and phenomenon under construction, family care needs to be explored both locally and through comparisons between different countries. Here the focus is on the former aspect as we have aimed to explore the position of elderly caregiving families in the Finnish society. Typically, the studies of family care shed light on one party of the care situation at a time – be it the person cared for, the caregiver or the service provider. In this chapter, the unit of analysis is the *situation* as a whole with a variety of private and professional actors. What, specifically, constitutes an actor on a given occasion may vary considerably. Sometimes it is the caregiver or the care recipient and sometimes it is the family as a unit. In the same way, the service system, or even "money", as seen earlier, may "act" as an anonymous entity but sometimes an individual professional is the originator of action. Furthermore, members of the broader social network might play a crucial part in the day-to day coping of a caregiving family. Therefore, recognizing the relevant actors on each occasion is an essential part of defining and managing family care.

The perspective adopted in this chapter provides insight into the cultural process and dynamics of family care in elderly families. The concepts of *microculture* and *cultural borderline* were introduced as vehicles for analyzing and interpreting the data consisting of observation and ethnographic interviews. We started with an initial assumption that family care consists of different microcultures and that to understand fully the challenge of family care it is important to identify cultural antagonisms resulting in different definitions of needs and conflicting ideas of how best to support the caregiving families. Using a discourse analytic orientation we tried to recognize these cultural antagonisms in three domains thought to be the most central ones in the everyday enterprise of family care: the domestic culture of the family, the broader social network of the family and the encounters between the family and the service system.

The changes in the domestic culture of an elderly family take place at least within two spheres: the family itself, which here means the elderly couple, and the home as the context of care. It seems obvious that the illness of the husband or wife results in a new division of responsibilities between the spouses. However, as we have shown, the re-division of labour is not just a series of practical choices but involves an ongoing process of negotiation of moral choices as well. Apart from the division of responsibilities, also the roles of the spouses are likely to undergo changes in the process of care. In addition to the roles of a wife and a husband, the spouses gradually find themselves acting as caregivers and care recipients. Often this happens without conscious or focused decision-making by anyone.

Our analysis illustrates the way in which the interpretations given to the home became important constituents of the family care situation. The desire to be at home for as long as possible was taken as given by all of our respondents. This meant that usually at least some physical alterations of the home were necessary in order to cope with the illness of one family member. These alterations were here examined in relation to the psychological theories of the home as a "shell of self" (see Csikszentmihalyi and Rochberg-Halton, 1981). Paradoxically, caring at home was sometimes only possible at the cost of transforming the home into a care setting. The illness and the care work practiced at home also seemed to create a need to reconsider the forms of social interplay inside the home. Here, it became obvious that the traditional cultural rules of family life may in fact contribute to the isolation of caregiving families.

According to our data, there was a considerable variation in the amount and quality of social contacts between different families. The ideal of a self-sufficient individual was brought up in many interviews but at the same time, the caregivers recounted situations where practical, emotional and moral help was welcomed. Specifically, relatives and professionals were employed to validate and justify difficult care decisions. Most of our respondents had experienced considerable changes in regard to their social networks during the care situation. Typically, the changes were interpreted as negative but from a cultural point of view, one clearly positive change was mentioned, namely the contacts with other caregivers. The family carers' support groups seemed to represent and create a kind of a microculture of its own.

With most elderly caregiving families in Finland, the support services or the lack thereof play an important part in shaping the care process. The contacts between the caregiving families and the service providers take place at different levels: sometimes only through the bureaucracy, for example when applying for caregiver allowances, and sometimes as face-to-face encounters outside or inside the home. With increasing professionalism in the domain of care, the monopoly over knowledge and competence is well established among specialists and authorities. Correspondingly, caregiving families are often faced with the dilemma of autonomy versus support. One critical source of tension between a family caregiver and a formal service provider is the issue of the caregiver having to adjust to the schedules of the professional. The stress of additional adjustment may sometimes cause more difficulties than the formal help actually contributes to care. For the caregiver, recognizing the disadvantageous aspects of a service can sometimes be too difficult, but in our data we did have at least one clear example of this.

We have tried to show that the many diverse meanings and microcultures of family care are displayed and constantly renegotiated in dialogue between different actors involved. Occasionally, these dialogues take place as face-to-face encounters, but mostly, people are not necessarily aware of the dialogues in which they are participating. Failing to recognize the borderlines between different microcultures may cause misunderstandings and ruptures of communication between different actors. Genuine co-operation between families and professionals would benefit from a shared understanding of the floating nature of the meanings attached to family care.

CONCLUSION

In this chapter, we have presented qualitative data that exemplifies the cultural dynamics of family care of the elderly. We used the concepts of microculture and cultural borderline to guide the analysis of the diverse meanings and interpretations given to care and related issues by the different actors involved in family care. The main focus of our analysis was the elderly family caregivers themselves and their conceptualizations of the process of care. We analyzed the caregivers' strategies in explaining and justifying their actions and experiences and identified some critical points where controversies and conflicts between different interpretations were manifested. The analysis was presented in three parts: the changes in the domestic culture of caregiving families, the social networks of the families and the encounters between the caregivers and service providers. The main findings highlight the role of the interpretations given to the care process in shaping the adjustment of the caregivers to the needs of the disabled spouse.

PRACTICAL CONSIDERATIONS AND RECOMMENDATIONS

- Cultural perspectives on family care provide useful insights into "microcultures" of home care.
- Family caregiving is still a phenomenon under construction as different stakeholders give different meanings to it.
- Caregivers are active contributors to their social networks and often provide support to others as well as receiving it.
- In a family care situation the home may become a centre of conflict instead of respite as care-related activities and professionals invade the privacy of the home.
- Cultural controversies were revealed especially in the relationships between the carers and the services system.
- Caregivers should be encouraged to maintain their feeling of home and adjust services with respect to these feelings.
- Caregivers need support in making decisions about choices of care.
- A caregiver's refusal of a particular support service should be respected and different services presented instead.
- The definition of a customer/service user should facilitate seeing the family as an entity with shared needs.
- Professionals working with family caregivers should be trained to be more sensitive to the needs of each family and individual caregivers.
- Recognizing the relevant actors on each occasion is an essential part of defining and managing family care.

TRANSCRIPT NOTATIONS

(.) a short pause
(…) a pause
__ emphasis
() quiet speech
[] researcher's clarification

REFERENCES

Ala-Nikkola, M. (2003). Sairaalassa, kotona vai vanhainkodissa? Etnografinen tutkimus vanhustenhuollon koti- ja laitoshoidon päätöksentekotodellisuudesta. [In hospital, at home or in institutional care? Ethnographic research on decision–making realities of old-age care]. Acta Universitatis Tamperensis 972. Tampere: Tampere University Press.

Albert, S. M. (1990). The Dependent Elderly, Home Health Care, and Strategies of Household Adaptation. In J. Gubrium, and A. Shankar (Eds.) *The Home Care Experience: Ethnography and Policy* (pp. 19-36). Newbury Park, CA: Sage.

Avlund, K., and Schultz-Larsen, K. (1991). What Do 70 Year-old Men and Women Actually Do? And What Are They Able to Do? From the Glostrup Survey in 1984. *Aging Clin Exp Res*, 3, 39-49.

Barker, J. C., Morrow, J., and Mitteness, L. S. (1998). Gender, Informal Social Support Networks, and Elderly Urban African Americans. *Journal of Aging Studies*, 12, 199-222.

Blaikie, A. (2002). The Secret World of Subcultural Ageing: What Unites and What Divides? In L. Anderson (Ed.) *Cultural Gerontology* (pp. 95-110). London: Auburn House.

Blieszner, R., and Adams, R. G. (1998). Problems with Friends in Old Age. *Journal of Aging Studies*, 12, 223-238.

Brewer, L. (2001). Gender Socialization and the Cultural Construction of Elder Caregivers. *Journal of Aging Studies*, 15, 217-235.

Bourgeois, M. S., Schultz, L., and Burgio, L. (1996). Interventions for caregivers of Patients with Alzheimer's Disease: A Review and Analysis of Content, Process, and Outcomes. *Int J Aging Hum Develop*, 43, 35-92.

Clark, P. G. (1989). The Philosophical Foundations of Empowerment. *Journal of Health and Aging*, 1(3), 267-285.

Clipp, C. C., and George L. K. (1990). Caregiver Needs and Patterns of Social Support. *Journal of Gerontology*, 45, 102-111.

Corbin, J. M., and Strauss, A. (1990). Making Arrangements: The Key to Home Care. In J. Gubrium, and A. Shankar (Eds.) *The Home Care Experience: Ethnography and Policy* (pp. 59-74). Newbury Park, CA: Sage.

Csikszentmihalyi, M., and Rochberg-Halton, E. (1981). *The Meaning of Things. Domestic Symbols and the Self.* Cambridge: Cambridge University Press.

Darlington, Y., and Scott, D. (2002). *Qualitative Research in Practice. Stories from the Field.* Buckingham, PA (Philadelphia): Open University Press.

Delamont, S., and Atkinson, P. (1995). *Fighting Familiarity: Essays on Education and Ethnography.* Cresskill, NJ: Hampton Press.

Eloviemi-Sulkava, U., Notkola, I-L., Hentinen M., Kivelä, S-L., Sivenius, J., Sulkava, R. (2001). Effects of Supporting Community-living Demented Patients and Their Caregivers: A Randomized Trial. *J Am Geriatr Soc,* 49, 1282-7.

Farran, C. J. (1997). Theoretical perspectives Concerning Positive Aspects of Caring for Elderly Persons with Dementia: Stress Adaptation and Existentialism. *Gerontologist,* 37, 250-256.

Flint A. J. (1995). Effects of Respite Care on Patients with Dementia and Their Caregivers. *International Psychogeriatrics,* 7, 505-517.

Gilleard, C., and Higgs, P. (2000). *Cultures of Ageing: Self, Citizen and the Body*. Harlow: Prentice Hall.

Gatz, M., Bengtson, V., Blum, M. (1990). Caregiving Families. In J. E. Birren and K. W. Schaie (Eds.) *Handbook of the Psychology of Aging* (pp. 404-26). San Diego: Academic Press.

Gordon, T., Holland, J., and Lahelma, E. (2001) Ethnographic Research in Educational Settings. In . P. Atkinson, A. Coffey, S. Delamont, J. Loftland, and L. Loftland (Eds.) *Handbook of Ethnography* (pp. 188-203). London: Sage.

Green, A., and Brodaty, H. (2002). Care-giver Interventions. In N. Qizilbash, L. S. Schneider, H. Chui, P. Tariot, H. Brodaty, J. Kaye, and T. Erkinjuntti (Eds.) *Evidence-based Dementia Practice.* Hong Kong: Blackwell Publishing.

Gubrium, J., and Shankar, A. (1990). *The Home Care Experience: Ethnography and Policy*. Newbury Park, CA: Sage.

Hyvärinen, M., Saarenheimo, M., Pitkälä, K., and Tilvis, R. (2003). Vanhusten omaishoitajat ja tukitoimet. [Supporting the Family Caregivers for the Elderly]. *Duodecim,* 119, *1949-7.*

Jutras S., and Lavoie, J. (1995) Living with an Impaired Elderly Person: The Informal Caregiver's Physical and Mental Health. *Journal of Aging and Health*, 7, 46-73.

Kirsi, T., Hervonen, A., and Jylhä, M. (2000). A Man's Gotta Do What a Man's Gotta Do: Husbands as Caregivers to Their Demented Wives: A Discourse Analysis Approach. *Journal of Aging Studies*, 14, 153-169.

Knight, B., Lutzky, S., and Macofsky-Urban, F. (1993). A Meta-analytic Review of interventions for Caregiver Stress: Recommendations for Future Research. *Gerontologist*, 33, 240-9.

Kramer, B. J. (1997) Gain in the Caregiving Experience: Where Are We? What next? *Gerontologist*, 37, 218-32.

Lawton, M. P., Kleban, M. H., and Moss M. et al. (1989). Measuring Caregiving Appraisal. *J Gerontol: Psychological Sciences*, 44, P61-P71.

Levine, C. (1999). Home Sweet Hospital: The Nature and Limits of Private Responsibilities for Home Health Care. *Journal of Aging and Health*, 11, 341-359.

Marin, M. (2003). Sosiaaliset verkostot. [Social Networks] In M. Marin, and S. Hakonen (Eds.) *Seniori- ja vanhustyö arjen kulttuurissa.* [Working with the Elderly in Everyday Context] (pp. 72-93). Juva: PS-Kustannus.

Mittelman M. S., Ferris S. H., Steinberg, G., Shulman, E., Mackell, J. A., Ambinder, A., Cohen, J. (1993). An Intervention that Delays Institutionalization of Alzheimer's Disease Patients: Treatment of Spouse-Caregivers. *Gerontologist,* 33, 730-40.

Mittelman M.S., Ferris, S. H., Shulman, E., Steinberg, G., Ambinder, A., Mackell, J. A., Cohen, J. (1995). A Comprehensive Support Program: Effect on Depression in Spouse-caregivers of AD Patients. *Gerontologist*, 35, 792-802.

Montgomery, R. J. V. (1999) The Family Role in the Context of Long-term Care. *Journal of Aging and Health*, 11, 383-416.

Neundorfer, M. M. (1991) Coping and Health Outcomes in Spouse Caregivers of persons with Dementia. *Nursing Research*, 40, 260-265.

Noelker, L. and Wallace, R. (1985). The Organization of Family Care for Impaired Elderly. *J Fam Iss*, 6, 23-44.

Pearlin, L., Aneschel, F., Mullan, J. T., Whitlatch, C. J. (1996). Caregiving and Its Social Support. In R. H. Binstock and L. K. George (Eds.) *Handbook of Aging and the Social Sciences*. (pp. 283-302). New York: Academic Press.

Phipps, E., Braitman, L. E., True, G., Harris, D., and Tester, W. (2003). Family Care Giving for Patients at Life´s End: Report form Cultural Variations Study (CVAS). *Palliative and Supporting Care*, 1, 165-170.

Rimmerman, A., and Muraver, M. (2001). Experiencing Undesired Daily Life Events, Instrumental Functioning, Social Support and Well-Being of Israeli Elderly Women: Comparison between Caregivers / Non-Caregivers for Adult Children with Mental Retardation. *Journal of Women and Aging*, 13, 57-69.

Rubinstein, R. L. (1991). Culture and Disorder in the Home Care Experience: The Home as Sickroom. In J. Gubrium, and A. Shankar (Eds.) *The Home Care Experience: Ethnography and Policy*. (pp. 37-58). Newbury Park, CA: Sage.

Sherman Heyl, B. (2001). Ethnographic Interviewing. In P. Atkinson, A. Coffey, S. Delamont, J. Loftland, and L. Loftland (Eds.) *Handbook of Ethnography* (pp. 369-83). London: Sage.

Schulz R., O'Brien A. T., Bookwala, J., and Fleissner, K. (1995). Psychiatric and Physical Morbidity Effects of Dementia Caregiving: Prevalence, Correlates, and Causes. *Gerontologist*, 35, 771-91.

Silverman M., and Huelsman E. (1990). The Dynamics of Long-Term Familial Caregiving. In J. Gubrium, and A. Shankar (Eds.) *The Home Care Experience: Ethnography and Policy*. (pp. 173-188). Newbury Park, CA: Sage.

Spindler, G., and Spindler, L. (1982). Roger Harkes and Schönhausen: From the Familiar to the Strange and Back. In G. Spindler (Ed.) *Doing the Ethnography of Schooling. Educational Anthropology in Action* (pp. 20-47). New York: Holt, Rinehart and Winston.

Spradley, J. P. (1980). *Participant Observation*. New York: Holt, Rinehart and Winston.

Tedre, S. (1999) Hoivan sanattomat sopimukset. Tutkimus vanhusten kotipalvelun työntekijöiden työstä. [The Unspoken Contracts in Social Care. A Case Study of Paid Workers in Finnish Municipal Home Help Services for the Elderly]. Publications in Social Sciences No 40. University of Joensuu.

Thompson, C., and Spilsbury, K. (2000) Support for Carers of People with Alzheimer's Type Dementia. Cochrane Review. The Cochrane Library. Oxford: Update Software Ltd.

Toseland, R. W., Smith, G., and McCallion, P. (2001). Family Caregivers of the Frail Elderly. In A. Gitterman (Ed.) *Handbook of Social Work Practice With Vulnerable and Resilient Population*. (pp. 548-81). New York. Columbia University Press.

Vitaliano, P. P., Scanlan, J. M., and Zhang, J. (2003) Is Caregiving Hazardous to One's Physical Health? A Meta-Analysis. *Psychological Bulletin*, 129, 946-972.

Wallsten, S. S. (2000). Effects of Caregiving, Gender, and Race on the Health, Mutuality and Social Supports of Older Couples. *Journal of Aging and Health,* 12, 90-111.

Wetherell, M., Taylor, S., Yates, S. J. (2001). *Discourse Theory and Practice.* London, Sage.

Zarit, S. H. and Leitsch, S. A. (2001). Developing and Evaluating Community Based Intervention Programs for Alzheimer's Patients and Their Caregivers. *Aging and Mental Health*, 5 (Supplement 1), S84-S98.

In: Family Caregiving for Older Disabled People
Editor: Isabella Paoletti, pp. 359-391
ISBN 1-59454-808-0

Chapter 17

CAREGIVERS AND COMMUNITY SERVICE NON-USE IN AUSTRALIA

Patricia Hill, Kimberly Fisher, Cathy Thomson and Michael Bittman
The University of New England
Armidale NSW 2351 Australia

INTRODUCTION

This chapter presents the findings of an Australian Research Council funded project which examined the 1998 *Australian Bureau of Statistics Survey of Disability Ageing and Carers* (SDAC) (ABS, 1999) in order to identify the characteristics of isolated or hidden carers not using community services[1]. In 1998 over 2.3 million people in Australia, representing approximately 13 per cent of the total population and including more women than men, provided informal care to an adult or child with impairments or to an elderly person (ABS, 1999). Twenty eight per cent of all Australian carers are providing care for people 65 years and over. Official estimates suggest approximately 46 per cent of Australians aged 65 years and over require some degree of help with the routine tasks of daily living, and the need for assistance significantly increases with age (ABS, 1999). Given the structural aging of the Australian population, the need for informal support for the elderly is likely to increase.

The need for support for those providing informal care to the elderly is not, in principle, different to the needs experienced by those who provide informal care to younger disabled adults or children. While many elements of Australian society support the care of non-

[1] Though the authors conducted the research reported here, the New South Wales Department for Women, the NSW Department of Ageing, Disability and Home Care, the NSW Department of Community Services, NSW Health and Carers NSW were partners in the larger project and provided advice and comment during this research. Nevertheless, the views expressed in this chapter are those of the authors and do not necessarily reflect the views of the above departments or the responsible Ministers including the Minister for Community Services, the Minister for Ageing, the Minister for Disability Services, Minister for Youth and the Minister for Health, or the NSW state government. The authors would also like to thank Isabella Paoletti for editorial advice, Ken Black from the ABS for advice on SDAC and Dr Jenny Chalmers and Kate Norris for comments on the statistical analysis. None of the above is responsible for any remaining errors or the views contained in this chapter.

disabled children - from state-sponsored education, to restaurants providing playing facilities for children and child menus, to child changing facilities in public toilets - comparable levels of support do not exist for people looking after adults needing care (Braithwaite 1990, Fine 1999). Some health problems experienced by adults needing care attract similar stigma regardless of age (Braithwaite 1990, Fine 1999). This chapter makes use of the limited large-scale data sources covering service use by carers. To retain a sample size sufficiently large for robust analysis, this study examines the factors relating to service non-use for all carers of adults in Australia and also considers whether the age of a care recipient influences the likelihood of the carer or the care recipient using services. One of our findings is that the age of the care recipient does influence the likelihood that adult carers will use some forms of services, however other factors are also important predictors of service non-use.

As has happened in many other industrialised countries, recent Australian public policy has striven to shift an increasing proportion of care from formal institutions to local communities (Bryson and Mowbray, 1981; Ungerson and Kember, 1997; Schofield et al, 1998; Fine, 1999). This increased emphasis on community care reflects concerns about the high cost of providing institutional care as well as the preference expressed by many people needing assistance to live at home (Dalley, 1988). At the same time, care in the community represents a transfer of responsibility for care from the state to the family, which in practice means care provided by women (Land, 1978; Ungerson and Kember, 1997). Consequently, the public discussion of informal care has simultaneously praised the financial savings and the social benefits to be gained from informal care, and expressed anxiety about the demands placed on women carers (Brody, 1981; Finch and Groves, 1983; Schofield, et al, 1998).

It is well documented that caring can place significant stress upon carers and their families. Carers often perform physically and mentally demanding tasks. They have low levels of social contact and little financial independence, and lower levels of employment, poorer health and higher levels of stress compared to non-carers of a comparable age in similar social circumstances (Brodaty and Hadzi-Pavlovic, 1990; Thomson, Fine and Brodaty, 1997; Scholfield et al, 1998: Watson and Mears, 1999). International research shows that community services designed to support carers can make a significant difference to their health and welfare (Thomson, Fine and Brodaty, 1997; Schofield et al, 1998; Braithwaite 1998; Zarit et al, 1998; Watson and Mears, 1999; Parker, 2000). Access to support and services may assist carers to preserve their health, wellbeing and social participation and enable them to sustain their caring role over a longer period of time. It may also help them to combine paid work with their caring activities. Maintaining labour force participation during working age not only preserves income security, it ensures greater independence over the whole course of a carer's life.

Despite the existence of formal services and the undoubted benefits to carers of using them, carers' service use remains low. The issue of support services to family caregiving and service non-use was pointed out by various authors in this book; for example Katila in chapter 2, describes the resistance in using formal services in the farming community in Finland, and in chapter 8, Watson points out the notably low use of support services by carers of people with Multiple Sclerosis. Understanding why carers do not take up services is a complex issue and could be the result of a number of inter-related factors, including the lack of need, targeting policies or the characteristics of the services themselves. Affordability, access issues and inflexible hours of operation may all contribute to low take-up of support services by carers (Beisecker, et al, 1996; Knapman and Waite, 1997; Thomson, Fine and Brodaty, 1997;

Brodaty et al, 2005). Moreover, there is reason to believe that services designed to support carers are not evenly distributed throughout Australia. Access to service provision is more difficult in regional and remote areas than in the capital cities, if for no other reason than the considerable distances involved.

One major reason for the low take-up of services, however, is the failure of carers to identify themselves as such. Research into the care of adults suggests that a sizeable part of the population of people providing care do not recognise themselves as carers, while others experience difficulty accepting that they have adopted a caring role (Braithwaite 1990; Misic 1996; Thomson, Fine and Brodaty, 1997; Bittman and Thomson 2000; Bittman et al, 2004; Brodaty et al, 2005).

Some insight into the reasons why carers do not view themselves as carers is given in Graham's (1983) celebrated distinction between 'caring for' and 'caring about'. 'Caring for' is related to the physical tasks associated with providing assistance, while 'caring about' involves the emotional relationship between the carer and care recipient. Among carers who do not self-identify as carers, the dimension of 'caring for' is subsumed and concealed by the dimension of 'caring about' (Dalley, 1988). As Parker has pointed out, 'the term "carer" tends to obscure the relationship that usually predates the situation which led to the need to provide care' (Parker, 2000: 3). While services are targeted at those most in need of assistance, a major factor limiting the take-up of services is the failure of carers to identify themselves as carers – a precursor to acknowledging a need for assistance. This failure even to be aware of the need for support services is tantamount to being 'isolated'. Without support and information on how to access services, carers may be unable to continue caring. The use of community services by the carer or care recipient may reduce the pressures on carers and assist them to maintain their caring role. It may also reduce the incidence of crisis in their care situation and hence the likelihood of inappropriate and premature institutionalisation of the care recipient.

Moreover, information on the types of carers who are not accessing formal services would help in the design of appropriate information campaigns and targeting of services. By identifying groups of carers and factors associated with service non-use, service providers would be able to improve the targeting of the resources available to support carers to enable disabled people in need of assistance to remain at home. Much of the research on carers and service use focuses on studying the characteristics of service users (Twigg and Atkin; 1994; Braithwaite, 1998; Gill, Hinrichsen and DiGiuseppe, 1998). But without information about carers who are not currently using services that they well may need, it is impossible to plan adequately for effective service delivery or equitable access to services. This chapter examines the characteristics of carers who do not use services. It begins by describing the method of data collection and the data analysis of the study. The chapter then outlines the use of different types of services, followed by the multivariate analysis used to assess the use and non-use of services by both carers and primary carers. The chapter next discusses the reasons carers and care recipients do not use services, and concludes by considering the recommendations and the policy implications of these findings.

THE STUDY

The Data

This investigation used the nationally representative *Survey of Disability, Ageing and Carers* (SDAC) conducted by the Australian Bureau of Statistics, Australia's official statistical organization, to identify the characteristics of carers not using community services (ABS, 1999). While considerable qualitative work in Australia has documented the experiences of individual carers, this dataset gives an overview of the size of the national population of carers and the distribution of carers from different backgrounds. The SDAC provides extensive information on many aspects of the care situation, including the need for assistance and the use of informal and formal support by care recipients. This information provides an opportunity to identify the categories of carers who are not using formal services, as well as the factors that impede or promote service use by carers and hence the major gaps in service delivery. Within the SDAC sample approximately 28 per cent of all carers are caring for elderly people. This proportion is slightly higher among carers who are caring more intensively as discussed below. This study provided an opportunity to identify differences in the service use of carers of older and younger people.

Sample of Carers

The sample was divided into two components: 1) the household component, which included people living in private dwellings (such as houses, home units and townhouses) and non-private dwellings (such as hotels, motels and boarding houses); 2) the 'cared accommodation' component, which included those living in hospitals, hostels, nursing homes and other homes. Multi-stage sampling techniques were used to select the sample which included a final sample of 36,951 people in the household component and 5,716 people in the cared for accommodation component. Information for the household component was collected by trained interviewers using computer assisted personal interviews (ABS, 1999). In this study we only examine the household component of the survey.

For this study, the Australian Bureaus of Statistics defined a carer as 'a person of any age who provides any informal assistance, in terms of help or supervision, to persons with disabilities or long-term conditions, or persons who are elderly. The assistance has to be ongoing, or likely to be ongoing, for at least six months'. For carers living in the same households as their care recipients, information is collected on the nine of the activities listed in Table 1 (ABS, 1999: 65).

The 1998 SDAC identified 4,727 carers (2,055 male and 2,672 female). Of these, around 75 percent (3,535 – 1,702 male and 1,833 female) were co-resident carers. The analysis for this study is confined to co-resident caring situations, as there is no information on the service use of care recipients who do not live with their carers. The literature suggests that co-resident carers may have lower levels of service use due to the targeting of services to carers and care recipients who live apart (Parker, 1990; Bebbington and Davies, 1993). The analysis for this study was conducted on a base sample of 3461 co-resident carers aged 10 years and over as

74 carers were excluded due to either the age of the carer or the limited information available on service use of the care recipient.

Table 1. Activities and tasks in SDAC 1998

Activity	Tasks
Communication	Understanding family/friends
	Being understood by family/friends
	Understanding strangers
	Being understood by strangers
Mobility	Getting into/out of bed/chair
	Moving about usual place of residence
	Moving about a place away from the usual residence
Self-care	Showering/bathing
	Dressing
	Eating
	Toileting
	Bladder/bowel control
Health care	Foot care
	Taking medications/administering injections
	Dressing wounds
	Using medical machinery
	Manipulating muscles or limbs
Paperwork	Reading/writing tasks such as :
	Checking bills/bank statements
	Writing letters
	Filling in forms
Transport	Going to places away from the usual place of residence
Housework	Household chores such as:
	Washing
	Vacuuming
	Dusting
Property maintenance	Changing light bulbs/tap washers/car registration stickers
	Making minor home repairs
	Mowing lawns/watering/pruning shrubs/light weeding/planting
	Removing rubbish
Meal preparation	Preparing ingredients
	Cooking food

Source: ABS, 1999: 59

The ABS distinguishes between *carers* and *primary carers*, a difference based on the intensity of the care given. A primary carer is defined as 'a person of any age who provides the most informal assistance, in terms of help or supervision, to a person with one or more disabilities. The assistance has to be ongoing, or likely to be ongoing, for at least six months and be provided for one or more of the core activities (communication, mobility and self-care)' (ABS, 1999: 71). Approximately 28 per cent of the carer sample and 34 per cent of the primary carer sample are caring for people aged 65 years and over. Further analysis of a subset of co-resident carers, comprising 723 co-residential primary carers, was also conducted as additional information on the need aspects of their care situation was available.[2]

Data on Service Use

In this study, we define service use or non-use in terms of whether care recipients reported accessing services in those areas where they indicated that they required assistance.[3] The list of activities, however, is not exhaustive; thus some forms of need and degree of use of services related to such needs falls outside the scope of analysis here.

The SDAC asked care recipients if they required assistance for each of nine activities (outlined in Table 1). In the analysis, carers are grouped according to the activities for which the formal services were required. For five of the nine activities – self-care, paperwork, housework, property maintenance and meal preparation – all care recipients required assistance. In this case the sample is one hundred percent of the SDAC sample of carers and primary carers respectively, and the activities have been grouped together into the one analysis. For the other four activities where only some care recipients needed assistance, the sample size is smaller – only that group of carers whose care recipients needed assistance has been selected for that particular analysis[4]. The next two tables report the percentage of carers (Table 2) and primary carers (Table 3) who helped care recipients who required assistance for each of the activities, as well as the sample size for each analysis and the percentage of carers whose care recipients needed assistance and did not use formal services for the activities.

Limitations of the Data

There are a number of important qualifications to the analysis that must be noted at the outset. Some problems arise from direct survey questions to identify carers and care activities. The people who provide care do not always recognise themselves as carers. In some circumstances, denying that they provide care or that the person they assist needs care serves as a coping strategy for the carer, while in other cases, where the care recipient's health has deteriorated gradually over time, the carer and care recipient may simply not recognise that such a relationship has developed between them (Bittman et. al. 2004). Additionally, carers do not always recognise caring activities as care, as the extra assistance with daily living can

---

[2] The 1998 SDAC also includes 918 primary carers, of whom 726 were co-resident. Three primary carers were deleted from the sample as their care recipients did not appear in the disability level file and thus there was no information on the care recipient's service use

[3] To analyse the SDAC data for this study, we constructed 'care units' comprised of carers and their care recipients living in the same household. This was a complex process, as within a household there can be more than one person caring for a care recipient, and one carer might provide assistance to more than one other household member. Moreover, carers themselves might be recipients of care from others within the household.

[4] However, the analysis does not consider the activity of communication assistance, as the sample size was too small for multivariate analysis). In the samples of primary carers, respite care is considered in addition to the use of other formal services by their care recipients, in order to identify those primary carers who were not receiving support from any formal services. Statistical analysis in this chapter was undertaken using SAS version 8.0.

have close parallels with standard domestic tasks (Bittman and Thomson 2000; Bittman et. al. 2004).

Table 2. Need for services, sample sizes and service non-use among care recipients of co-resident carers

Carers			
Activity	Percentage that needs assistance with task	Sample size for analysis	Percentage that needs assistance and does not use services
Five activities*	100	3461	79.1
Health care	47.9	1653	54.4
Mobility	44.6	1525	75.3
Transport	44.6	1508	83.4
Communication	14.9	516	39.5

Source: ABS, 1999
*The five activities are housework, meal preparation, paperwork, property maintenance, and self-care
All percentages estimates are weighted by carer weights

Table 3. Need for services, sample sizes and service non-use among care recipients of co-resident primary carers

Primary carers			
Activity	Percentage that needs assistance with task	Sample size for analysis	Percentage that needs assistance and does not use services (carer also does not use respite services)
Five activities*	100	723	62.1
Health care	76.0	538	46.0
Mobility	79.9	572	63.7
Transport	65.3	463	69.4
Communication	28.3	204	27.5

Source: ABS, 1999
*The five activities are housework, meal preparation, paperwork, property maintenance, and self-care
All percentages estimates are weighted by carer weights

As an example, carers of people with special dietary requirements can be hard-pressed to estimate the precise proportion of their food preparation tasks which they have to undertake for their household, if no one required help, compared to the proportion which constitutes the extra care required by the care recipient. In this research project, we conducted preliminary analysis using time use data to develop a profile the daily patterns of care providers. Using this profile we identified persons who claim not to be carers but whose daily activities resemble the activity profile of carers and who live in circumstances where another person needs assistance. This analysis suggests that the true population of care providers is at least one third higher than the estimate derived from studies where respondents self-identify as carers or non-carers (Bittman et al, 2003; Bittman et al, 2004).

Another important qualification is that the SDAC sample size is not large enough to allow a detailed analysis of Aboriginal and Torres Strait Islander people or people from linguistic or ethnic minority groups, as the number of people in these groups in the sample is small despite being proportional to the population. Finally, readers should note that the SDAC only measures the take-up of a service. We do not have data on how long or how frequently people used services, nor do we have information on the degree to which these services proved useful. These limitations aside, the SDAC remains the most comprehensive data covering care and service use in Australia, and we are able to draw a number of conclusions from analysis of this data. As little published academic work on care in Australia makes use of large dataset information, this study provides some sense of the scale of the experiences documented in the widely published qualitative research (one exception is a study by Brodaty et al, 2005). This chapter next describes the method of data analysis.

Method of Data Analysis

Multivariate Analysis of the Overall Use of Different Types of Services

Bivariate analyses were used to identify those factors likely to have an influence on service use and non-use, and hence those population subgroups who were more likely not to use formal services. This produced a range of 23 potential variables for multivariate analysis (see Table 4).

The factors were classified according to a conceptual framework suggested by Andersen and Newman (1973) into 'predisposing', 'enabling' or 'need' variables. Within this framework, the characteristics of the total informal care situation, including carer and care recipient characteristics, are considered as potential influences on the use of community services. *Predisposing* variables are socio-demographic characteristics existing prior to the onset of the care situation that may predispose the carer to use or to not use services, such as the age or sex of the carer. *Enabling* variables represent characteristics that facilitate or inhibit the use of services, such as income and employment. *Need* variables represent characteristics specific to the care situation, such as the degree of disability or the level of caregiver burden. The analysis examines each of these factors in turn.

More detailed analysis was conducted for primary co-residential carers using the additional the information gathered from them. The SDAC study asked only primary carers to complete a supplementary questionnaire about their experiences of the care situation and also the SF-12 self-assessment health questionnaire. As well as providing extra variables for the analysis of primary carers (indicated in Table 4), the supplement allowed us to create two indices - a 'carer burden' index to reflect the presence, and if present, the degree of burden carers experience as a result of their caring role; and an index of 'poor health'.

Table 4. Potential independent variables for the multivariate analyses

Category	Variable
The predisposing variables (characteristics that exist prior to onset of caring relationship and may predispose the carer to use services) are:	1.Sex of carer 2.Age of carer 3.Marital status of carer 4.Household composition 5.Birthplace of carer 6.Highest educational qualification of carer 7.Disability status of carer 8.Whether carer has a long–term health condition 9.Relationship of carer to care recipient 10.Whether carer speaks to care recipient in English **
The enabling variables (characteristics that facilitate the use of services) are:	11.Personal income of the carer 12.Main source of cash income of the carer 13.Index of relative socio-economic disadvantage of the carer's local area 14.Employment status of carer 15.Geographical location of carer
The need variables (characteristics that are specific to the care situation) are:	16.Sex of the care recipient 17.Age of the youngest care recipient 18.Highest disability level of care recipients in household 19.Number of care recipients 20.Hours spent actively caring** 21.Whether carer has a fall-back informal carer** 22.Whether carer reports a relatively high level of 'carer burden'** 23.Whether carer reports having relatively poor health (physical and emotional)**

Notes: Variables marked with ** are available for the primary carers only

CARER BURDEN

The SDAC data include 18 potential indicators of carer burden (see Appendix Table A1 for the complete list of variables), 15 of which were included in the final index. Carers were regarded as experiencing a relatively high burden if they selected the burdened option on five or more of these fifteen indicators. While this was an arbitrary decision, the sensitivity of this threshold was tested by using different thresholds in the regression models. The results were similar for thresholds ranging from 3 to 6 indicators, and thus the decision was considered relatively robust. Fifty percent of primary carers scored five or more on the index. They are thus classified as experiencing a relatively high burden.

CARER HEALTH

The physical and mental component summary scores given in SDAC have also been included in the index of poor health (with all individual items listed in the Appendix, Table A2). Cronbach's alpha for this group of indicators is 0.88. Carers were considered to have relatively poor health if they selected the poor health option on three or more of the indicators. (The sensitivity of this decision was tested as described for the 'burden' index and found to be robust for thresholds ranging from 2 to 4 indicators). Around sixty percent of primary carers scored three or more on the index. After testing these indices, we found more robust results from reducing the indices to dichotomous variables marking whether the primary carer reported a relatively high burden of caring or relatively poor health.

The following analysis first provides an overview of the need for and use of services by all carers and care recipients. Next, bivariate analysis provides an indication of whether carers supporting the elderly are more or less likely than other carers to use services for different activities. The multivariate analysis then examines the predisposing and enabling characteristics that are strongly associated with service non-use after controlling for need characteristics in the care situation. This permits consideration of whether the age of the care recipient influences the use of services when other factors are taken into account. The analysis then discusses the need factors showing strong associations with service use and non-use, followed by a description of the socio-demographic characteristics that were significantly associated with service non-use. Finally, the chapter examines the reasons given by co-residential primary carers for not using respite services.

ANALYSIS OF RESULTS

Overview of the Need for Support and Types of Services Used

The following section examines the need for support and the types of services used. Overall the analysis showed that the majority of primary carers were not using community services except when the care recipient needed assistance with activities such as communication and health heed. Figure 1 shows the percentages of co-resident carers who had care recipients needing assistance, and of those whose care recipients did use community services. They are grouped within each of the nine activities (listed in Table 1). The first bar in each activity group indicates the percentage of carers with care recipients who actually needed assistance for that activity, and the second bar shows the percentage who used formal services.

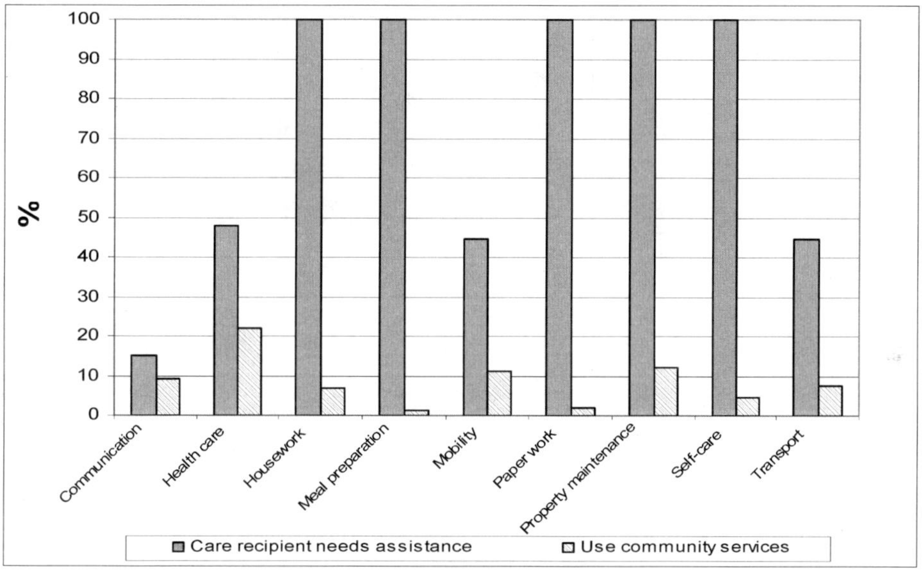

Figure 1. Proportion of carers with care recipients needing assistance for each activity, and who use community services

It is clear that, for all activities except for those related to communication, the majority of co-resident carers had care recipients who did not use formal services. In the case of assistance with communication, 15 percent of carers had care recipients who needed assistance for this activity and over half of these used formal support services, but this was the exception. The activity for which most care recipients used formal services was health care – this included such tasks as taking medications, dressing wounds or using medical machinery. Around 48 percent of all carers had care recipients who need help for this task and nearly half of this group used formal services.

Figure 2 displays the community service use of primary carers. As with Figure 1, the first bar in each group shows the proportion of primary carers with care recipients who needed assistance for that activity, and the second bar shows the proportion of primary carers who had care recipients who used formal services. The third bar in Figure 2 shows the proportion of primary carers who either used respite care themselves or had a care recipient who used formal services, and hence shows the total community service use for the care situation. Figure 2 also shows that, even with respite added to the other community services (the third bar in each group), the majority of primary carers did not seek formal assistance for most activities, with the exception of communication and health care. Overall, only 13 percent of primary carers had ever used respite care.

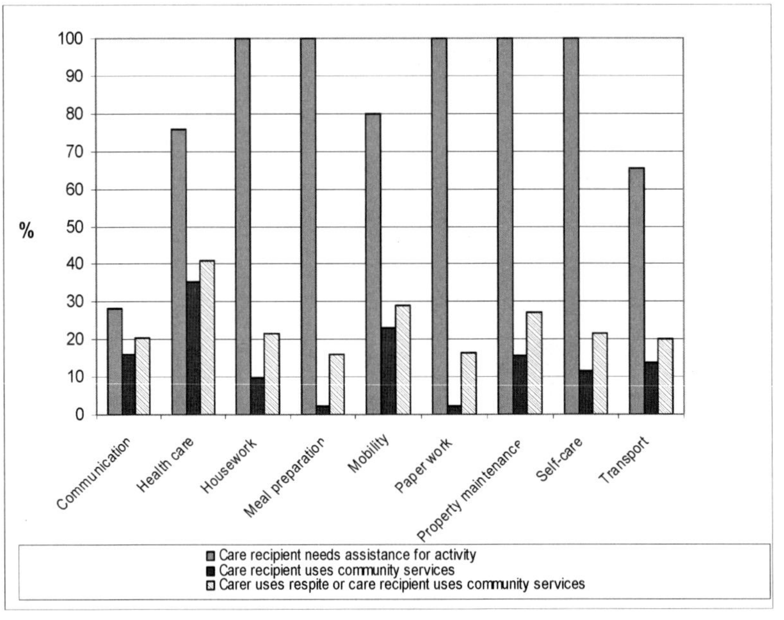

Figure 2. Proportion of primary carers with care recipients needing assistance for each activity, and who use community services and/or respite.

Approximately half of the primary carers who responded to the SDAC spent more than 40 hours per week caring for someone with a profound or severe handicap. Primary carers had care recipients with higher levels of need than carers. They were nearly twice as likely as non-primary carers to have care recipients who needed assistance for communication, health care, mobility and transport; and they were also more likely to have care recipients who used community services for these activities. However, for the five activities for which all care recipients required assistance, only in the case of self-care were primary carers more likely than carers to have a care recipient who received support from community services. In the other four tasks – housework, meal preparation, paperwork, and property maintenance – they did not receive proportionally more support from community services than did carers.

Bi-Variate Analysis of Service Use by Primary Carers by the Age of their Care Recipient

One of the need factors considered, as a potential independent variable in the multivariate analyses, was the age of the care recipient. Table 5 reports the bi-variate results of the proportion of primary carers with care recipients of different ages who use services for the different activities.

Primary carers who were only caring for elderly care recipients were more likely than other primary carers to use formal services for the five activities – housework, meal preparation, paperwork, property maintenance and self-care. Primary carers caring for people who had very young care recipients (under 25 years) and primary carers with elderly care recipients were the two groups most likely to use health care services. Primary carers of the elderly were, however, less likely than primary carers of younger people (aged under 45 years) to use formal services for mobility and transport services.

Table 5. Bi-variate analysis of service non-use by primary carers by the age of the care recipient

	Services not used			
	Five services and respite	**Health care and respite**	**Mobility and respite**	**Transport and respite**
Age of youngest care recipient in household				
Under 25 years	66.6	38.4	29.9	46.7
25-44 years	66.1	49.1	62.7	61.2
45-64 years	70.4	57.5	84.9	83.4
65 years and over	50.6	42.1	71.3	75.2

These findings were qualitatively similar for carers who were not primary carers. While there are differences in the service use for carers of the elderly and non-elderly reported here, the multivariate analysis below indicates whether the age of a care recipient significantly influences service use once we controlled for other factors.

Multivariate Analysis of Factors Relating to Community Service Non-Use

The following tables examine the factors associated with service use, classified according to the conceptual framework suggested by Andersen and Newman (1973). This framework includes 'predisposing (socio-demographic characteristics e.g. sex or age), 'enabling (factors that facilitate or inhibit service use e.g. income or employment' and 'need (factors specific to the care situation e.g. level of disability or carer burden)' variables. Each of these factors is considered for carers and primary carers.

Tables 6 and 7 provide a summary of the predisposing, enabling and need factors, for carers and for primary carers respectively, identified in the multivariate analysis that are significantly associated with service non-use. The complete logistic regression results can be found in the Appendix, Tables A3 to A10. Table 6 provides an overview of the characteristics associated with service non-use by the care recipients of carers[5].

Table 7 provides an overview of the characteristics associated with service non-use by the care recipients of primary carers, as well as the non-use of respite services by the primary carer.

[5] There was less information available on the care situations of carers than of primary carers because primary carers filled in the self-completion questionnaire and carers did not, so it was not possible to control for a number of factors, including the number of hours spent caring, the 'burden' level reported by the carer, the carer's self-assessed health status, whether there was a fall-back carer available, and whether the language spoken to the care recipient was English. The results for carers must be interpreted with that limitation in mind.

There are four columns in Tables 6, one column each for: the group of five activities (housework, meal preparation, paperwork, property maintenance and self care), health care, mobility and transport activities. Taking all other factors included in the multivariate analysis into account Table 6 shows that carers with elderly care recipients are more likely to use health care services. This finding also holds for primary carers.

Table 7 reveals that primary carers with older care recipients or with care recipients aged under 25 are more likely to use health care services than other primary carers. However, primary carers with older care recipients (aged over 45 years) were less likely to use mobility and transport services. In contrast to the bivariate analysis, the age of the care recipient was not a significant independent predictor for the use of the five services by primary carers. The analysis now examines the factors related to service use and non-use by the need, then predisposing, then enabling factors identified in Andersen and Newman's (1973) conceptual framework.

Services Use and Non-Use

Need Factors and Service Use

Need factors are those characteristics specific to the care situation such as the degree of disability or the level of caregiver stress. The results show that the higher the level of need in the care situation the more likely it was that services would be accessed for assistance. Carers were more likely to use community services when they had a care recipient with a higher level of disability, or were caring for more than one care recipient.

Four factors increased the likelihood that primary carers and their care recipients would use community services. The more time primary carers spent looking after another person, the more likely they were to use services. Primary carers caring for 40 hours per week and above were more likely to use services than those caring for 20 hours per week or less. Having a fallback carer available also consistently predicted service use for all activities, apart from health care. The fact that the presence or absence of a fallback carer had no influence in the case of health care suggests that support in health care activities may need to be provided by trained professionals rather than informally. For the other activities apart from health care, the presence of someone else to provide informal care in the care situation decreased the probability of using services.

Carers who themselves had greatest need for services were more likely to access them. The variables used in this analysis to identify burdened carers and carers with poor health (and thus a higher need for support) also showed significant associations with higher levels of service use, primarily for the five activities (housework, meal preparation, paperwork, property maintenance and self-care). It would seem that carers who experience greater difficulty in their care situations are only slightly more likely to access services than carers who do not. Also, when carers in high need access services, they tend only to make use of services for activities that may be considered to be domestic tasks.

Table 6. Carers and service non-use

Factors	Five activities*	Health care	Transport	Mobility
Predisposing	Carer is male Carer under 65 years Carer does not live in a lone parent household Carer born in country other than Australia or north western Europe Carer has year 10 or less or vocational qualifications Carer does not have a long-term health condition	Carer born in country other than Australia or north-western Europe Carer does not have vocational qualification	Lives in couple or lone parent household	Carer is female
Enabling	Carer's personal income level is not in the top quintile Lives in a more socio-economically disadvantaged area Lives in a capital city	Lives in a more socio-economically disadvantaged area Carer's main source of income is government pension or benefit	Carer's main source of income is wage/salary or private income	Lives outside a capital city
Need	Youngest care recipient under 25 Care recipient has a severe or a lower level of disability	Care recipient is female Youngest care recipient under 65 years Care recipient has mild or lower level of disability One care recipient	Care recipient is over 25 years Care recipient has moderate disability One care recipient	Care recipient is female Care recipient is 45-64 years old Care recipient has severe disability One care recipient

Housework, meal preparation, paperwork, property maintenance and self-care.

Table 7. Primary carers and service non-use

Factors	Five activities* and respite	Health care and respite	Transport and respite	Mobility and respite
Predisposing	Carer under 45	Carer born in country other than Australia or north-western Europe Carer does not have long term health condition	Carer is a spouse, parent or other relative of the care recipient	Carer is a spouse, other relative or friend of care recipient
Enabling	Lives in a more socio-economically disadvantaged area	Carer's main source of income is government pension or benefit		Lives in a more socio-economically disadvantaged area
Need	Care recipient has a severe or a moderate disability Carer cares for less than 40 hours per week Carer has relatively low 'carer burden' levels Fall-back carer available Carer has relatively good health	Youngest care recipient is 25-64 years old Carer cares for less than 20 hours per week One care recipient	Youngest care recipient is over 45 years Cares for less than 20 hours One care recipient Fall-back carer available	Youngest care recipient is over 45 years Carer cares for less than 40 hours per week One care recipient Fall-back carer available Carer has relatively low 'carer burden' levels

* Housework, meal preparation, paperwork, property maintenance and self-care.

PREDISPOSING FACTORS AND SERVICE USE

Predisposing factors exist prior to the onset of the care situation, such as age, sex, country of birth, and may predispose carers to access community services. When need factors were controlled for in the regression analysis, it was found that there were a number of factors that tended to be strongly associated with the non-use of community services. These are listed in the top rows of Tables 6 and 7. The analysis indicated that the predisposing factors such as age and gender that affect the probability of service use are weaker predictors of service non-use than need factors. Factors that have effects on the use of the majority of services are discussed below.

Younger carers were less likely on the whole to use services than older carers. Carers aged under 65, and primary carers under 45, were, respectively less likely to use services to support their care situation than older carers. This may be because services are targeted to carers who are older and have poor health.

Male carers were slightly less likely than female carers to access services for the five activities. There may be a number of reasons for this. Male carers may have fewer informal networks from which they can derive information about services. They may be caring for their spouses who may not wish to have services for these activities. Possibly, men may not perceive that they need services.

The most consistent predisposing factor predicting service non-use was birth in Africa, the Americas, Asia, or south-eastern Europe. Carers born in these regions were less likely to access services than Australian-born carers, particularly for health care activities. Primary carers born in these countries were also less likely to use health care services than the Australian-born carers. This suggests that carers and primary carers born abroad either lacked knowledge of health care services, or found these services inaccessible or culturally inappropriate. The language spoken at home was not a key predictor of service non-use, suggesting that immigrant status may be more important than language spoken, particularly in relation to the use of health care services.

Other factors with small but significant effects on the probability of not accessing services for the five activities in the case of carers (but not primary carers) were the absence of a long-term health condition, and not living in a lone parent household. Carers who did not have a long-term health condition were less likely to use services than those who did; and carers not in lone parent households were less likely to use services for the five activities than carers in lone parent households. Carers with relatively low levels of education (year 10 or less or vocational qualifications) were less likely to use services for the five activities.

ENABLING FACTORS AND SERVICE USE

Enabling factors are those factors, such as income or employment status, that can facilitate or impede the use of community services. Some clear findings relating to enabling factors emerge. Primary carers, who lived in relatively disadvantaged socio-economic areas (that is, those living in areas the Australian Bureau of Statistics ranked in the bottom 40 percent on an Index of Relative Socio-Economic Disadvantage), were least likely to use community services. Whether this was because carers in these areas could not afford services, or whether there were fewer services available in these areas, is not known.

Personal income showed an association with service use only for non-primary carers. Carers who had personal incomes in the top quintile were slightly more likely to use services for the five activities than carers in other income brackets. This may indicate that these carers are more able to pay for services such as housework or property maintenance.

If they relied on government benefits as a main source of income, both primary and non-primary carers were less likely to access support from formal health care services than carers who mainly derived income from wages, salaries or a private income. Primary carers reliant on benefits are particularly disadvantaged and are less likely than wage earning primary carers to use health care services. On the other hand, in the case of transport, carers in receipt of welfare benefits were slightly more likely than wage earners to use services.

Non-primary carers were less likely to access formal services for the five activities if they lived in a capital city rather than elsewhere in a state, although this factor was not significant for primary carers. The lower level of service use in the capital cities may indicate that there is greater pressure on resources in the capital cities, or it may be an artefact of the limited categories of the geographic information available in the data set. Other research has suggested that a more useful distinction would be between cities, regions and remote areas, but it was not possible to investigate this from the information contained in SDAC.

Understanding the reasons for service non-use is also important to assist in designing strategies to increase access to support services. The next section examines this issue.

Reasons for Service Non-Use

The following analysis of the reasons for service non-use found that the majority of carers and care recipients stated they did not need services. However, there were carers and care recipients who were unaware of available support services.

Reasons Primary Carers Do Not Use Respite Services

There is relatively little information in SDAC on why it is that the majority of carers do not use community services to support them in their caring role. However, there is information about the reasons why primary carers do not use respite services.

Figure 3 shows that the majority (55 percent) said that they did not use respite care because they perceived that they did not need this service. Only 13 percent had ever used respite care. There were six percent who said they did not use it because they did not want to, and another six percent who said their care recipient did not want to receive respite care. A further 12 percent said they either 'did not know about it' or 'had not heard of it', while four percent reported availability barriers. The data thus suggest that about a third of primary carers who perceive they need respite care use such services. The findings also indicate that efforts could be made to address information and accessibility issues for the small proportion of primary carers (16 percent) who gave these factors as reasons for not accessing respite care.

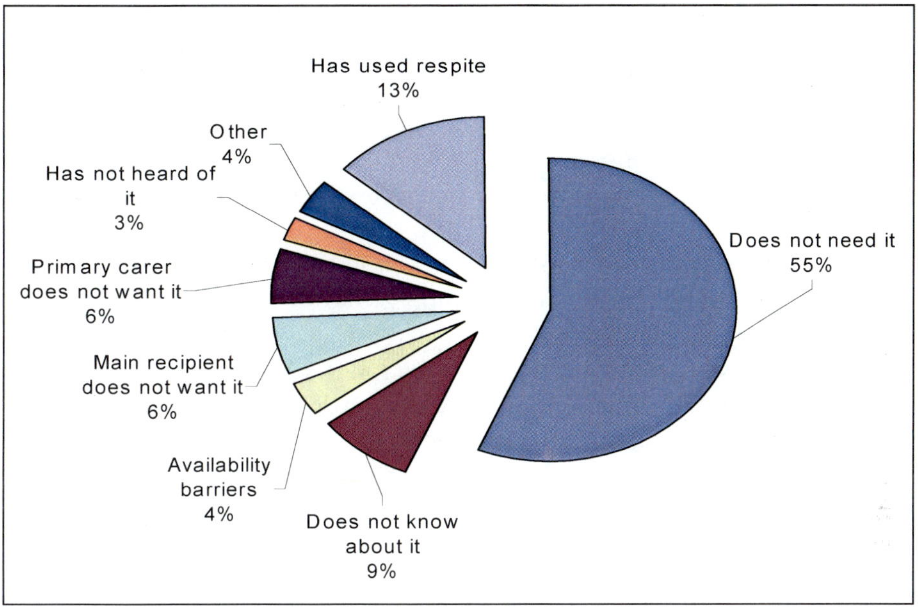

Figure 3. Reasons why primary carers do not use respite services.

Reasons Care Recipients Do Not Use Services

Care recipients who needed assistance with any activity were asked if they received sufficient support for performing that activity, or if they required additional assistance. Care recipients were then asked a follow-up question about the main reason that they did not receive more help from formal services. For all the activities except communication, fewer than 20 percent of those care recipients who needed more assistance for a task reported an unmet need for formal services. In the case of communication activities, 30 percent of care recipients reported an unmet need. Attitudinal barriers (refusing access to services on account of pride or feeling that their need is not sufficiently important to require services) accounted for part of this unmet need. Barriers that government agencies could more easily address accounted for another element of unmet need (not knowing of the existence of the service or reporting that the service costs too much).

Discussion

Considerable research has demonstrated that carers can better maintain their caring role when they use appropriate support services (Bebbington and Davies 1993; Schofield et. al. 1998). Identifying carers who do not use services can assist policy-makers to design and target services more effectively.

There are two clear findings from the analysis of community service use in Australia. First, carers and care recipients who have high needs (such as high levels of disability), carers reporting high levels of burden and those providing more intensive amounts of care are most likely to use services. This may reflect the current targeting of services to carers who have higher needs or may suggest that carers themselves only seek help when their level of need is relatively high and perhaps at a crisis point. Second, the factors associated with the non-use of services - including youth, minority ethnicity, a low level of education, low income, receipt of government benefits, and living in relatively socio-economically disadvantaged areas – also tend to be associated with dimensions of social disadvantage. The study suggests carers with high needs and who are socially and economically disadvantaged are less likely to access support services.

The question of the age of the care recipient as a factor influencing service non-use was also considered in this study. Carers of older people are more likely to use healthcare services suggesting a high level of need for specialised medical assistance. These carers appear less likely to be accessing support for mobility and transport services possibly reflecting lower levels of participation by elderly people in activities outside the home. Overall other factors such as those discussed above were as significant in predicting service non-use as the age of the care recipient.

The study found that carers and care recipients are more likely to use services as the level of need increases (indicated by carer's poor health, carer burden and care recipients with profound levels of disability). However these carers are only slightly more likely to access services than other carers. These carers often experience great difficulties in their situation but mostly access services that assist with domestic tasks. Thus carers who experience relatively high burden and relatively poor health may be two groups who need to be targeted for increased support from services.

Also primary carers experiencing poor health who were supporting care recipients with moderate levels of disability were less likely to use formal services than those whose care recipients have a 'profound' disability. This group may be of particular concern to policy makers as they are potentially vulnerable to being unable to continue in their caring role due to ill health or physical restrictions. The provision of services either to the carer or to the care recipient may be especially effective in supporting these carers.

More information about respite and other community services needs to be disseminated in Australia, as there is a small but not insignificant group of carers and care recipients who are unaware of these services. The accessibility and affordability of community services also needs to be addressed. Further analysis might be able to reveal which groups of carers find access and affordability a particular problem. A general effort to encourage care recipients to view community services as appropriate forms of support could also help those carers least likely to use services in Australia.

CONCLUSIONS

The analysis shows that a high level of need in the care situation leads to a greater likelihood of service use. This includes such factors as caring for a person with profound and severe levels of disability, providing intensive levels of support and experiencing high levels of carer burden. Low service use by carers was associated with disadvantage including youth, ethnic and linguistic minority backgrounds, low levels of education, low income, receipt of government benefit and living in relatively socio-economically disadvantaged areas. The findings of the study also indicated that patterns of service use were different for carers of elderly people who were more likely than other carers to use healthcare services and less likely to use transport and mobility services. The reason given by the majority of carers for not using respite services was a lack of need. Other carers stated either they or the care recipient did not want to use services, while still others were unaware of support services.

RECOMMENDATIONS

- Further investigation of why carers are not using community services is needed. This investigation should focus on three groups of carers who are less likely to be accessing community services:
    - younger carers (under 45 years of age);
    - carers from ethnic and linguistic minority backgrounds; and
    - carers who live in relatively more socio-economically disadvantaged areas.
- More information about respite and other community services needs to be disseminated to a small but significant group of carers and care recipients who are unaware of support services.
- Access to, and affordability of, community services needs to be addressed. Further analysis might be able to reveal which groups of carers find access and affordability a particular problem.
- There needs to be a general effort to encourage carers and care recipients to view community services as appropriate forms of support and investigate why they are regarded as inappropriate.
- Raising awareness and understanding about the issues involved in caring will assist carers to self-identify.

REFERENCES

Andersen, R., and J.F. Newman (1973) ‘Societal and individual determinants of medical care utilization in the United States’ *Milbank Quarterly* 51, 95-124.

Australian Bureau of Statistics. (1998) *Time use survey Australia: User’s guide*, 1997 Catalogue No. 4150.0, Canberra: ABS.

Australian Bureau of Statistics. (1999) *1998 Disability, ageing and carers: Summary of findings* Cat. No. 4430.0, Canberra: ABS.

Bebbington, A., and B. Davies. (1993) ‘Efficient targeting of community care: The case of the home help service’ *Journal of Social Policy* 22(3), 373-391.

Beisecker, A., Wright, L., Chrisman, S. and J. Ashworth. (1996) ‘Family caregiver perceptions of benefit and barriers to the use of adult day care for individuals with Alzheimer’s disease’ *Research on Aging* 18(4), 430-450

Bittman, M., Fast, J.E., Fisher, K., and C. Thomson. (2004) “Making the invisible visible: The life and time(s) of informal caregivers” in M. Bittman and N. Folbre (Eds.), *Family time: The social organisation of care* (pp. 69-89). London: Routledge.

Bittman, M., Fisher, K., Hill, P., Thompson, D., and C. Thomson. (2003) *Identifying isolated carers: Final report*. Submitted to the New South Wales Department for Women, the

NSW Department of, Ageing, Disabilityand Home Care, the NSW Department of Community Services, NSW Health and Carers NSW.

Bittman, M., and C. Thomson (2000) 'Invisible support', in J. Warburton and M. Oppenheimer (Eds.) *Volunteers and volunteering* (pp.98-112). Sydney: Federation Press.

Braithwaite, V. (1990) *Bound to care*, Sydney: Allen and Unwin.

Braithwaite, V. (1998) 'Institutional respite care: breaking chores or breaking social bonds' *The Gerontologist* 38(5), 610-617

Brodaty, H. and D. Hadzi-Pavlovic (1990) 'Psychosocial effects on carers of living with persons with dementia' *Australian and New Zealand Journal of Psychiatry* 24, 351-61.

Brodaty, H., Thomson C., Thompson C., and M. Fine (2005), 'Why caregivers of people with dementia and memory loss don't use services', International Jounral of Geriatric Psychiarity, 20, 537-546.

Brody, E. (1981) 'Women in the middle and family help to older people' *The Gerontologist* 21(5), 471-479.

Bryson L., and M. Mowbray. (1981) 'Community: the spray-on solution' *Australian Journal of Social Issues* 16(4), 255-267.

Commonwealth Department of Family and Community Services. (2002) *Young carers research project: Final report*. Canberra: Commonwealth Department of Family and Community Services.

Dalley, G. (1988) *Ideologies of caring: Rethinking community and collectivism* London: Macmillan.

Finch, J., and D. Groves. (Eds.) (1983) *A labour of love: Women, work and caring* London: Routledge and Kegan Paul.

Fine, M. (1999) *The responsibility for child and aged care: Shaping policies for the future* SPRC Discussion Paper, No.105, Kensington: Social Policy Research Centre, University of New South Wales.

Gill, C., Hinrichsen, G. and R. DiGiuseppe. (1998) 'Factors associated with formal service use by family members of patients with dementia' *Journal of Applied Gerontology* 17(1), 38-50

Graham. H. (1983) 'Caring: a labour of love' in J. Finch and D. Groves (Eds.) *A labour of love: Women, work and caring* (pp.13-30). London: Routledge and Kegan Paul.

Land, H. (1978) 'Who cares for the family?' *Journal of Social Policy* 7(3), 257-284.

Misic, A. (1996) *The hidden society: A study of non-English speaking background carer issues in the Western Sydney Region* Sydney: The Carers Association of New South Wales, Inc.

Knapman, C. and H. Waite (1997) 'Rights, relationships and dementia care', in Caltabiano, R. and R. Frangos (Eds.) *Achieving Inclusion: Exploring Issues in Disability* Centre for Social and Welfare Research, James Cook University of North Queensland, 199-217

Parker, G. (2000) 'Disability and caring: the cutting edge' a keynote address at the 2nd Annual International Conference on Caring, 'Sharing the Care: A Critical Time for Decision Makers Around the Globe' 29-31 March 2000, Brisbane, Australia.

Parker, G. (1990) *With due care and attention: A review of research on informal care, 2nd ed*. Occasional Paper No. 2, London: Family Policy Studies Centre.

Schofield, E., Bloch, S., Herrman, H., Murphy, B., Nankervis, J., and B. Singh. (Eds.) (1998) *Family caregivers: Disability, illness and ageing* Sydney: Allen and Unwin.

Thomson, C., Fine, M. and H. Brodaty. (1997) *Carers' Support Needs Project: Dementia Carers and the Non-Use of Community Services: Report on the Literature Review*, Commissioned by the Ageing and Disability Department, Social Policy Research Centre, University of New South Wales, Sydney

Twigg, J. and K. Atkin. (1994) *Carers Perceived: Policy and Practice in Informal Care* Buckingham: Open University Press

Ungerson, C., and M. Kember. (Eds.) (1997) *Women and social policy* London: Macmillan.

Watson, E., and J. Mears. (1999) *Women, Work and Care of the Elderly* Sydney: Ashgate

Zarit, S.H., Stephens, M.A.P., Townsend, A. and R. Greene. (1998) 'Stress reduction for family caregivers: effects of adult day care use' *The Journals of Gerontology, Series B* 53(5), September, 267-278.

APPENDIX – VARIABLES USED IN THE CARER BURDEN, CARER POOR HEALTH INDICES AND COMPLETE REGRESSION ANALYSIS RESULTS

Table A1. Carer burden indicators

Domain	Indicator (due to the caring role)
Emotional	The carer had been diagnosed with a stress-related illness.
	The carer frequently felt weary or lacked energy.
	The carer frequently felt worried or depressed.
	The carer frequently felt angry or resentful.
	The carer did not feel satisfied.
Social/Time	The carer had lost touch or was losing touch with friends.
	The relationship between carer and care recipient had become strained.
	The carer had less time for relationships with co-resident family members or the relationships with family members had become strained.
	The carer had less time for relationships with spouse/partner or the relationship with spouse/partner had become strained.
Financial	The carer's income had decreased or the carer had extra expenses.
	The carer had difficulty with everyday living costs.
Physical/emotional	The carer's physical or emotional wellbeing had changed.
	The carer needed more support in caring role.
	The carer had sleep interrupted by caring role (frequently, occasionally or frequency not stated)
	Sleep interrupted interfered with normal daily activities frequently or occasionally
Variables considered but not included in the burden index after assessment were:	Carer had difficulty or was unable to take public transport when accompanied by care recipient.
	Carer regularly paid a significant part of the recipient's living costs.
	The caring role was the main reason carer was not working.

Table A2. Poor health indicators

Self-assessment indicators	General health assessment – health fair to poor
	Limited a lot in moderate activities
	Limited a lot in climbing stairs
	Accomplished less than would have liked to, due to physical problems in the last four weeks
	Limited in work/regular activities due to physical health
	Accomplished less than would have liked to, due to emotional problems in the last four weeks
	Work/activities not as careful as usual due to emotional problems
	Pain interfered with work moderately, quite a bit or extremely in the last four weeks
	Felt down a good bit of the time, most of the time or all of the time in the last four weeks
	Felt calm some of the time, a little of the time or none of the time in the last four weeks
	Had a lot of energy some of the time, a little of the time or none of the time in the last four weeks
	Physical/emotional problems interfered with social life a good bit of the time, most of the time or all of the time in the last four weeks
	Physical health score is less than the median for this group
	Mental health score is less than the median for this group

Table A3. Logistic regression: co-resident primary carers and non-use of five formal services and respite

Parameter	Significance	Estimate	Standard Error	Chi-Square	Probabilities
					Baseline probability 0.5908
					Average marginal probability
Intercept		0.367	0.276	1.773	
Age of carer					
Aged under 45	***	0.627	0.201	9.774	0.1375
Aged 65 and over		-0.266	0.215	1.529	-0.0616
Socio-economic status of carer's local area					
2nd quintile		-0.139	0.241	0.332	-0.0320
3rd quintile		-0.039	0.250	0.024	-0.0089
4th quintile		-0.252	0.259	0.946	-0.0585
5th quintile	***	-0.919	0.275	11.189	-0.2213
Care recipient's level of disability					
Severe	**	0.439	0.190	5.362	0.0977
Moderate or less	***	1.280	0.485	6.974	0.2281
Hours spent actively caring					
Hours not stated		0.353	0.396	0.794	0.0759
Less than 20 hours	***	0.769	0.222	12.022	0.1660
Between 20 and 39 hours	***	0.691	0.239	8.382	0.1443
Burden index score >5	***	-0.515	0.192	7.229	-0.1164
Health index score .>3	**	-0.428	0.186	5.325	-0.0956
Has fall-back carer available	**	0.396	0.173	5.275	0.0902
					Average probability of sample 0.6505
Predicted correct 67.2					
Sensitivity 82.3					
Specificity 41.9					
McFadden's pseudo r^2= 0.12					

Table A4. Logistic regression: primary carers and the non-use of health care and respite service

Parameter	Significance	Estimate	Standard Error	Chi-Square	Probabilities
					Baseline probability 0.4736
					Average marginal probability
Intercept		-0.106	0.253	0.176	
Country of birth					
North Western Europe		0.315	0.278	1.286	0.0784
Other country	***	0.780	0.291	7.177	0.1923
Has long term health Condition	**	-0.439	0.201	4.778	-0.1085
Main source of income is private	***	-0.970	0.214	20.526	-0.2305
Age of youngest care recipient					
Under 25 years		0.428	0.270	2.516	0.1063
25 to 44 years	**	0.690	0.296	5.431	0.1707
45 to 64 years	***	0.657	0.246	7.112	0.1626
Number of care recipients					
More than one care recipient	***	-1.025	0.254	16.237	-0.2361
Hours spent actively caring					
Hours not stated		0.233	0.420	0.308	0.0579
Less than 20 hours	***	0.634	0.228	7.722	0.1569
Between 20 and 39 hours		0.149	0.263	0.318	0.0369
					Average probability of sample 0.4451
Predicted correct 62.6					
Sensitivity 53.1					
Specificity 70.5					
McFadden's pseudo r^2= 0.08					

Table A5. Logistic Regression: Primary carers and the non-use of mobility and respite services

Parameter	Significance	Estimate	Standard Error	Chi-Square	Probabilities
					Baseline probability 0.7787
					Average marginal probability
Intercept	***	1.258	0.307	16.760	
Relationship of carer to care recipient					
Parent	**	-0.665	0.382	3.028	-0.1492
Child	***	-0.973	0.308	9.977	-0.2266
Other relative		-0.308	0.455	0.457	-0.0686
Socio-economic status of carer's area					
2nd quintile		-0.185	0.296	0.390	-0.0401
3rd quintile	*	0.561	0.329	2.912	0.1108
4th quintile		-0.109	0.328	0.110	-0.0235
5th quintile	***	-0.891	0.340	6.875	-0.2071
Age of youngest care recipient					
Under 25 years	***	-1.708	0.439	15.147	-0.3914
25 to 44 years	**	-0.746	0.345	4.668	-0.1710
45 to 64 years		0.449	0.322	1.952	0.0913
Care recipient's level of disability					
Severe or moderate	*	0.479	0.261	3.374	0.0992
Number of care recipients					
More than one care recipient	***	-0.759	0.269	7.968	-0.1723
Hours spent actively caring					
Hours not stated	*	-0.839	0.472	3.165	-0.1978
Less than 20	***	1.043	0.299	12.138	0.2020
Between 20 and 39	**	0.668	0.300	4.970	0.1291
Has fall-back carer available	**	0.475	0.229	4.296	0.1014
Burden index score>5	**	-0.517	0.230	5.047	-0.1087
					Average probability of sample 0.6923
Predicted correct 75.7					
Sensitivity 87.5					
Specificity 54.6					
McFadden's pseudo r^2= 0.26					

Table A6. Logistic regression: Primary carers and the non-use of transport and respite services

Parameter	Significance	Estimate	Standard Error	Chi-Square	Probabilities
					Baseline probability 0.7548
					Average marginal probability
Intercept	***	1.124	0.246	20.892	
Relationship of carer to care recipient					
Parent		-0.445	0.400	1.240	-0.1104
Child	***	-1.206	0.327	13.635	-0.2816
Other relative		0.110	0.564	0.038	0.0274
Age of care recipient					
Aged less than 25 years	***	-1.306	0.472	7.668	-0.3050
Between 25 and 44 years	***	-0.956	0.369	6.703	-0.2289
Between 45 and 65 years		0.042	0.336	0.015	0.0104
Number of care recipients					
More than one care recipient	***	-0.830	0.282	8.675	-0.2017
Hours spent actively caring					
Hours not stated		-0.377	0.486	0.602	-0.0934
Less than 20 hours	***	1.352	0.331	16.678	0.3178
Between 20 and 39 hours		0.495	0.301	2.702	0.1223
Has fall-back carer available	***	0.727	0.240	9.143	0.1797
					Average probability of sample 0.7358
Predicted correct 74.3 Sensitivity 88.8 Specificity 41.5 McFadden's pseudo r^2= 0.17					

Table A7. Logistic regression: Co-resident carers and the non-use of five services

Parameter	Significance	Estimate	Standard Error	Chi-Square	Probabilities
					Baseline probability 0.9013
					Average marginal probability
Intercept	***	2.211	0.206	115.527	
Male	***	0.272	0.093	8.546	0.0414
Carer aged 15 to 24		0.093	0.178	0.275	0.0139
Carer aged 25 to 44	*	0.244	0.131	3.494	0.0362
Carer aged 65 and over	***	-0.590	0.141	17.624	-0.1004
Couple household		-0.143	0.134	1.140	-0.0223
Lone parent household	***	-0.579	0.151	14.593	-0.1011
Other household		0.140	0.141	0.975	0.0207
Country of birth					
North Western Europe		0.067	0.140	0.227	0.0100
Other country	**	0.293	0.137	4.573	0.0418
Highest educational qualification					
Bachelor degree	***	-0.623	0.169	13.541	-0.1108
Diploma	***	-0.512	0.172	8.861	-0.0889
Vocational qualification		-0.130	0.115	1.275	-0.0202
Year 11 or 12	***	-0.520	0.149	12.188	-0.0895
Has long term health condition	***	-0.272	0.101	7.234	-0.0412
Carer's personal income					
Quintile unknown	***	-0.538	0.162	11.027	-0.0929
1st quintile		-0.204	0.144	2.002	-0.0324
3rd quintile		-0.180	0.138	1.709	-0.0285
4th quintile		-0.081	0.158	0.265	-0.0126
5th quintile	**	-0.449	0.181	6.151	-0.0762
Socio-economic status of carer's local area					
2nd quintile		0.108	0.144	0.563	0.0162
3rd quintile	**	-0.300	0.138	4.746	-0.0483
4th quintile	***	-0.418	0.141	8.767	-0.0689
5th quintile	***	-0.718	0.151	22.498	-0.1261
Geographical location					
Lives in rest of state	***	-0.290	0.100	8.395	-0.0455

Table A7. Continued

Parameter	Significance	Estimate	Standard Error	Chi-Square	Probabilities
Age of youngest care recipient	***	0.972	0.164	35.191	
Less than 25 years		0.094	0.136	0.477	0.1238
25 to 44 years		-0.059	0.131	0.204	0.0141
65 years and over					-0.0091
Highest level of disability in household	***	-0.901	0.119	57.587	
Profound		0.043	0.138	0.097	-0.1568
Moderate					0.0065
Mild/or employment /schooling restriction/or no restriction		0.170	0.123	1.910	0.0253
Predicted correct 78.9					Average probability of sample
Sensitivity 97.8					0.8118
Specificity 10.0					
McFadden's pseudo r^2=0.09					

Table A8. Logistic regression: co-resident carers and the non-use of health care services

Parameter	Significance	Estimate	Standard Error	Chi-Square	Probabilities
					Baseline probability 0.7495 Average marginal probability
Intercept	***	1.096	0.176	38.708	
Highest educational qualifications					
Bachelor degree		-0.232	0.216	1.159	-0.0580
Diploma		-0.142	0.224	0.401	-0.0354
Vocational qualification	***	-0.435	0.135	10.372	-0.1083
Year 11 or 12		-0.144	0.178	0.652	-0.0359
Country of birth					
North Western Europe		0.168	0.176	0.906	0.0416
Other country	***	0.692	0.165	17.543	0.1659
Socio-economic status of carer's local area					
2nd Quintile		-0.039	0.163	0.056	-0.0096
3rd quintile		-0.131	0.160	0.670	-0.0327
4th quintile		-0.236	0.163	2.093	-0.0589
5th quintile	***	-0.541	0.183	8.784	-0.1342

Table A8. (Continued)

Parameter	Significance	Estimate	Standard Error	Chi-Square	Probabilities
Main source of income					
Wages/salaries or private income	***	-0.364	0.116	9.900	-0.0904
Sex of first care recipient					
Female	***	-0.490	0.108	20.513	-0.1215
Age of youngest care recipient					
Less than 25 years	*	0.289	0.160	3.273	0.0714
25 to 44 years		0.093	0.162	0.326	0.0230
65 years and over	***	-0.685	0.146	22.058	-0.1697
Highest level of disability of care recipients					
Profound		0.028	0.129	0.047	0.0070
Moderate		-0.251	0.174	2.092	-0.0628
Mild/employment schooling restriction/ No restriction	**	0.388	0.182	4.558	0.0950
Number of care recipients					
Two care recipients	***	-1.601	0.166	92.675	-0.3643
Three care recipients	***	-1.630	0.341	22.861	-0.3532
					Average probability of sample
Predicted correct 65.0 Sensitivity 71.9 Specificity 57.2 McFadden's pseudo r^2=0.10					0.5286

Table A9. Logistic regression: Co-resident carers and the non-use of mobility services

Parameter	Significance	Estimate	Standard Error	Chi-Square	Probabilities
					Baseline Probabilities 0.9444
					Average marginal
Intercept	***	2.832	0.216	172.154	probability
Sex of carer					
Male	**	-0.347	0.152	5.244	-0.0533
Geographical residence of carer					
Does not live in capital city	***	0.632	0.157	16.201	0.0911

Table A9. Continued

Parameter	Significance	Estimate	Standard Error	Chi-Square	Probabilities
Sex of care recipient					
Female care recipient	**	0.323	0.151	4.554	0.0495
Age of care recipient					
Under 25 years	***	-2.129	0.206	106.333	-0.4168
25 to 44 years	***	-0.809	0.231	12.332	-0.1425
65 years and over	**	-0.564	0.222	6.481	-0.0933
Disability level of care recipient					
Profound	***	-1.042	0.152	47.316	-0.1612
Number of care recipients					
Two care recipients	***	-1.725	0.172	100.511	-0.3475
Three care recipients	**	-0.706	0.345	4.186	-0.1297
					Average probability of sample
Predicted correct 80.4 Sensitivity 91.3 Specificity 47.9 McFadden's pseudo r^2=0.29					0.8125

Table A10. Logistic regression: Co-resident carers and the non-use of transport services

Parameter	sig	Estimate	Standard Error	Chi-Square	Probabilities
					Baseline probability 0.8992 Average marginal probability
Intercept	***	2.189	0.249	77.418	
Household type					
Couple	***	0.780	0.261	8.931	0.0702
Lone parent	**	0.602	0.287	4.396	0.0510
Other household		0.282	0.218	1.675	0.0270
Main source of income					
Wages, salary or other private income	**	0.384	0.163	5.529	0.0394
Age of youngest care recipient					

Table A10. Continued

Parameter	sig	Estimate	Standard Error	Chi-Square	Probabilities
Under 25 years	***	-0.996	0.238	17.569	-0.1307
25 to 44 years		-0.144	0.248	0.336	-0.0151
65 years and over		-0.225	0.235	0.920	-0.0236
Highest disability level of care recipients					
Profound	***	-0.893	0.184	23.641	-0.0986
Moderate	**	0.885	0.402	4.841	0.0699
Mild/employment or schooling Restriction/or no restriction		0.534	0.344	2.406	0.0469
Number of care recipients					
Two care recipients	***	-1.718	0.181	90.122	-0.2687
Three care recipients		-0.489	0.414	1.399	-0.0593
					Average probability of sample
Predicted correct 85.3%					
Sensitivity 96.3%					
Specificity 29.6%					
McFadden's pseudo r2=0.21					0.8852

In: Family Caregiving for Older Disabled People
Editor: Isabella Paoletti, pp. 393-405
ISBN 1-59454-808-0

Chapter 18

ETHNICITY AND CAREGIVING: A CASE STUDY IN ENGLAND

Katharine Jeary and Olive Stevenson
University of Nottingham, UK.

INTRODUCTION

This chapter aims to explore the complexities and professional challenges found to arise within the context of the provision of personal care to an elderly person from a minority ethnic background when there are also concerns that the elderly person is possibly subject to abuse. The case study, which forms the core of this chapter, is drawn from a qualitative research project undertaken in 2001-2002 by the University of Nottingham, England, and funded by the Nuffield Foundation.

The context of the study will be outlined, in terms of current policies and practice in relation to elder abuse in England. There is a brief overview of some of the literature which underpins these, relating both to elder abuse generally and to the increasing population of elderly people from ethnic minority backgrounds. Following a brief description of the research project, the case study will be detailed, focusing on issues arising from the formal provision of personal care to an elderly, disabled woman from an ethnic minority, where the professionals involved have concerns that she is possibly being abused. The complexities and ethical issues inherent in this case, and indeed more generally, including differing cultural expectations, communication difficulties, and so on, will then be reflected upon. The chapter aims to illustrate some of the complexities, subtleties and sensitivities inherent in formal caregiving in a situation where age, ethnicity and possible elder abuse are all key factors. It also aims to give food for thought to those responsible for policy-making or the development of practice in these areas.

THE CONTEXT OF THE STUDY

The research was timely, as in 2000 the Department of Health, London, published 'No Secrets', a guidance document relating to the development and implementation of multi-agency policies and procedures to protect vulnerable adults from abuse. This was a landmark document placing a formal requirement on statutory health and social care authorities to work closely together in the identification and investigation of alleged adult abuse, and in ensuring the protection of victims. 'No Secrets' defines the main forms of adult abuse as physical, sexual, psychological, financial, neglect and discriminatory. Abuse may consist of a single or repeated acts, and it may occur in any relationship. It may result in significant harm to, or exploitation of, the person subjected to the abuse. The importance of the publication of 'No Secrets' lies in the acknowledgement at governmental level that the abuse of vulnerable adults in the United Kingdom needs to be addressed strategically. Those working in this field, who were interviewed for this research, voiced the hope that this may be a sign of intent that a more effective protective legislative framework and dedicated resourcing may follow.

'No Secrets' requires a structured inter-agency, information-sharing approach to the protection of vulnerable adults. It ascribes the lead role to local authority Social Services departments and requires cooperation and collaboration between all organisations, whether statutory, voluntary or private sector, when an allegation of adult abuse is made. Within that framework, details of structure and responsibilities may vary locally, but many authorities have chosen to adopt processes and procedures similar to those already in place for child protection. This was the case in the city in which this study was undertaken. In brief, an allegation of adult abuse would be followed by a strategy meeting, at which the details of an investigation would be planned. The outcome of the investigation would then be presented to a case conference, chaired by a manager from the lead authority. This meeting would be attended by a range of managers and practitioners from involved agencies and organisations, including social services, healthcare, criminal justice, contracted care providers, and so on. In this particular authority, there was an expectation that the victim of the alleged abuse, or their chosen advocate, should also be invited. The case conference had two specific objectives. These were firstly, by sharing and discussing all available information, to establish whether or not abuse had occurred, and secondly, to compile a detailed protection plan to prevent further abuse, where required.

The existence, nature and frequency of the abuse of vulnerable adults had been gaining increasing recognition and concern in England during the late 1980s and 1990s, as had acknowledgement of the need for the development of protective services. These issues were highlighted both in relation to adults with learning disabilities (ARC and NAPSAC, 1993; Brown, 1999) and to elderly people (Stevenson, 1989; Bennett and Kingston, 1993; Hughes, 1995; Baumhover and Beall, 1996). Issues concerning the protection of children from abuse had been on the national agenda for considerably longer and, notwithstanding the differing legal rights of adults and children, there were lessons to be learned from that experience when developing policies and practice in relation to vulnerable adults (Stevenson, 1996). During the 1990s too considerable work was being undertaken concerning issues of 'mental incapacity' and 'ability to consent' (Law Commission, 1995; Lord Chancellor's Dept. 1999) in the context of protecting vulnerable adults.

Against this background, this chapter focuses specifically on elder abuse, ethnicity and caregiving, exploring issues which may arise when adult abuse is suspected or alleged within a family from an ethnic minority background and formal adult protection procedures are invoked. An understanding of such issues is particularly important not only in view of general demographic trends indicating an increasing proportion of the United Kingdom population being elderly, but also in terms of the relevant and sensitive provision of domiciliary and residential care for elderly people from ethnic minority backgrounds. Currently within the United Kingdom the ethnic groups have a younger age structure than the 'White' population, with some differences between these groups, but the Office for National Statistics (ONS, 2002) anticipates 'progressive ageing of the minority ethnic population in the future'.

The disadvantages experienced by ageing members of ethnic minority groups have been described as 'double jeopardy', a shorthand description of the two-fold disadvantages of age and race discrimination, (Dowd and Bengston, 1978), and subsequently as 'triple jeopardy', which adds the disadvantage of social class (Jackson et al., 1982), or of services not being accessible to them (Norman, 1985). Research has tended to focus more on the numerically larger ethnic minority groups in the United Kingdom, notably those from Afro-Caribbean and Asian backgrounds (Norman, 1985; Blakemore and Boneham, 1994). When considering the appropriate provision of care for elderly people, the heterogeneity of the older population within ethnic minority groups should not be overlooked. Many of those now requiring care, whether provided by the family or more formally, are among the first of their community to be growing old in the United Kingdom. Their reasons for coming to this country will have been very varied, as will the levels at which they will have wished and been able to integrate with the indigenous population and to come to understand aspects of the culture of their new homeland.

Many of these factors are illustrated by the following case study, which concerns Sumeera M., a 67 year old Black African woman living in a city in northern England. Before looking in detail at how Sumeera was cared for, both within her family and by paid carers, it is relevant to view her ethnic background within the context of her local community. Whilst official statistics (ONS, 2001) indicate a substantial proportion of people from ethnic minority groups within the region of England in which Sumeera lived, by far the largest group is of Pakistani origin, with Bangladeshi, other Asian, Black Caribbean and Chinese also being substantially represented. The Black African population within the region is very small in comparison, and indeed in actual numbers. Thus those charged with the provision of culturally sensitive and accessible care for elderly members of ethnic minority groups have a very broad range factors to consider, together with the added complexity of the heterogeneity within each of the individual ethnic groups, with differences stemming, for example, from their social or other status in their country of origin, expectations of kinship networks, and so on (Sokolovsky, 1990; Dandekar, 1996). The following section outlines the main steps of our research project.

The Study: Its Objectives and Methodology

The primary objective of the study was to contribute positively to the development of policy and professional practice in relation to the protection of vulnerable adults against abuse, highlighting particularly the inter-agency dimensions of this. In order to achieve this, the central focus of the study was the case conference element of the adult protection process, as described above. The investigation of the process, content and dynamics of adult protection case conferences, augmented by the views of participants and policy-makers, offered insights into issues affecting risk assessment, the formulation of responses to alleged abuse, factors which assist or hinder realistic planning, ethical dilemmas facing those involved, and the causes and impact of tensions in multi-disciplinary and inter-agency working. This was an 18-month study, based in a northern English city.

The study included data from 50 adult protection case conferences. The methodology encompassed observation and audio-recording of meetings which covered a wide spectrum of alleged abuse in terms of type, location and abuser-victim relationships. The transcripts were thematically analysed. 58 semi-structured, audio-recorded interviews with case conference participants were undertaken, including representatives of the public, private and voluntary sectors, covering social care, social work, healthcare, police, and so on. Interviews averaged 1.5 hours' duration, and again the transcripts were thematically analysed. The researcher was also given access to formal documentation and records about each case for textual analysis.

The case study described and discussed in this chapter was observed and audio-recorded at the case conference stage. Five participants of the meeting were subsequently interviewed, namely the elderly woman's social worker, a community nurse, the manager of the domiciliary care providing organisation, the social worker's line manager and the senior manager who chaired the case conference. Whilst the case study describes an actual case, the names of those concerned have been changed in the interests of confidentiality. In the next section we present the case study in detail.

CASE STUDY: SUMEERA M

Sumeera: A Brief History

In the early 1970s Sumeera left her homeland in north Africa to begin a new life in a northern English city. Her husband's cousin had settled in the same city a few years previously. Envisaging a better quality of life for his family, Sumeera's husband brought his wife and two daughters, in their late teens, to England. At that stage Mr M spoke some English, but his wife and daughters did not. With assistance Mr M secured a home for his family and employment for himself. The elder daughter, Irfit, soon entered a pre-arranged marriage and lived with her husband in the same locality as her parents. Apart from routine contacts with medical, housing or other agencies, Sumeera and her husband led quietly industrious lives for the following two decades. Mr M, made some links with others from their ethnic background, particularly through the mosque, but none of these acquaintances lived in the immediate neighbourhood. Sumeera and her husband mixed very little with the local community, which was predominantly Pakistani, and they relied mainly on other family members for social contact. By this stage Irfit had several children who regularly visited their grandparents. Her younger sister had also married but had moved to another town.

In the mid-1990s Mr M died after a short illness. Sumeera continued to live alone in the flat the couple had rented from the local housing authority. Having been dependent on her husband in respect of the practicalities of life, such as financial matters, housing repairs, company when going out, and so on, Sumeera began to find life difficult, as well as lonely. Her life had been family-centred, and Sumeera had learned very little English in the intervening years.

Irfit's eldest two children moved in with their grandmother. This had two-fold benefits, in that it gave Sumeera assistance and company, and at the same time it relieved the overcrowding in Irfit's home, as she and her husband had their five children living with them. Like her mother, Irfit had a family-centred life, mixed very little with the local community other than in her husband's company, and her spoken English remained very limited.

Two years after Mr M died, Sumeera had her first stroke. Several months later she had another and was admitted to hospital. At this stage the local social services were asked to assess Sumeera's needs and wishes, as it was clear that she would not be able to live independently without considerable input from family or paid caregivers. The eventual outcome was that Sumeera moved into her daughter's home, with Irfit and the three youngest children, and the other family members moved to Sumeera's former home. Nursing care was provided, as needed, to deal with problems such as pressure sores, leg ulcers, and so on. Paid caregivers went into Sumeera's home three times a day to provide personal care. Whilst efforts had originally been made to find caregivers from a similar ethnic background to Sumeera, this had not proved possible, and her current nursing and social care needs were all provided for by White English female caregivers.

Adult Protection Proceedings and Multi-Agency Concerns

The 'care package' described above had been in place for several months. Occasionally the caregivers had voiced concerns about the family's care of Sumeera to the social worker overseeing the case. As the frequency of these concerns increased and Sumeera's quality of life and health were seen to deteriorate, the social worker decided to invoke formal adult protection procedures. There were two threads to the reasons behind this decision. Firstly, paid caregivers who worked with Sumeera reported that her care and welfare were being neglected by family members, and that her physical and mental health were deteriorating unnecessarily due to this neglect. Secondly, the paid carers were on the point of withdrawing their services from Sumeera because of the abuse they considered they were subjected to whilst carrying out their duties within Sumeera's home.

A multi-agency case conference was therefore convened which, in line with local formal procedures, had two specific purposes. Firstly the meeting was required to establish whether or not there was any substance to the allegations of abuse by neglect, and secondly, to put in place agreed protective measures to ensure the appropriate care and safety of Sumeera in future. Eight representatives of statutory (Social Services, healthcare) and private sector organisations (domiciliary care-providers) involved in Sumeera's care attended the meeting. In terms of their ethnic backgrounds, all were White English except one who was Black English. No members of Sumeera's family were present, nor an advocate on her behalf; it subsequently transpired that they had not been informed of the meeting (contrary to local policy). The researcher observed and audio-recorded the meeting, but took no other part in it.

By way of observation, it was interesting how the conduct, tone and general dynamics of the meeting appeared to mirror the factors which were being highlighted about Sumeera's family. There were descriptions of how the multitude of difficulties within the family seemed to be overwhelming them, and of how attention to Sumeera's care was therefore becoming 'lost' in the morass. There was much concern expressed about Sumeera, as well as the goodwill to provide appropriate care for her, but there was an accompanying air of frustration and almost despair. Within the meeting many of the difficulties identified were attributed to 'misunderstandings' between the professionals, Sumeera and her family caregivers, arising from the lack of a mutual language in which to communicate effectively and from a lack of knowledge of each other's cultural contexts and expectations.

The Alleged Neglect

'No Secrets' describes the form of abuse termed 'neglect and acts of omission' as including 'ignoring medical or physical care needs, failure to provide access to appropriate health, social care or educational services, the withholding of the necessities of life, such as medication, adequate nutrition and heating' (para. 2.7).

The paid caregivers involved with Sumeera, both healthcare and social care providers, voiced concerns that Irfit and other family members neglected her within the terms of this definition. In respect of medication, for example, it was known that tablets prescribed by the doctor for Sumeera were not collected from the pharmacist and therefore not given to her as required. Irfit was reminded about this by the caregivers, but the problem persisted. Out of concern for Sumeera's well-being the caregivers occasionally went to the pharmacy themselves and brought the tablets to Sumeera's home, but this was outside their contracted duties. There remained concerns, though, about whether or not Sumeera was given the medication in the correct doses at the right times.

One form of medication prescribed for Sumeera was a diuretic. The paid caregivers had tried to reinforce to Irfit the doctor's explanation that the medication would make Sumeera thirsty and that she should be given adequate fluids to drink. There were signs, however, that Sumeera was often distressed and in real need of a drink of water when they visited.

Sumeera suffered from urinary incontinence and wore pads both during the day and at night. These were available free of charge through the health services, but they had to be collected from the same pharmacy as the medication. Again the family failed to comply with this expectation, and there were regularly no pads available for the caregivers undertaking Sumeera's personal care. On one occasion it was found that the youngest of Irfit's children was wearing one of the pads intended for her grandmother.

Another act of 'neglect' or 'omission' related to the provision by the family of clean bedlinen and clothing for Sumeera, and to the provision of soap for the caregivers to use when washing Sumeera. All of these items were frequently not available.

A different form of neglect, which concerned the professionals working to maintain Sumeera's health and quality of life, consisted of the family depriving her of the use of equipment provided for her comfort or assistance. For example, Sumeera was given a particular type of mattress for her bed, which was designed to prevent or ease pressure sores. A short time later the caregivers noticed, on one of their daily visits, that the mattress had been removed from Sumeera's bed and was on the floor in another room clearly for use by another family member.

The Alleged Abuse of the Paid Caregivers

At the time of the adult protection case conference the private sector agency employing Sumeera's caregivers was threatening to withdraw its workers from this particular contract, under which two caregivers went into her home for half an hour three times a day. Their duties were solely to assist Sumeera with her personal care and dressing. The caregivers were described as being 'at the end of their tether'.

The ways in which the paid caregivers perceived themselves as being abused fell into two distinct categories. Firstly they were physically abused by Sumeera herself, and secondly they felt that their professional role was abused by Irfit and other family members. The caregivers' manager, who attended the adult protection meeting, was keen to emphasise that her workers had been committed to giving Sumeera sensitive and appropriate care, but they were reaching a point at which they were no longer willing to tolerate the treatment they received within her home.

The physical abuse of which the caregivers complained consisted of Sumeera often lashing out at them with her fists, scratching them, spitting and attempting to bite them whilst they were washing, toileting or dressing her. Sumeera, although having severe mobility problems, was said to have the strength to hit her carers quite hard, causing bruising. This situation created dilemmas for the caregivers in terms of what constitutes an ethical level of restraint of the elderly person in such circumstances. Equally concerning for them, however, were the health implications of the spitting and biting, particularly as members of Sumeera's family were known to have been treated in the recent past for tuberculosis.

In some ways, though, the caregivers found the physical abuse from Sumeera easier to accept than the 'abusive' attitudes displayed by Irfit and her children. They appreciated that Sumeera was frequently in pain, was frustrated by the lack of meaningful communication with them, and was generally an unhappy woman. As far as Irfit was concerned, though, the caregivers felt that they were treated as servants rather than as professionals employed to fulfill specific tasks at specified times. The caregivers had anticipated working in partnership with Irfit, to maximise Sumeera's quality of life, both by the care provided and by relieving some of the pressures on Irfit. Rather than a partnership, however, frustrations were building up in the caregivers at the family's neglect of Sumeera, as described above, by the misappropriation of items provided for Sumeera and the lack of other essential items at the required times. Expectations were placed upon the caregivers by the family to 'fetch and carry', particularly when items were needed from the local pharmacy. The caregivers felt that the family would not appreciate that they had designated tasks and time-slots, and that they then had to move on to their next client. The caregivers asked both the family and themselves, 'Why can't the grandchildren do simple tasks for their grandmother, such as collecting items from a pharmacy?' Some of them were teenagers, after all. The caregivers felt baffled by this. The tensions emerging between the support services and Sumeera's family will be discussed in the next section.

Reflections on Complex and Professionally Challenging Issues Arising from this Case Study

Although the central issues which are discussed here emerged within the context of formal adult protection procedures, the over-riding emotion evident within the multi-agency meeting was that of frustration at the fact that formally provided care for Sumeera was being effective neither at protecting her from potential (and perhaps unintentional) harm nor at improving her quality of life. There were also expressions of frustration that Sumeera's family were obstructing rather than assisting the formally provided care, and that the family were not seen as 'pulling their weight' in respect of Sumeera's care. The underlying reasons for this apparent lack of cooperation remained unexplored, however. There was a pervading inability to probe beneath the surface and get to grips with the cultural context and relationships in the case, leaving the door wide open to misunderstandings.

The Language Problem

One very obvious difficulty was the lack of a common language between Sumeera and her paid caregivers. Like her mother, Irfit had spent most of her adult life within the family setting, caring for her husband and five children, and her English appeared to be very limited too. The third generation, Irfit's children, were all bi-lingual, speaking their family's language in the home and English at school. From the paid caregivers' perspective, it was their usual practice to chat with their clients as they dealt with their personal care, trying to elicit their preferences when there were different ways of performing tasks, and so on. Attempts to use gestures or facial expressions seemed to result in aggressive responses. Initially Sumeera would speak to the caregivers in her own language, but she clearly found it exasperating that they could not understand. The caregivers occasionally asked the children to interpret, to explain things to either Sumeera or Irfit, or to tell them why their grandmother was reacting in a particular way, but the children were reluctant to cooperate and tended to give monosyllabic answers. Thus on a day-to-day basis the frustrations and the concerns about Sumeera would continue.

For more formal, periodic assessments and reviews of Sumeera's social care needs, an interpreter would be used. As mentioned previously, however, there were relatively few people from Sumeera's ethnic background living in that region and thus finding an accredited interpreter for her particular language was not easy. There was clear reluctance from Irfit to having a member of her local ethnic community as an interpreter in her home, seemingly as it might evoke censure of her within that community if the family's problems became known. Thus an interpreter had to be sought further afield, and this was also a costly resource which had to be used sparingly. The health and social care professionals who had used an interpreter with Sumeera's family voiced concerns about how much was translation of the family's responses and how much was 'interpretation'. These professionals were conscious of the fact that cultural and attitudinal factors, which were remaining tacit, might be influencing both Irfit's responses and Sumeera's behaviour. It became apparent at one point, although never made explicit by Irfit, that a suggested period of 'respite care' for Sumeera of a week in an elderly people's home, intended to give Irfit a break, might be regarded by her ethnic minority community as Irfit shirking her duties and thereby 'losing face'.

The Cultural Considerations in Caregiving

This explanation of Irfit's rejection of 'respite care' for her mother was accepted at face-value by the professionals seeking to protect Sumeera. There was no deeper exploration of the relationship between daughter and mother, nor of any cultural considerations concerning expectations relating to parental care. Nothing appeared to be known, for example, about the traditions within their particular culture which may have had a bearing on a daughter's willingness to care for her elderly mother. Another perspective, which was also not explored at the case conference, was the possibility of Irfit's reluctance to accept 'respite care' being rooted in fear of what might come to light if her mother were cared for over a period of time elsewhere. The possibility of a problematic dynamic between daughter and mother, as may occur in any ethnic group, was not considered, although it may have been relevant. There was nothing to suggest that other family members were routinely 'neglected'.

Thus the 'misunderstandings' arising in this case extended well beyond difficulties in verbal communication. The initial assessment of need and subsequent reviews all required a sensitivity to cultural issues relevant to the elderly person and an understanding of their experience of the environment and culture within which they now live. The research interviews with several professionals involved in arranging and resourcing Sumeera's health and social care suggested that little more was known about Sumeera's personal history than has been outlined in this paper. She was, however, someone who had spent her formative years, and indeed half her life thus far, in a very different culture and environment. Nothing was really known about the reasons for Mr M bringing Sumeera and their daughters to England, which may have been economic, political, due to persecution, or whatever. There were no real indications of whether Sumeera had become integrated into the small local community from her own ethnic background or whether she retained any contact with them. Any of these factors could be impacting on Sumeera's and Irfit's attitudes towards and feelings about state provision of personal care for Sumeera. In reality, of course, much of the history of those within the indigenous elderly community remains a mystery when assessments are made for provision of care, but more often than not the assessors are from a similar cultural background, are able to discuss plans with the elderly person or his/her relatives, and can fairly quickly tune into any special circumstances or requirements. This is not to suggest that in such cases the assessors always 'get it right', but there may be fewer variables to consider.

It is often a routine part of a paid caregiver's role to assist with the washing and toileting of an elderly person, as indeed in Sumeera's case. These are intensely personal activities, however, which, if sensitively undertaken, require an understanding of the elderly person's attitudes towards his or her body and its appropriate care. These may of course be intertwined with religious beliefs and expectations. In fact, there are cultural differences to consider too. For example Lam, in chapter 4, points out how in the Chinese traditional culture it is not appropriate that close kin provide personal care: they would feel embarrassed about having any physical contact with their elderly. If the dignity and integrity of the elderly person are to be respected, these are issues which need detailed enquiry and discussion prior to the commencement of formal care. If insufficient attention is paid to this, caregivers may inadvertently cause offence, or indeed be considered abusive, and so initial assessments of need should explore specific actions and expectations in all aspects of the personal care to be provided.

Sumeera's case exemplifies many of the tensions and difficulties arising from the provision of personal care to elderly people from ethnic minority groups, particularly perhaps where that group is very small within the local community. A key-player in this case was, of course, the primary caregiver, Irfit. Hers was a pivotal and complex role. Although the majority of her adult life had been spent in England, she, like her mother, had spent her formative years in a very different environment and culture. At the time of this study Irfit's acceptance of her role as the main caregiver to her mother had wide-ranging implications for her, both in practical and emotional terms. Those assessing and providing for Sumeera's care needs were unaware, however, of the real emotional impact on Irfit of being the main caregiver. Did she, for example, resent having to look after her mother on a full-time basis? What were her feelings for her mother? How did she feel about her sister apparently making no contribution to their mother's daily care? Such issues were not explored and therefore not taken into account. On a practical level, being her mother's main caregiver involved Irfit in the bureaucracy and idiosyncracies of state-provided care in a culture in which she was living but which remained largely peripheral to her day-to-day life.

Although the limitations of the verbal communication between the paid caregivers and Irfit meant that her feelings about having primary responsibility for the care of her mother, and the consequent major changes for her nuclear family, remained only speculative, the physical impact on Irfit was apparent, as she frequently seemed exhausted. During the day she had caring responsibility for a lively pre-school child, (and for ensuring that the other children went to school). She had the paid caregivers coming into her home three times a day, and caring responsibility for her mother during the remainder of each 24 hours. Nothing was known about Irfit's responsibilities in relation to her husband and their two children living with him. The social services' response to Irfit's evident exhaustion was the offer of 'respite care', which, as mentioned previously, she refused.

As with family caregivers from many cultural backgrounds, Irfit was in a position of trying to accommodate and respond to the needs of family members from both the older and younger generations. A particular factor for Irfit, and others in her position, were the tensions between the traditional expectations and values of their ethnic group and the sometimes differing expectations and values of the culture within which her children were growing up. Hers were the first children in the family to have been born in the United Kingdom and to be going through its education system, thereby potentially becoming decreasingly ethnically embedded. From a broader perspective this raises a raft of problematic issues, requiring further debate in a more formal political arena, about the extent to which society encourages multiculturalism and genuinely values diversity and the extent to which ethnic minority groups settling in the United Kingdom are expected to adapt and conform to local culture.

Such tensions come into focus when considering the invoking of adult protection procedures in Sumeera's case. The local procedures, based on the 'No Secrets' guidance, required that the subject of an adult protection case conference, or his/her chosen advocate, should be invited to attend the meeting. In this particular case, however, it was evident that neither Sumeera nor Irfit were informed of the meeting, nor indeed of the procedures generally. It is perhaps all too easy for professionals, in a case such as this, to rationalise the exclusion of the people most centrally concerned. There are the obvious communication difficulties, concepts such as 'neglect' and 'abuse' would need to be explained and understood, and so on, but such factors, whilst time-consuming, are not insuperable hurdles. The rationalisations should be weighed against the benefits of involving Sumeera (whose mental capacity and levels of understanding were surmised, rather than established) and Irfit. There were so many areas of uncertainty in relation to the care of Sumeera that the involvement in the adult protection procedures of Irfit, at least, may have offered the potential to bring some clarity and to discuss seeming misunderstandings. It might also have brought home to Irfit the seriousness with which the problems relating to her mother's care were viewed by the care providers. Her attendance would however have needed to be sensitively prepared and handled, as it could have been a threatening experience for her, and criticism of her care of Sumeera could have reinforced barriers to cooperation rather than improved Sumeera's situation.

Thus the alleged neglect of Sumeera by the family and the threatened withdrawal of care by the paid caregivers were the subject of a lengthy meeting of professionals, but the central characters' perspectives and feelings were not represented, other than by the professionals. The descriptions of the allegedly abusive situation, of Sumeera's behaviour, of family members' attitudes, and so on, were therefore all 'filtered' through those most closely involved in Sumeera's daily care. Whilst they were genuinely trying to represent and think through all aspects of the situation, the considerable gaps in understanding could only be effectively filled by the involvement of Irfit or Sumeera's chosen advocate. Their role would have been one of clarifying issues from their cultural and personal perspectives, and of listening to, and discussing, the professionals' concerns. The study suggests that this lack of relevant perspectives is by no means unique in adult protection case conferences; only 15% of the meetings studied were attended by the subject or a chosen advocate. However, in cases where the alleged abuse involves an elderly person from an ethnic minority family the potential for culturally-based assumptions and misunderstandings is increased, and the relevance and effectiveness of protective planning may be lessened. There are of course significant resource implications in fully involving people from a different cultural background and with little knowledge of the local language in meetings about very sensitive and personal issues, particularly if they feel that their actions are being viewed critically. It may however be argued that it is ethically incumbent on those invoking adult protection procedures to ensure that people from ethnic minorities are as fully informed as possible about what is happening and provided with relevant assistance to maximise their understanding and participation. In the case of Sumeera, the case conference highlighted a raft of problematic issues concerning Sumeera herself, Irfit and the caregivers; the meeting sought solutions to some practicalities of care, and placed great hope (though little confidence) in finding some caregivers from the same ethnic background as Sumeera. There was no discussion about informing Sumeera and Irfit of the case conference. Some months later there were still no caregivers from a similar ethnic background. It had however been learned that Irfit's sister, who had scarcely been mentioned in the discussions about Sumeera's care, lived within easy travelling distance of her mother and spoke good English.

Conclusions

This case study illustrates some of the myriad of complexities and ethical issues inherent in the formal provision of personal care to an elderly woman from an ethnic minority background living with two younger generations of her family in an English city. Other cases of 'caregiving and ethnicity' will undoubtedly raise different and additional issues, and not all, of course, will involve concerns about abuse, as in Sumeera's case. There are however points of general applicability which may be drawn from this case study and which have relevance for both practitioners and policy-makers; some recommendations are presented below.

The intention of this paper has been to highlight some of the issues found in one actual case of ethnicity and caregiving, in which there were many (possibly not unusual) problems, and to reflect more broadly upon the practice and policy implications of these issues. A recurring theme throughout the case study is that of the importance of effective communication. Where that is achieved the provision of personal care may move away from the perception of 'active caregiver' and 'passive recipient', whatever the ethnic background of those involved in the interaction.

Recommendations

- In all cases in which the personal care needs of a vulnerable adult from an ethnic minority are being professionally assessed, every reasonable effort should be made to enquire about and understand the customs and traditions which are important to the care recipient and which may impact on the appropriate provision of care. Investment of time and resources at this stage may help to preclude inadvertent offence and misunderstandings later. It also creates an informed context within which mutually acceptable compromises may be negotiated, where necessary.
- Sensitivity to cultural considerations should not preclude a thorough assessment of the nature and quality of intra-familial relationships in situations where the main caregiver is a blood-relative of the vulnerable adult. Where abuse is suspected, the possibility of a pathological relationship may exist, and 'political correctness' should not inhibit exploration of this. As stated in 'No Secrets', the abuse of a vulnerable adult may occur in any relationship. Caregivers, whether paid or informal, may also be abusers.
- Looking at the broad picture of ethnicity and caregiving, there are clearly significant training issues which should be addressed. The case study illustrates how formally provided personal care may be undermined by a quite basic lack of knowledge and understanding, which may in turn lead to an emotionally charged atmosphere.
- It is important to acknowledge the diversity among and between the many ethnic minority groups in the United Kingdom. In terms of formal care provision there are significant differences in expectations and preferences, such as the ethnic background of the caregivers. The provision of appropriate care for the smaller ethnic minority groups, such as Sumeera's, may have particular implications for service-providers.

- In the United Kingdom, the heterogeneity of the population and the anticipated increase in elderly people from ethnic minority backgrounds, (as well as a general increase in the elderly population), are fundamental issues requiring attention from policy-makers in terms of care provision and protection of the elderly from abuse. This will be an ongoing situation as new waves of settlers arrive for different reasons. There are political tensions between 'valuing diversity' and having the resources to provide only a 'one size fits all' approach to formal caregiving. There are also unresolved social issues concerning the extent to which ethnic minority groups are expected to adapt and conform to local culture.

REFERENCES

ARC and NAPSAC (Eds.). (1993). *It could never happen here!* Bradford: Thornton and Pearson

Baumhover, LA and Beall, SC. (1996). *Abuse, Neglect and Exploitation of Older Persons. Strategies for Assessment and Intervention.* London: Jessica Kingsley

Bennett, G and Kingston, P. (1993). *Elder Abuse. Concepts, Theories and Interventions.* London, Chapman and Hall

Blakemore, K and Boneham, M. (1994). *Age, Race and Ethnicity. A comparative approach.* Buckingham, Open University Press

Brown, H. (1999). Abuse of people with learning disabilities – layers of concern and analysis. In Stanley, Manthorpe and Penhale (Eds.), *Institutional Abuse. Perspectives across the life course* (pp. 89-109). London, Routledge

Dandekar, K. (1996). *The Elderly in India.* New Delhi, Sage

Department of Health (2000). *No Secrets : guidance on developing and implementing multi-agency policies and procedures to protect vulnerable adults from abuse.* London, DoH

Dowd JJ and Bengston VL. (1978). Aging in minority populations – an examination of the double jeopardy hypothesis. *Journal of Gerontology, **33**, 427-36*

Hughes, B. (1995). *Older people and community care – critical theory and practice.* Buckingham, Open University Press

Jackson M., Kolody B. and Wood JL. (1982). To be old and black : the case for double jeopardy on income and health. In Manuel RC (Ed): *Minority Aging.* (pp. 77-82). Connecticut, Greenwood Press

Law Commission (1995). *Mental Incapacity.* London, HMSO

Lord Chancellor's Department, Cm4465 (1999). *Making Decisions.* London, The Stationery Office Ltd.

Norman, A. (1985). *Triple Jeopardy : growing old in a second homeland.* London, Centre for Policy on Ageing

Office for National Statistics (2001). *Regional distribution of the minority ethnic population, April 2001.* London, ONS

Office for National Statistics (2002). : *Annual Local Labour Force Survey 2001/2.* London, ONS

Sokolovsky, J. (1990). *The Cultural Context of Aging.* New York, Bergin and Garvey

Stevenson, O. (1989). *Age and Vulnerability. A guide to better care.* London, Edward Arnold

Stevenson, O. (1996). *Elder Protection in the Community. What can we learn from Child Protection?* London, Department of Health

INDEX

A

B

C

D

E

F

G

H

I

J

K

L

M

N

O

P

Q

R

S

T

U

V